Serono Symposia USA
Norwell, Massachusetts

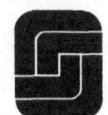

Springer
New York
Berlin
Heidelberg
Barcelona
Hong Kong
London
Milan
Paris
Singapore
Tokyo

PROCEEDINGS IN THE SERONO SYMPOSIA USA SERIES

Continued after Index

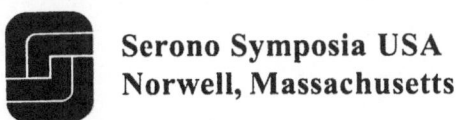

Serono Symposia USA
Norwell, Massachusetts

Erwin Goldberg

Editor

The Testis
From Stem Cell
to Sperm Function

With 39 Figures

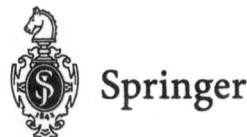

Springer

Erwin Goldberg, Ph.D.
Department of Biochemistry,
  Molecular Biology and Cell Biology
Northwestern University
Evanston, IL 60208-3500
USA
erv@nwu.edu

Proceedings of the XVth Testis Workshop on The Testis: From Stem Cell to Sperm Function, sponsored by Serono Symposia USA, Inc., held April 7 to 10, 1999, in Louisville, Kentucky.

For information on previous volumes, contact Serono Symposia USA, Inc.

Library of Congress Cataloging-in-Publication Data
The testis : from stem cell to sperm function / edited by Erwin Goldberg.
      p. cm.
      "Serono symposia, USA."
      Includes bibliographical references and index.
      ISBN-13: 978-1-4612-7416-2   e-ISBN-13: 978-1-4612-2106-7
      DOI: 10.1007/978-1-4612-2106-7

      1. Testis—Congresses.   I. Goldberg, Erwin.
QP255 .T49 2000
573.6'55—dc21   00-023804

Production coordinated by Chernow Editorial Services, Inc., and managed by Francine McNeill; manufacturing supervised by Jeffrey Taub.
Typeset by KP Company, Brooklyn, NY.

9 8 7 6 5 4 3 2 1

SPIN 10762947

Springer-Verlag New York Berlin Heidelberg
A member of BertelsmannSpringer Science+Business Media GmbH

XVth TESTIS WORKSHOP ON THE TESTIS: FROM STEM CELL TO SPERM FUNCTION

Scientific Committee

Erwin Goldberg, Ph.D., Chair
William J. Bremner, M.D., Ph.D.
Richard Bronson, M.D.
Edward M. Eddy, Ph.D.
David L. Garbers, Ph.D.
Matthew Hardy, Ph.D.
Norman B. Hecht, Ph.D.
Barry T. Hinton, Ph.D.
John D. Kirby, Ph.D.
Patricia L. Morris, Ph.D.
Bernard Robaire, Ph.D.
Barbara M. Sanborn, Ph.D.
J. Lisa Tenover, M.D., Ph.D.
Jacquetta M. Trasler, M.D., Ph.D.
Christina Wang, M.D.
Barry R. Zirkin, Ph.D.

Organizing Secretary

Leslie Nies
Serono Symposia USA, Inc.
100 Longwater Circle
Norwell, Massachusetts

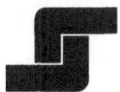

Preface

This volume contains the proceedings of the XVth North American Testis Workshop, held in Louisville, Kentucky, April 7 to 10, 1999, to describe current advances in testis biology. The first two chapters provide a useful historical perspective of testis physiology and formulate compelling research questions about important aspects of sperm formation and function. This prologue sets the scene for the remainder of the volume that follows a logical progression, as the title implies, from stem cell to cell function, but that is necessarily preceded by sex determination, the quintessential requirement for there being a testis in the first place.

The program for this XVth Testis Workshop evolved from recommendations of the scientific committee and their advice on the selection of invited speakers. The XVth Testis Workshop has a strong comparative flavor with contributions on worms (*Caenorhabditis*), flies (*Drosophila*), and chickens, which are models that permit and thereby reveal the power of genetic analyses of the molecular mechanisms involved in spermatogenesis. A glimpse into the future is provided with information from EST, protein, and genome databases that already have an impact on progress in our understanding of the male germ cell. Although there is heavy emphasis in these chapters on cellular and molecular events, database mining and translational profiling relevant to testis function and dysfunction and assisted reproduction technologies are not overlooked. As a result, this volume contains something for everyone from the bench scientist to the clinical practitioner and should remain a valuable reference resource at the cutting edge of male reproduction.

From my perspective, organizing this symposium and editing these proceedings have been relatively painless thanks to the cooperation of the invited speakers, and most of all to Leslie Nies, president of Serono Symposia USA, Inc., and her staff, including Dianne Ferreira, who selected the magnificent Seelbach Hotel for the meeting, Carole Mulkern and Pauline Bentley, who handled the registration desk, catering, and so on, with competence and charm, and Judy Donahue, the driving force for production of this book. I am especially grateful to Drs. Michael McClure and Donna Vogel for advice and guidance on submitting a conference grant proposal. Funding from NICHD, NCRR, and NIA made possible the attendance of new investigators. With the prospect of continued support from Serono Symposia USA, the Testis Workshop has a bright future in the twenty-first century.

ERWIN GOLDBERG

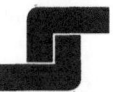

Contents

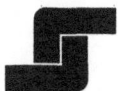

Contributors

ROBERT W. BAILEY, Department of Biochemistry and Biophysics, Washington State University, Pullman, Washington, USA.

JAMES R. BARTLES, Department of Cell and Molecular Biology, Northwestern University Medical School, Chicago, Illinois, USA.

MARISA S. BARTOLOMEI, Department of Cell and Developmental Biology, University of Pennsylvania, Philadelphia, Pennsylvania, USA.

IGLIKA N. BATOVA, Department of Cell Biology and Anatomy, The University of North Carolina at Chapel Hill, Chapel Hill, North Carolina, USA.

DIDI D.M. BRAAT, Department of Obstetrics and Gynecology, University Hospital of Nijmegen, Nijmegen, The Netherlands.

BLANCHE CAPEL, Department of Cell Biology, Duke University Medical Center, Durham, North Carolina, USA.

BIN CHEN, Department of Cell and Molecular Biology, Northwestern University Medical School, Chicago, Illinois, USA.

ANN CLARK, Ontogeny, Inc., Cambridge, Massachusetts, USA.

MARIA P. DE MIGUEL, Kimmel Cancer Center, Thomas Jefferson University, Philadelphia, Pennsylvania, USA.

DIRK G. DE ROOIJ, Department of Cell Biology, Utrecht University Medical School, Utrecht, The Netherlands.

ADAM S. DOHERTY, Department of Cell and Developmental Biology, University of Pennsylvania, Philadelphia, Pennsylvania, USA.

PETER J. DONOVAN, Kimmel Cancer Center, Thomas Jefferson University, Philadelphia, Pennsylvania, USA.

EDWARD M. EDDY, Laboratory of Reproductive and Developmental Toxicology, National Institute of Environmental Health Sciences, National Institutes of Health, Research Triangle Park, North Carolina, USA.

MARK J. FEDERSPIEL, Molecular Medicine Program, Mayo Clinic and Mayo Foundation, Rochester, Minnesota, USA.

DAVID P. FROMAN, Department of Animal Sciences, Oregon State University, Corvallis, Oregon, USA.

MARGARET T. FULLER, Department of Developmental Biology, Stanford University School of Medicine, Stanford, California, USA.

DAVID L. GARBERS, Howard Hughes Medical Institute and Department of Pharmacology, University of Texas Southwestern Medical Center, Dallas, Texas, USA.

MICHAEL D. GRISWOLD, Department of Biochemistry and Biophysics, Washington State University, Pullman, Washington, USA.

NORMAN B. HECHT, Center for Research on Reproduction and Women's Health and Department of Obstetrics and Gynecology, University of Pennsylvania School of Medicine, Philadelphia, Pennsylvania, USA.

BARRY T. HINTON, Department of Cell Biology, University of Virginia Health Sciences Center, Charlottesville, Virginia, USA.

JOHN D. KIRBY, Division of Agriculture, University of Arkansas, Fayetteville, Arkansas, USA.

JAN A.M. KREMER, Department of Obstetrics and Gynecology, University Hospital of Nijmegen, Nijmegen, The Netherlands.

JACQUELYN C. LABUS, Department of Cell Biology, University of Virginia Health Sciences Center, Charlottesville, Virginia, USA.

ZI JIAN LAN, Department of Cell Biology, Baylor College of Medicine, Houston, Texas, USA.

MARY MIN-CHIN LEE, Pediatric Endocrine Unit and Department of Pediatrics, Massachusetts General Hospital and Harvard Medical School, Boston, Massachusetts, USA.

STEVEN W. L'HERNAULT, Department of Biology, Emory University, Atlanta, Georgia, USA.

TING-YI LIN, Department of Developmental Biology, Stanford University School of Medicine, Stanford, California, USA.

R. JOHN LYE, Department of Cell Biology, University of Virginia Health Sciences Center, Charlottesville, Virginia, USA.

ELENA LYMAR, Department of Biochemistry and Biophysics, Washington State University, Pullman, Washington, USA.

MARVIN L. MEISTRICH, Department of Experimental Radiation Oncology, University of Texas M.D. Anderson Cancer Center, Houston, Texas, USA.

ERIC J.H. MEULEMAN, Department of Urology, University Hospital of Nijmegen, Nijmegen, The Netherlands.

KIYOSHI MIKI, Laboratory of Reproductive and Developmental Toxicology, National Institute of Environmental Health Sciences, National Institutes of Health, Research Triangle Park, North Carolina, USA.

CHISATO MORI, Department of Anatomy and Developmental Biology, Faculty of Medicine, Kyoto University, Kyoto, Japan.

YOSHITAKE NISHIMUNE, Research Institute for Microbial Diseases, Osaka University, Osaka, Japan.

MASARU OKABE, Genome Information Research Center, Osaka University, Osaka, Japan.

MICHAEL G. O'RAND, Department of Cell Biology and Anatomy, The University of North Carolina at Chapel Hill, Chapel Hill, North Carolina, USA.

ROGER A. PEDERSEN, Department of Obstetrics, Gynecology and Reproductive Sciences, University of California, San Francisco, San Francisco, California, USA.

M. JODEANE PRINGLE, Department of Developmental Biology, Stanford University School of Medicine, Stanford, California, USA.

TIMOTHY A. QUILL, Howard Hughes Medical Institute and Department of Pharmacology, University of Texas Southwestern Medical Center, Dallas, Texas, USA.

RENEE A. REIJO PERA, Department of Obstetrics, Gynecology and Reproductive Sciences, and Departments of Physiology and Urology, University of California, San Francisco, San Francisco, California, USA.

DOUGLAS D. RHOADS, Department of Biological Sciences, University of Arkansas, Fayetteville, Arkansas, USA.

RICHARD T. RICHARDSON, Department of Cell Biology and Anatomy, The University of North Carolina at Chapel Hill, Chapel Hill, North Carolina, USA.

BERNARD ROBAIRE, Departments of Pharmacology and Therapeutics and of Obstetrics and Gynecology, McGill University, Montreal, Quebec, Canada.

BIANCA H.G.J. SCHRANS-STASSEN, Department of Cell Biology, Utrecht University Medical School, Utrecht, The Netherlands.

RICHARD M. SCHULTZ, Department of Biology, University of Pennsylvania, Philadelphia, Pennsylvania, USA.

VALERIE SERRE, Department of Pharmacology and Therapeutics, McGill University, Montreal, Quebec, Canada.

FAY L. SHAMANSKI, Department of Obstetrics, Gynecology and Reproductive Sciences, Reproductive Genetics Division, University of California, San Francisco, San Francisco, California, USA.

GLADIS A. SHUTTLESWORTH, Department of Experimental Radiation Oncology, University of Texas M.D. Anderson Cancer Center, Houston, Texas, USA.

ANDREW W. SINGSON, Department of Biology, Emory University, Atlanta, Georgia, USA.

J. LISA TENOVER, Department of Medicine, Emory University School of Medicine, Atlanta, Georgia, USA.

KIMBERLY D. TREMBLAY, Department of Cell and Molecular Biology, Harvard University, Cambridge, Massachusetts, USA.

WALTER A. TRIBLEY, Department of Biochemistry and Biophysics, Washington State University, Pullman, Washington, USA.

JOEP H.A.M. TUERLINGS, Department of Human Genetics, University Hospital of Nijmegen, Nijmegen, The Netherlands.

PAUL J. TUREK, Department of Urology, University of California, San Francisco, San Francisco, California, USA.

RON VAN GOLDE, Department of Obstetrics and Gynecology, University Hospital of Nijmegen, Nijmegen, The Netherlands.

ANS M.M. VAN PELT, Department of Cell Biology, Utrecht University Medical School, Utrecht, The Netherlands.

MIN WANG, Department of Cell and Molecular Biology, Northwestern University Medical School, Chicago, Illinois, USA.

WILLIAM D. WILLIS, Laboratory of Reproductive and Developmental Toxicology, National Institute of Environmental Health Sciences, National Institutes of Health, Research Triangle Park, North Carolina, USA.

FREDERICK C.W. WU, Department of Endocrinology, Manchester Royal Infirmary, Manchester, United Kingdom.

LILI ZHENG, Department of Cell and Molecular Biology, Northwestern University Medical School, Chicago, Illinois, USA.

BARRY R. ZIRKIN, Division of Reproductive Biology, Department of Biochemistry, Johns Hopkins University, School of Hygiene and Public Health, Baltimore, Maryland, USA.

Prologue

1

Unlocking the Mysteries of Male Reproductive Function: How Far Have We Come and Where Are We Going?

BARRY R. ZIRKIN AND BERNARD ROBAIRE

Even casual perusal of the history of male reproduction reveals an obvious truth, one that undoubtedly applies to scientific discovery in general: Major leaps in understanding and insight have typically followed dramatic technological/methodological advances. The major objectives of this chapter are twofold. The first is to provide an overview of major advances in our understanding of male reproduction over the past 300 years in relationship to the technical breakthroughs that have led to them. The second is to speculate (fantasize?) about the promise of the remarkable new technologies that have either burst on the scene in the past few years or are about to do so in the near future, and the consequent breathtakingly increased pace of modern scientific discovery. By design this chapter is long on "blue sky" and short on referenced literature. A brief suggested reading list that includes both key historical references and some pivotal articles is included at the end of this chapter. For information regarding new molecular approaches and their promise to relate the genome to health and disease, please refer to the National Center for Biotechnology Information (www.ncbi.nlm.gov).

The Age of Microscopy

More than 300 years ago, Leeuwenhoek developed the microscope and was the first to describe spermatozoa. Establishing the function of spermatozoa, however, occurred nearly a century later when, in 1780, Spallanzani showed that removal of sperm from semen prevented fertilization. It was not until the mid-1800s that it was first shown that spermatozoa are cells, that they originate in the seminiferous tubules of the testis, and that a sequence of changes in germ cells lining seminiferous tubules occurs to form them. This was 200 years after de Graaf had described the testicle as consisting of tubules. Finally, in 1875, Hertwig demonstrated that fertilization involves the union of sperm and egg. Thus, two centuries elapsed between the first description of spermatozoa and the acceptance of the role of this cell in reproduction.

The mid-to-late 1800s represented a period of remarkable discovery, and it was largely based on improved light microscopy. In 1865, Sertoli first described cells, with nuclei near the base of the seminiferous tubules, that surround germ cells; these cells were subsequently named after him. At about the same time, the germ cells at the periphery of the seminiferous tubules, between the Sertoli cells, were identified as the stem cells from which all subsequent stages of spermatogenesis were derived, and the meiotic divisions and the differentiation of spermatids were described. Thus, by 1900, thanks to observations made with the light microscope, the principal events of spermatogenesis were recognized. Fifty years later, the application of periodic-acid Schiff staining method for the carbohydrates of the developing acrosome and the use of newly developed autoradiographic methods allowed Leblond and Clermont to establish the cyclic nature of the seminiferous epithelium and the duration of the stages of spermatogenesis.

The introduction of the electron microscope in the 1950s, along with new developments in tissue fixation, embedding, and sectioning, made it possible for all the membranous organelles of cells to be examined at high resolution. Exploitation of electron microscopy in the early 1960s brought fundamental changes in our understanding of the organization of the seminiferous tubules. In particular, new concepts were introduced regarding how testicular cells communicate with each other via gap junctions, and the occluding junctions between Sertoli cells became recognized as the basis for the blood–testis barrier.

During the 1980s and 1990s the presence and exact cellular localization of many proteins in tissues of the male reproductive tract became possible through the use of new tools for preparing selective antibodies, and powerful new immunolocalization techniques. Immunolocalization was initially done only at the light microscope level. With innovations such as the immunogold technique, however, it became possible to localize proteins within specific subcellular organelles, and this has allowed for new insight into structure-function relationships in cells. The 1990s saw growing applications of confocal microscopy to the male reproductive tract. The application of this methodology should soon make it possible to monitor in situ how physiological perturbations, drugs, or environmental chemicals result in alterations of the three-dimensional organization of complex structures such as seminiferous and epididymal tubules.

Interest in the morphological events of spermatogenesis paralleled an understanding of the regulation of this process. Leydig cells were first observed between the seminiferous tubules in 1850; however, it was again some 50 years later before further morphological observation suggested that these cells were secretory and thus possibly involved in reproduction and in maintaining secondary sex characteristics. The intimate relationship between Leydig cell structure and steroidogenic function was recognized in the 1970s and 1980s, after the introduction of electron microscopy and when it became possible to examine testicular secretions by biochemical methods.

The Age of Biochemical Analysis of Hormones

The first demonstration that testicular secretions were able to prevent the regressive effects of castration was made in the rooster by Berthold in 1849. Measurement of androgenic hormone activity, however, awaited the development of a bioassay for male sex hormone about 80 years later. Shortly thereafter, in the early 1930s, androsterone was the first androgen to be crystallized, with the starting point of approximately 15,000 L of male urine. Testosterone itself was synthesized 4 years later in 1935. This, and the synthesis of progesterone at around the same time, led to an explosion of interest in steroid biochemistry over the next three decades.

Analytical and separation methods such as gas–liquid and thin-layer chromatography, mass spectrometry, and nuclear magnetic resonance allowed researchers to isolate and quantify minuscule amounts of steroids. The development of radioimmunoassay in the later 1950s, however, led to a revolution in the ability of both researchers and clinicians to quantify the hormones that regulate the male reproductive system accurately, and reproducibly rapidly, whether secreted by the testis or the pituitary. Combined with in situ testicular perfusion techniques developed and refined by Eik-Nes and Ewing, the biosynthetic pathways, metabolism, and physiological regulation of androgen synthesis in the testis were elucidated.

Dramatic advances occurred in our understanding of the hypothalamic and pituitary hormones that regulate gonadal functions in parallel with developments in steroid biochemistry. Among these discoveries, perhaps the most significant, made in the mid-1920s, was that the reproductive systems of both males and females are regulated in some way by the anterior pituitary. In the early 1930s, evidence was presented that the pituitary secretes two hormones, follicle stimulating hormone (FSH) and leuteinizing hormone (LH), and, importantly, that pituitary function is itself regulated at least in part by the negative feedback effects of gonadal hormones. Leydig cells were shown to be the primary, if not the sole, source of testicular androgen, and these cells were shown to be regulated by LH. The intratesticular concentration of testosterone was found to be many times that seen in the circulation, and an elevated testosterone concentration was found to be essential for normal spermatogenesis. Injection of androgens into intact male rats was unexpectedly found to reduce testis size. It was subsequently shown that testosterone administration lowered the LH content of the pituitary. These important observations led to attempts, which started in the 1970s and are still ongoing, to use testosterone for male contraception.

The Age of Cell and Molecular Biology

Whereas most explanations for how spermatogenesis was regulated were in terms of the endocrine environment of germ cells before 1960, the subsequent recognition that cells within the seminiferous epithelium communicate, as do those between the seminiferous tubules and the interstitium, made it plausible that there were short-loop interactions between cell types that also played a role in regulation. The development of methods for isolating and purifying Leydig, Sertoli, peritubular, and specific germ cells in the 1970s, combined with the introduction of a technique for studying whole mounts of intact seminiferous tubules, led to renewed study of stem cells within the seminiferous epithelium and to new insight into cell–cell communication and the maturation of spermatozoa.

In the 1980s, study of isolated cells in conjunction with molecular analyses of the RNA and protein content and synthesis by cells of the male reproductive tract led to new understanding of genetic inactivation, haploid gene expression, and long-lived mRNAs. More detailed understanding will require the ability to isolate and culture germ cells under conditions that will promote their division and maturation, as well as the development of a wider range of stable testicular and epididymal somatic cell lines. With such methods, it will be possible to identify the products of these cells, the biosynthetic pathways involved, and control mechanisms.

Our understanding of the function of the epididymis has followed a slower course than understanding of the testis. By the 1930s, it was known that sperm undergo maturation and acquire their fertilizing capacity in the epididymis. At that time and for many years thereafter, however, these changes in sperm were believed to be dependent on the passage of time and not on any specific function of the epididymis. Indeed, as late as the mid-1950s, the epididymis was thought simply to concentrate the sperm that emanated from the testis, serving as a site of sperm accumulation and storage. That view has changed dramatically, with the understanding now that epididymal structure and function are regulated by androgen, and that epididymal epithelial cells synthesize many essential products required by sperm for their motility and fertility.

During the 1980s and 1990s a series of factors, mostly proteins, have been shown to be synthesized in, and/or to have receptors on, different testicular and epididymal cell types. The precise roles of factors such as inhibin, activin, IGF, NGF, FGF, and NO in regulating steroidgenesis, spermatogenesis, and sperm maturation in the epididymis remain to be elucidated. The advent of in vitro culture systems in which the interactions of multiple cell types can be monitored would make it possible to resolve many of these questions.

Perspective

The period of the 1960s–1980s was remarkably rich in discovery and insight. The stages of the cycle were defined for the human, the syncytial nature of developing germ cells was recognized; the blood–testis barrier was described, the pathway of testosterone biosynthesis and its localization to specific organelles of Leydig cells were elucidated, receptors for LH and FSH were demonstrated on Leydig and Sertoli cells; the mechanism of action of LH on its target cell was elucidated, some of the biochemical effects of FSH on Sertoli cells were identified; the composition of intratesticular fluid was shown; the control of epididymal function and the role of the epididymis in sperm maturation were confirmed, and the ultrastructure of spermatozoa was elucidated. These discoveries set the stage for the remarkable advances made possible by the introduction of sophisticated biochemical and molecular biological methods of the 1980s and thereafter, as well as the explosion in the identification of germ cell and Sertoli cell products and their regulation that these methods have made possible. Chapter 2 in this volume will focus on these advances.

Where Are We Going?

The introduction of highly sophisticated tools designed for large-scale DNA sequencing are in the process of revolutionizing the way science is done, and they will fundamentally change the way in which we think about the reproductive processes. The use of the new tools will require teams of scientists from different disciplines working together and sharing techniques and information in ways that we have not done before. Such collaborative interactions will allow sharing of DNA sequencing data, expensive microarray/chip facilities, and sophisticated data analysis. It will be necessary to link databases in order to relate the functions of macromolecules to sequences and to the three-dimensional structures of proteins. There will be a need to integrate information about individual genes with our growing understanding of the structure and functions of cells and tissues forming the reproductive system.

The complete genomic sequences of close to 20 organisms are available already, and the mapping and sequencing phases of the Human Genome Project are rapidly moving forward. As yet, however, the function, expression, and regulation of most of the genes so far catalogued are not known. A major focus for the near future will be to relate DNA sequence data to biological function. Clues as to gene function already can be derived from gene knockout, knockdown and knock-in studies, as well as from studies designed to detect and quantitate gene expression patterns. There are a variety of powerful methods already in common use for assessing gene expression, including northern blots, S1 nuclease protection, differential display, mRNA amplification, and sequencing of cDNA libraries. cDNA- and oligonucle-otide-based array technologies have begun to augment these approaches. With these techniques, it is possible to monitor gene expression in multiple (hundreds to thousands) genes simultaneously by direct hybridization of to-tal RNA to high-density DNA arrays. It is becoming possible to do this with a single cell as starting material. These powerful new tools will allow us to begin to determine how cellular components work together to regulate and carry out complex cellular processes, which is essentially a physiologist's approach to molecular issues.

In the past few years, two breakthroughs relating to the male germ cell are particularly noteworthy for the future impact they will have on reproductive biology in particular, and on the biological sciences in general. The first is the ability to transplant spermatogonia between syngeneic animals as well as be-tween species. The implications of this discovery for understanding stem-cell renewal and differentiation are far-reaching both for basic understanding and for potential clinical applications (e.g., preserving stem cells for later use by patients). The second is the development of efficient mammalian transgenesis using intracytoplasmic sperm injection (ICSI). This method should allow for much greater efficiency of incorporation of retroviral constructs and thus for transgenesis in a variety of species.

The rapid sequence of breakthroughs that is taking place in the field of cloning is forcing a reexamination of some of the basic tenets in re-productive biology. The role of spermatozoa-specific information (e.g., DNA methylation patterns and imprinting) in determining the parental-specific inheritance can now be reexamined in a new light. Questions regarding the role played by chromosomal elements (e.g., methylation patterns and length of telomeres) can be asked in a strucutured and sys-tematic manner.

Where are these new technologies leading us? Biological research will increasingly expand from the comfort of the reductionist approaches with which we all are familiar to the integration of molecular information into physiological systems. The counterpart of genes identified in our experi-mental species of choice can easily be looked for in the human genome. If it is found, hypotheses about function can be tested experimentally in the experimental systems. Some key questions for us to consider as a community are: How far do we go with these new technologies? How might they be applied to basic research and/or to the application of basic research to infertility and/or contraception in populations or individuals? Should we place any limitations on their application to humans? If so, which limitations and who should decide? Can we "customize" (for the individual person) the diagnoses that are made and/or the treatments that are offered? Will university-based research take the lead, or will the major advances be made by the private sector? If, as seems likely, syn-ergy between universities and industry will provide for the greatest and best-balanced advances, how can this be achieved?

We have only begun to use the new technologies and approaches to understand how cellular components work together to regulate and carry out cellular processes. The prospects seem overwhelming, and the pace of discovery is breathtaking. At the same time, the promise seems limitless for those among us willing and able to look beyond what is comfortable.

Suggested Reading

Berthold AA. Transplantation der hoden. Arch Anat Physiol Wiss Med 1849;16:42–46.

Brinster RL, Nagano M. Spermatogonial stem cell transplantation, cryopreservation and culture. Sem Cell Develop Biol 1998;9:401–9.

Campbell KH, McWhir J, Ritchie WA, Wilmut I. Sheep cloned by nuclear transfer from a cultured cell line. Nature 1996;380:64–66.

Clermont Y. Kinetics of spermatogenesis in mammals: seminiferous epithelium cycle and spermatogonial renewal. Physiol Rev 1972;52:198–236.

Ewing LL, Zirkin B. Leydig cell structure and steroidogenic function. Rec Prog Horm Res 1983;39:599–635.

Greep RO, Koblinsky MA, Jaffe FS. Reproduction and human welfare: a challenge to research. Cambridge: MIT Press, 1976.

Perry ACF, Wakayama T, Kishikawa H, Kasai T, Okabe M, Toyoda Y, Yanagimachi R. Mammalian transgenesis by intracytoplasmic sperm injection. Science 1999; 284:1180–83.

Sertoli E. Dell'esistenza di particolari cellule ramificate nei canalicoli seminiferi del testicolo umano. Morgagni 1865;7:31–40.

2

Spermatogenesis After the Millennium

Norman B. Hecht

As predicted for the Macintosh computer, spermatogenesis will continue after Y2K. In fact, continued overpopulation and high levels of infertility, as well as discoveries such as Viagra, lend great importance to improved understanding of the mechanisms that regulate male reproduction. In this chapter, I will discuss a few areas of research that should be vigorously pursued in the coming years. The topics to be discussed are restricted to the testis, and represent only a limited vision for future research in andrology as seen by one with the bias of a molecular biologist.

Spermatogenesis can be loosely divided into three stages: spermatogonial proliferation and differentiation, meiosis, and spermiogenesis. Each will be discussed with a focus on their unique processes and some important questions that deserve attention in the coming years. I shall then discuss several other perceived breakthrough areas that merit research in the near future.

Spermatogonia

A detailed understanding of the mechanisms regulating spermatogonial differentiation would provide an opportunity to control spermatogenesis with precision. During the spermatogonial proliferation phase, spermatogonial type A stem cells actively divide, producing three populations of spermatogonia with very different destinies (1). One group of spermatogonia represents presumably identical copies of a pool of stem cells, a second group enters a pathway of differentiation and become spermatozoa, and a sizable number of other spermatogonia undergo cell death by apoptosis. Once starting along the differentiation pathway, the type A spermatogonia become intermediate and type B spermatogonia, and begin the long sequence of morphological and biochemical changes that lead to haploid spermatozoa. The cellular programming events appear to be irreversible because the differentiating spermatogonia are believed to be incapable of re-entering the pathway that produces stem cells. That a significant number of the spermatogonia undergo apoptosis suggests a sophisticated monitoring system is operating within these cells.

Type A spermatogonia represent a diverse population of cells, often designated type A_0, A_1, A_2, A_3, or A_4 spermatogonia. In this group of cells, the identity of the "true" stem cell needs to be definitively established. Although controversy exists among stem-cell renewal models, two models merit discussion. One model proposes that type A_0 spermatogonia represent a reserve population of stem cells that divide slowly and are the cells that repopulate the testis after chemical or radiation insults (2). In this model, the types A_1–A_4 spermatogonia are proposed to be the renewing stem cells that are capable of maintaining the fertility of an individual. An alternate model suggests that types A_1–A_4 spermatogonia are differentiated and type A_0 spermatogonia are the stem cells (3,4). The possibility exists that both models are correct, depending upon the species analyzed. Regardless of the correctness of each model, a crucial question for reproductive biology research is: What are the regulatory factors that lead spermatogonia down each of three distinct pathways? For instance, if the cycling type A spermatogonia could be prevented from entering the pathway that produces spermatozoa, this would allow the temporary suppression of spermatogenesis while maintaining possibilities for future fertility. An understanding of why and how certain spermatogonia are targeted for apoptosis whereas others survive would have implications far beyond reproductive biology.

To date, populations of spermatogonia can be isolated and maintained in culture, but our ability to induce these cells to divide and differentiate is limited. We also have not identified the "true" stem cell of the testis. The technical problems of identifying and isolating specific type A spermatogonia are substantial. Once isolated, defining the environment needed for spermatogonia to continue their "in vivo" programs of recycling or differentiating is equally formidable. The ability to culture and manipulate spermatogonial "stem cells" would have great implications for studies where genomic modifications are planned. Although progress has begun to be made to identify spermatogonial markers such as the c-kit receptor, additional biochemical markers for individual subpopulations of spermatogonia are needed. Directed gene targeting of essential spermatogonial proteins, as has been conducted with the RNA-binding protein, TIAR (5), needs to be actively pursued. On the other hand, specific mutations that influence early stages of germ-cell development [e.g., the juvenile spermatogonial depletion (jsd) mutant in mice] need to be creatively utilized to help to define the mechanisms of type A spermatogonial renewal and differentiation (6). In the jsd mutant, homozygous male mice undergo a normal wave of spermatogenesis when they are 3–10 weeks old, but subsequently become sterile. Their mutation leads to failure to maintain mitotic proliferation of type A spermatogonia by an unknown mechanism. The identification of additional mutants affecting spermatogonia should prove useful in understanding the processes of stem-cell renewal and differentiation.

Meiosis

Understanding the mechanisms of chromosome pairing and genetic recombination must represent a major goal for reproductive biologists in the next century. Meiosis is crucial for the survival of a species because it allows genetic recombination, producing the biological diversity of a species as well as providing a mechanism to create haploid gametes. The importance of meiosis is seen in the highly conserved events of chromosome pairing, recombination, and the two subsequent cellular divisions leading to haploid gametes that occur in both single-cell eukaryotes and metazoans.

As male germ cells enter meiosis, they undergo one last semi-conservative DNA replication cycle, although they will divide twice more. Chromosomes begin to condense and homologous chromosomes pair, producing a unique and highly conserved germ-cell structure, the *synaptinemal complex*. Gene expression is extensive during meiosis and many germ-cell–specific proteins [e.g., lactate dehydrogenase C4, phosphoglycerate kinase 2, cytochrome c_T, and the heat shock protein 70-2 (HSP 70-2)] are initially transcribed in meiotic germ cells (reviewed in Ref. 7). Why do meiotic and postmeiotic male germ cells require the expression of so many testis-specific isoproteins for commonly expressed proteins? How is their expression temporally regulated?

Gene targeting is providing an increasing number of animals that exhibit spermatogenic arrest during meiosis (Table 2.1). The elegant gene targeting of HSP 70-2 and cyclin A1 are especially informative. Disruption of the spermatocyte-specific HSP 70-2 results in failed meiosis, apoptosis, and male infertility (8). The absence of the HSP 70-2 protein disrupts CDC2/cyclin

TABLE 2.1. Genes whose deletion in the mouse generate defects in meiosis and male fertility.

Gene disrupted	Phenotype	Female phenotype
PMS2	Partial arrest in meiosis	Fertile
MLH-1	Arrest in meiosis	Sterile
ATM	Arrest in meiosis	Sterile
BAX	Arrest in meiosis	Fertile
RXRβ	Partial arrest in meiosis	Fertile
HSP 70-2	Partial arrest in meiosis	Fertile
Microrchidia (morc)	Arrest in early meiosis	Fertile
Cyclin Al	Arrest at end of meiotic prophase	Fertile

B1 assembly, preventing development of CDC2 kinase activity (9). Gene targeting of cyclin A1 in mice leads to increased male germ-cell apoptosis, desynapsis abnormalities and spermatocytes that do not pass into the first meiotic division (10). It is of interest that inactivation of cyclin A1 does not impede meiosis or affect fertility in female mice.

New insights into the regulatory mechanisms of meiosis will be achieved by investigators who combine genetic and evolutionary approaches. Numerous genes have been identified that are essential for normal meiosis in yeast, where it is estimated that 15% of the yeast genome (~1000 genes) is active during sporulation (11). In addition to gene targeting in mice as a means to create meiotic mutants, the natural "mutation"—men and women—also should not be overlooked. In the postpubertal male, spermatogenesis is a continuous process, and meiosis occurs without interruption. In contrast, the germ cells in the adult female arrest in the diplotene stage of meiotic prophase 1. Factors that prevent meiotic arrest in males or arrest meiosis in females need to be identified.

Spermiogenesis

During spermiogenesis, the round spermatid differentiates into the highly polarized spermatozoon under the control of a haploid genome that ceases transcription early in the process. Many of the events that occur during spermiogenesis are novel among eukaryotic cells. Major cellular architectural changes occur, including the creation of an acrosome, an axoneme, and a complex sperm tail, while the nucleus transforms from a nucleosomal structure to a tightly compacted and biochemically unique structure. At the end of spermiogenesis, most of the cytoplasm of the elongated spermatid is removed as the residual body is pinched off. The species-specific–shaped spermatozoa contain little cytoplasm, no cytoplasmic ribosomes, and a distinct form of mitochondria. Many of the proteins synthesized during spermiogenesis are transcribed from the haploid nucleus and/or are translated from stored mRNAs. During spermiogenesis, the cessation of nuclear transcription requires hundreds of sperm proteins to be synthesized from stored "paternal" mRNAs (reviewed in Ref. 12). Many questions arise from these unique events. For instance, how does transcription terminate? Why do the chromatin changes require histone replacement by the intermediary transition proteins 1 and 2, rather than a direct replacement of histones by protamines? Is there a defined order of chromatin change leading to a temporal compaction of genes? Why do sperm-head shapes of each species differ and what determines their shape?

Although many structural proteins [e.g., DNA-binding proteins (transition proteins 1 and 2 and protamines 1 and 2), mitochondrial proteins, outer dense fiber proteins, and fibrous sheath proteins] are expressed in spermatids, proteins such as olfactory receptors, a spliced form of the cystic fibrosis transmembrane receptor, a growth hormone-releasing hormonelike factor, and a tumor necrosis factor are also expressed. These apparently "ectopically expressed" genes lead some investigators to conclude that the haploid genome is "out of control" and the entire genome is randomly transcribed as the chromatin changes. Others argue that the presumed ectopically expressed genes are simply misnamed and have necessary functions during spermatogenesis. For instance, a smooth muscle actin, olfactory receptors, and transmembrane proteins related to snake toxins are synthesized in round spermatids. Because male germ cells are not a smooth muscle, do not detect odor, or do not poison animals, it is likely that these proteins are misnamed. It seems unlikely that evolution would allow gametes promiscuously to express large numbers of unneeded genes because expression of random proteins in gametes could have deleterious effects on gamete function and survival of the species.

Spermiogenesis provides an optimal environment to examine posttranscriptional regulation of gene expression because of the termination of transcription, the need for protein synthesis, and the numerous marker molecules expressed in spermatids (13). Following transcription, introns must be removed from mRNAs, some mRNAs are differentially spliced or processed in their 5' or 3' untranslated regions, and all mRNAs must be transported from the nucleus to the cytoplasm. For X or Y chromosome-linked genes that encode proteins essential for all spermatozoa, their products must be shared equally among all spermatids. This transfer has been shown for protamine 1, whose mRNAs are shared among spermatids by transport through intercellular bridges (14). Our overall understanding of posttranscriptional mechanisms in male germ cells is unfortunately equivalent to airplane design at the time of the Wright brothers. A major effort needs to be undertaken to decipher the mechanisms of mRNA processing and splicing in germ cells because they often produce extended or truncated forms of mRNAs that are also expressed in somatic cells. Studies of the mechanisms of novel promoter usage in germ cells and/or the use of secondary polyadenylation sites are needed. The mammalian testis is an especially rich source of RNA-binding proteins. The identification and characterization of several testicular RNA-binding proteins has begun to help decipher translational activation and repression and mRNA transport in the mammalian testes. The question, What stabilizes stored mRNAs for up to 7 days in the cytoplasm, merits investigation.

Somatic Cell–Germ Cell Interactions

The importance of Sertoli cells in germ-cell development has been known for a long time (14). The many unsuccessful efforts to culture male germ cells has demonstrated that germ cells are heavily dependent on chemical and probably physical associations with the Sertoli cell (15,16). A barrier created by Sertoli cells in the seminiferous tubule also maintains a critical physiological separation between premeiotic and postmeiotic germ cells and provides a means of bidirectional movement of factors between Sertoli cells and the developing germ cells. A large number of proteins, including activin, inhibin, interleukin-1, interleukin-6, transferrin, ceruloplasmin, cathepsin L, α2-macroglobulin, androgen-binding protein, retinol-binding protein, sulfated glycoproteins 1 and 2, and testibumin are secreted by Sertoli cells and are likely to influence germ-cell development. Germ-cell products (e.g., nerve growth factor and basic fibroblast growth factors) are likely in turn to influence Sertoli cell function and may be contributing factors to the distinct differentiated states of Sertoli cells. Transplantation studies, however, have revolutionized our thinking of germ-cell dependence. Although germ cells may be dependent upon Sertoli cells for nutritional support, they appear to function highly autonomously upon transplantation. When Brinster and colleagues repopulated sterile mouse testes with populations of donor testicular cells, they found that although transplanted mouse and rat testicular cells developed into morphologically normal spermatozoa (17,18), the rat germ cells differentiated at the rate of a rat germ cell. This indicates that mouse Sertoli cells can support rat germ-cell differentiation, but cannot regulate their cycle. Germ-cell transplantation offers many research opportunities for the future. The introduction of genetically altered populations of cells into testes promises to revolutionize animal husbandry. Should this technology be used to help infertile men? The limits that need to be placed on this technology raise numerous ethical concerns that must be resolved soon.

Genetic Causes of Infertility

Many cases of idiopathic male infertility have a genetic base. The cause of about 7% of male infertility has been attributed to submicroscopic deletions of the Y chromosome that delete two RNA-binding protein gene families, the RNA-binding motif-containing genes (RBM) and the deleted in azoospermia genes (DAZ) (19–21). Defects in other Y chromosome genes, autosomal genes, and X-linked genes will also lead to male infertility. In light of the estimated 15% of yeast genes involved in sporulation, the number of mammalian genes needed for normal spermatogenesis should be in the thousands.

Most medical procedures that are routinely used on humans have been extensively studied first in animal model systems. Although true for many of the techniques employed in assisted reproductive technologies for humans, there are disturbing examples where this is not so. In this rapidly moving area of medicine, many questions need to be answered.

First, how does one choose a "good" sperm for ICSI? The criterion currently used [i.e., a sperm that looks morphologically normal (or as normal as possible) is normal] begs the question of genetics. It ignores the fact that a single base-pair change in a critical region of a gene would still produce normal-appearing spermatoza! In the coming years, procedures need to be developed to evaluate individual sperm for genetic defects. This is a pressing need because it has been established that infertile men carrying Y chromosome microdeletions pass this defect onto sons produced by ICSI.

Second, can the procedures of round spermatid injection (ROSI) and/or round spermatid nuclear injection (ROSNI) be used for humans? To date, a few mice have been produced using this approach by a premier research laboratory (22). Live progeny were born that appeared normal. The success of ROSNI or ROSI in mice demonstrates that, although spermiogenesis is essential for the reorganization of the male germ cell to become a motile cell, it is not needed for fertilization or development. The genetic ramifications of this are profound because we do not know when genomic imprinting in the male gamete is completed (DNA methylation of sperm has been reported to occur in the epididymis). Moreover, selecting one round spermatid for injection is even more difficult than selecting one sperm for ICSI because it is exceptionally difficult to identify unstained round spermatids after they have been dissociated from seminiferous tubules. The likelihood that most of the germ cells obtained from a biopsy of an infertile man are morphologically abnormal confounds the problem. If ROSI is to be pursued in humans, procedures to evaluate and select round spermatids need to be developed! A major research effort must be undertaken with the model system of choice (i.e., mice) in which a large population of progeny are produced by ROSNI and ROSI. We know from many gene-targeting studies that an apparently normal phenotype often becomes an "interesting" model with subtle defects upon more detailed examination. Using humans as an experimental system for ROSNI and ROSI is not acceptable!

Gene Therapy and Somatic Cell Cloning

The rapidly advancing fields of somatic cell gene therapy and somatic cell cloning promise to add a new dimension to the quality of human health in the twenty-first century. Although it is not likely that somatic cells will replace spermatozoa as the male gamete of choice, many of the techniques being developed for somatic cell modification can be applied to germ cells. A dialogue among diverse members of society needs to define where limits should be placed. The rapid strides in vector technology promise to provide procedures that can ameliorate many sources of somatic cell deficiencies. Under what conditions should these technologies be applied to germ cells? Do we want to "cure" an individual only to see the defect reappear in his or her children? The excitement and fun that the study of biology has provided to us in the past will continue into the twenty-first century.

Acknowledgments. The author thanks members of his laboratory for valuable comments on this chapter and J. Wood for her excellent secretarial assistance.

References

1. Dym M. Spermatogonial stem cells of the testis. Proc Natl Acad Sci USA 1994;91:11287–89.
2. Dym M, Clermont Y. Role of spermatogonia in the repair of the seminiferous epithelium following x-irradiation of the rat testis. Am J Anat 1970;128:265–82.
3. Huckins C. The spermatogonial stem cell population in rats. Anat Rec 1971;169:533–58.
4. Oakberg EF. Spermatogonial stem cell renewal in the mouse. Am J Anat 1971;169:515–32.
5. Beck A, Miller I, Anderson P, Streuli M. RNA-binding protein, TIAR, is essential for primordial germ cell development. Proc Natl Acad Sci USA 1998;95:2331–36.
6. Beamer WG, Cunliffe-Beamer TL, Shultz KL, Langley SH, Roderick TH. Juvenile spermatogonial depletion (jsd): a genetic defect of germ cell proliferation of male mice. Biol Reprod 1988;38:899–908.
7. Eddy EM, O'Brien DA. Gene expression during mammalian meiosis. Curr Top Dev Biol 1997;37:141–200.
8. Dix DJ, Allen JW, Collins BW, Mori C, Nakamura N, Poorman-Allen P, et al. Targeted gene disruption of *Hsp-70-2* results in failed meiosis, germ cell apoptosis, and male infertility. Proc Natl Acad Sci USA 1996;93:3264–68.
9. Zhu, D, Dix DJ, Eddy, EM. HSP70-2 is required for CDC2 kinase activity in meiosis I of mouse spermatocytes. Development 1997;124:3007–14.
10. Liu D, Matzuk M, Sung WK, Guo Q, Wang P, Wolgemuth D. Cyclin A1 is required for meiosis in the male mouse. Nat Genet 1988;20:377–80.
11. Chu S, DeRisi J, Eisen M, Mulholland J, Botstein D, Brown P, et al. The transcriptional program of sporulation in budding yeast. Science 1998;282:699–705.
12. Hecht NB. Molecular mechanism of male germ cell differentiation. BioEssays 1998;20:555–61.
13. Sertoli E. Dell'esistenza di particolari cellule ramificate nei canalicoli seminiferi del testicolo umano. Morgagni 1865;7:31–40.
14. Calderwood, KA, Handel MA. Protamine transcript sharing among postmeiotic spermatids. Proc Natl Acad Sci USA 1991;88:2407–11.
15. Griswold MD. Interactions between Sertoli cells and germ cells in the testis. Biol Reprod 1995;52:211–16.
16. Jegou B. The Sertoli-germ cell communication network in mammals. Int Rev Cytol 1993;147:25–96.
17. Brinster R, Zimmermann J. Spermatogenesis following male germ-cell transplantation. Dev Biol 1994;91:11298–302.
18. Franca L, Ogawa T, Avarbock M, Brinster R, Russell L. Germ cell genotype controls cell cycle during spermatogenesis in the rat. Biol Reprod 1998;59:1371–77.
19. Ma K, Inglis JD, Bickmore S, Bickmore WA, Speed RM, Thomson EJ, et al. A Y chromosome gene family with RNA-binding protein homology: candidates for the azoospermia factor AZF controlling human spermatogenesis. Cell 1993;75:1287–95.

20. Reijo R, Lee T-Y, Salo P, Alagappan R, Brown LG, Rosenberg M, et al. Diverse spermatogenic defects in humans caused by Y chromosome deletions encompassing a novel RNA-binding protein gene. Nat Genet 1995;10:383–93.
21. Pryor JL, KentFirst M, Muallem A, VanBergen AH, Nolten WE, Meisner L. Microdeletions in the Y chromosome of infertile men. N Engl J Med 1997;336: 534–39.
22. Ogura A, Matsuda J, Yanagimachi R. Birth of normal young after electrofusion of mouse oocytes with round spermatids. Proc Natl Acad Sci USA 1994;91:7460–62.

Part I

Testis Development and Differentiation

3

Sry and the Testis: Molecular Pathways of Organogenesis

BLANCHE CAPEL

A fundamental goal in developmental biology is to understand how regulatory genes initiate cellular processes and control the patterning and differentiation of tissues. Such processes include cell proliferation and cell movements that reorganize tissue and generate novel cell-signaling relationships that play important roles in the morphogenesis of organs. Our lab is investigating how one important regulatory gene, the mammalian sex-determining gene, *Sry,* initiates the cellular changes that give rise to a testis rather than an ovary from the bipotential gonad.

Gonads of XX and XY embryos initially arise as identical bipotential primordia. In mammals, primary sex determination occurs when development of the bipotential gonad diverges toward the testis or ovarian pathway. Differentiation of secondary sex characteristics is subsequently controlled by hormonal secretions of the testis or ovary (1). Initiation of testis development depends on expression of the Y-linked gene, *Sry.* Proof was provided by gain and loss of function experiments: Expression of an *Sry* transgene in an XX mouse results in testis development (2,3), whereas deletion of *Sry* from the Y chromosome in the XY*^{Tdym1}* mouse results in ovary development (4,5).

In the mouse, *Sry* expression is detected near midgestation [between 10.5 and 12.5 days postcoitus (dpc)], exclusively in the XY gonadal primordium (6–8). The Sry protein belongs to a large family of HMG-type DNA-binding proteins. Some members of the family, including Sry, can bind specific sequences; all members of the family appear both to induce and to recognize chromatin conformation (9–11). Work on other members of the HMG family has shown that HMG proteins move to the nucleus (12), where they bind DNA inducing a 60-degree bend in chromatin, which leads to the juxtaposition of other transcription factors bound at distant sites (13,14). Hence, Sry may not act as a simple transcription factor (15), which offers some explanation of why direct gene targets of Sry have been difficult to discover.

Following *Sry* expression in XY embryos, both cellular differentiation and morphological development of the gonad diverge toward the testis pathway. *Sry* is thought to act within Sertoli cell precursors to specify the Sertoli cell lineage. It also must initiate the reorganization of cells coordinately to specify characteristic testis architecture. One of the first obvious changes distinguishing male gonad differentiation is the development of testis cords, which become visible by 12.5 dpc in the mouse. Testis cords consist of germ cells enclosed by epithelialized Sertoli cells surrounded by a basal lamina and a layer of peritubular myoid cells.

Little is known about the nature of signaling events downstream of *Sry* that specify the origin and differentiation of Sertoli cells or direct their organization into testis cord structures. In this chapter, we will describe several *Sry*-dependent pathways that characterize the initiation of testis development and elucidate the function of this key regulatory gene. The identification of these pathways will be an important tool in the discovery of the molecular targets of *Sry*.

Sertoli Cells Arise from the Coelomic Epithelium

Sertoli cells are thought to express *Sry* and serve as an organizing center in the gonad, although evidence for this hypothesis is indirect. Studies of XX↔XY chimeras indicated that Sertoli cells are the only cell type in the testis for which the presence of a Y chromosome is important (16). In XX↔XY chimeric gonads, Leydig, germ cells, and peritubular myoid cells could be XX or XY with equal probability; however, 90% of Sertoli cells were XY, demonstrating a strong bias for the XY cells of the chimera to differentiate as Sertoli cells. The fact that other cell types in the gonad showed no bias for the presence of a Y chromosome implies that expression of the *Sry* gene is only important in the pre-Sertoli cell; unfortunately, in the absence of an antibody against the mouse protein or an efficient transgenic reporter construct driven by the *Sry* promoter, the early cell type(s) expressing *Sry* have not been directly confirmed.

The origin of Sertoli cells has been a subject of interest for most of the twentieth century. Two main sources have been proposed: the coelomic epithelium and the mesonephros (17–20). Based on microscopy and immunocytochemical experiments in which the coelomic epithelium appeared to be labile during early gonad development (21), we tested the hypothesis that Sertoli cells arise from this source. We performed lineage-tracing experiments by labeling coelomic epithelial cells with the fluorescent lipophilic dye, DiI, and culturing for 48 hours. We have established an organ culture system in which cord formation routinely occurs in XY gonads explanted to culture after 15 tail somites (ts; 15 ts corresponds to 11.25 dpc as defined in Ref. 7) and cultured for 2 days in a shallow trench atop an agar block (22). Using this system, we found that descendants of coelomic epithelial cells gave rise to both Sertoli cells and other somatic cells of the testis (23). Coelomic epithelial cells moved to the interior of the gonad, where some DiI positive cells could be found inside testis cords abutting the basal lamina, as delineated by laminin-1 staining. Direct labeling of DiI positive cells with a Sertoli cell-specific antibody marker, Müllerian inhibiting substance (MIS), confirmed their identity. DiI positive cells were also found between cords, in the interstitial space.

To determine whether different coelomic epithelial cells have different fates, or if a single coelomic epithelial cell could give rise to Sertoli as well as interstitial cells, a single cell of the coelomic epithelium was labeled with DiI. Any gonad with more than one labeled cell was discarded. In experiments where a single cell was labeled at the 15–17 ts stage, multiple labeled cells could be found inside as well as outside testis cords after culture. In all cases DiI positive cells inside cords were found to abut the basement membrane and display a structural morphology characteristic of Sertoli cells. The identity of DiI positive cells found outside testis cords is under investigation. Cells found in the interstitial space were negative for the endothelial cell marker, PECAM, and for the Leydig cell marker; SF1. These cells may be precursors not yet expressing these lineage-specific markers, they may belong to other connective tissue lineages that are not yet defined by specific markers, and they may represent more than one cell type.

These experiments revealed that the ability of the coelomic epithelium to give rise to Sertoli cells was developmentally regulated. While cells labeled at 15–17 ts stages gave rise to Sertoli and other lineages, cells labeled at 18–20 ts stages were found exclusively outside testis cords. The developmental restriction of the fate of coelomic epithelial cells may be a result of changes in a signaling event over time. Movement to the interior of the gonad gradually decreased and ended as the tunica albuginea formed in the XY gonad, around 12.5 dpc (23).

Biphasic Proliferation of the Coelomic Epithelium Depends on *Sry*

It has long been appreciated that the XY gonad increases in size faster than the XX gonad. A parallel line of investigation in the lab revealed that one mechanism involved in testis organogenesis downstream of *Sry* is the upregulation of proliferation in the XY gonad. Coelomic epithelial cells undergo biphasic, male-specific proliferation beginning just before the peak of *Sry* expression (as reported in Ref. 7). Experiments to explore the possibility that proliferation pathways lie downstream of *Sry* were conducted by injecting a pregnant female with bromodeoxyuridine (BrdU) 2 hours prior to dissection. Individual embryos were sexed, the gonad/mesonephros complex was dissected, and whole samples were fixed and labeled with antibodies to detect BrdU, which is incorporated into the nuclei of dividing cells.

Two other antibodies were used to identify cell types and illuminate the structure of the gonad: steroidogenic factor 1 (SF1), which is believed to label both pre-Sertoli and pre-Leydig cells at 11.5–12.5 dpc, and PECAM, which labels endothelial and germ cells in the gonad at this stage. A detailed timecourse conducted between 13 ts (shortly after 10.5 dpc, when *Sry* expression initiates) and 34 ts (close to 13.5 dpc), revealed that proliferation of total somatic cells, and of cells in the coelomic epithelium in particular, is upregulated in a biphasic manner. The first significant divergence in proliferation occurs near 16 ts in coelomic epithelial cells that are SF1 positive. A second, more striking phase of male-specific proliferation is evident between 19 and 22 ts, in coelomic epithelial cells no longer positive for SF1 (unpublished observations).

To prove that proliferation in the coelomic epithelium depends on *Sry* and not on some other gene on the Y chromosome or on X chromosome dosage, similar experiments were conducted to examine proliferation in an XX mouse carrying *Sry* as a transgene [known to form a normal testis (3)], and in a mouse carrying a weak allele of *Sry*, XY[POS] [known to give rise to a high percentage of ovaries and ovotestes (24)]. Examination of the proliferation profiles in these mice revealed that XX carriers of the *Sry* transgene showed a proliferation pattern similar to normal XY males, whereas XY[POS] gonads showed a proliferation pattern indistinguishable from XX females (unpublished observations). These experiments indicate that proliferation differences detected between XY and XX gonads depend on *Sry* and represent a pathway initiated directly or indirectly by the male sex-determining gene. In all cases examined, upregulation of proliferation is strongly correlated with differentiation of the testis.

Sertoli Cells Are Derived from the First Phase of Proliferation in the Coelomic Epithelium

Further experiments using a BrdU pulse/chase-labeling method confirmed the stage of coelomic epithelial proliferation that gives rise to Sertoli cells. To determine which cell types arise from the stages of proliferation, pregnant females were pulsed for 1 hour with BrdU between 11.0 and 11.5 dpc (15–18 ts). They were then chased with excess thymidine and allowed to develop either for 6 hours or for 2 additional days. On the other hand pregnant females were pulsed during the period between 11.5–12.0 dpc (18–22 dpc), and treated similarly. Samples were collected, fixed, cryosectioned, and stained with antibodies against BrdU and laminin. Laminin-1 reveals testis cord structure and, therefore, the localization of BrdU-positive cells either inside or outside testis cords. These experiments confirmed the results from DiI-labeling experiments: Sertoli cells arise from a population of cells proliferating prior to 18 ts. When pulsed gonads were dissected 6 hours into the chase, proliferating cells in the coelomic epithelium could be seen to have moved beneath the coelomic epithelium at both stages of development. When pulsed gonads are dissected 2 days after the chase, however, Sertoli cells carry the BrdU label only if the mother was pulsed prior to midday on day 11.5 (18 ts). Prior to 18 ts, both Sertoli cells and cells that reside in the interstitium are derived from the proliferating population. After 18 ts, proliferating cells still give rise to an unidentified interstitial population, but no longer to Sertoli cells (unpublished observations). Our current hypothesis is that *Sry* is required in a cell-autonomous manner for the first phase of proliferation in Sertoli precursors. The second phase of proliferation that gives rise to interstitial cells may be a non–cell-autonomous effect of *Sry*.

Migration of Somatic Cells from the Mesonephros Plays a Role in Testis Cord Formation and Sertoli Cell Differentiation

A second mechanism involved in testis organogenesis shown to depend on *Sry* is the male-specific induction of somatic-cell migration from the mesonephros into the gonad. We combined our culture system with a tissue recombination assay, apposing mesonephroi from ROSA26 (B6,129-TgR (ROSA26)26Sor) (25) (blue) mice and gonads from wild type CD1 (white) mice. This assay revealed that cells from the mesonephros migrate into an XY gonad, but not into an XX gonad. Further experiments using gonads from XX mice carrying *Sry* as a transgene, and XY mice carrying a Y chromosome deleted for the *Sry* gene, proved that mesonephric cell migration depends on the presence of the *Sry* gene.

At least three cell types in the XY gonad are derived from the mesonephros. These include (1) cells surrounding Sertoli cell cords, in the position of peritubular myoid cells, (2) endothelial cells, and (3) another cell type associated with the endothelium, but negative for the endothelial marker PECAM. Recruitment of mesenchymal cells and their interactions with an epithelium are known to be important for development of many organs. The identity of the cell types migrating into the XY gonad raised the possibility that interactions between these cells and the pre-Sertoli cell could lead to the epithelialization of pre-Sertoli cells and their organization into testis cords. Buehr et al. had shown that blocking cell migration into XY gonads impaired cord formation (26). We extended these experiments by examining the effect of separating the mesonephros and gonad at successively earlier stages of development. At the earliest stage when separation has proved possible (16 ts), cord formation was completely blocked (unpublished observations). This experiment, however, was difficult to interpret because the viability of 16 ts gonads in culture was severely reduced, the frequency of cord formation even in unseparated controls dropped to ~70%, and damage to gonads during separation was likely to occur. We therefore sought a better way to study the role of migration in testis cord formation.

Cell migration does not normally occur into an XX gonad, but it can be induced to occur by placing a small piece of an XY gonad on the surface of an XX gonad in a "sandwich" arrangement. When somatic-cell migration is induced from the mesonephros into an 11.5 dpc XX gonad, germ-cell organization (revealed by staining for alkaline phosphatase) and laminin deposition (revealed by staining with an antibody against laminin-1) took on a malelike pattern. When XX and XY gonads were apposed and cultured in the absence of a mesonephros or with a 0.1 μm membrane barrier positioned between the mesonephros and the gonad, no organization was seen (unpublished observations). These experiments indicate that migration of somatic cells from the mesonephros is critical for testis cord formation. We cannot rule out the possibility that an additional factor present in the XY portion of the graft is also important for induction of cords in the XX tissue; however, if so, this factor alone is not sufficient to induce cord formation in the absence of migrating cells from the mesonephros.

When migration was induced into 11.5 dpc XX gonads, Sertoli cell differentiation was initiated. During normal development, *Sox9* is expressed at early stages in XX and XY gonads, but by 12.5 dpc, expression of *Sox9* is downregulated in XX gonads and strongly upregulated in XY gonads, specifically in Sertoli cells. In a reciprocal manner, *Dax1* is downregulated in XY gonads and upregulated in XX gonads. When migration of somatic cells from the mesonephros is induced into the XX gonad in sandwich cultures, *Sox9* expression is strongly upregulated inside the forming cords and *Dax1* is downregulated in a pattern similar to normal XY gonads. XY gonads separated from their mesonephroi prior to 16 ts and cultured for 2 days show little to no expression of *Sox9* (unpublished observations), which suggests that migration of mesonephric cells is critical for the initiation or maintenance of Sertoli cell differentiation in XY gonads. It is striking that migrating mesonephric cells can induce Sertoli cell differentiation in XX gonads in the absence of the *Sry* gene. It is not known whether Sertoli cell differentiation in XX gonads is initiated by the deposition of a basal lamina between pre-Sertoli and peritubular myoid cells, or by other signals between pre-Sertoli and migrating cells.

Induction of Cord Formation and Sertoli Differentiation Is Stage Specific

We have also shown that mesonephric cell migration is required for testis cord formation in XX and XY gonads in a stage-specific manner. When sandwich gonads were assembled at 12.5 dpc or later, migration could still be induced into the XX gonad, but cord formation did not occur. To determine whether this effect reflected a change in the inducing or responding tissue, tissue recombinations were assembled between components at different stages. The results of these heterochronic experiments indicated that both the XY-inducing tissue and the XX-responding tissue must be obtained and assembled prior to 12.5 dpc, but the stage of the mesonephros could be older than 12.5 dpc. Although endothelial and endothelial-associated cells continued to migrate until at least 16.5 dpc (the latest stage at which recombinant organ culture experiments have been successful), cord formation in the XX responding tissue could not be induced after 12.5 dpc (unpublished observations). With respect to the inducing tissue, one hypothetical explanation for this finding is that the signal for a critical migrating cell type (e.g., the peritubular myoid cell) is limited to a narrow window of development prior to 12.5 dpc. Experiments in which the mesonephros was from a 12.5 dpc XY donor suggested that it is depleted of an important cell type relative to the XX mesonephros. The lack of an antibody that can specifically identify early peritubular myoid cells is an impediment to progress in this direction. With respect to the responding tissue, it also seems likely that the bipotential phase of the XX gonad comes to an end near 12.5 dpc such that it can no longer respond to signals to enter the male pathway. After this time, critical interactions with germ cells or other developmental signals between somatic cells may limit its potential.

Summary

The overall goal of our lab is to develop paradigms of how genes control organogenesis. In mammals the primary step in male sex determination is the initiation of testis development in the bipotential gonad primordium. This step depends on the Y-linked male sex-determining gene, *Sry,* which is expressed between 10.5 and 12.5 dpc in the mouse. Elucidating the function of *Sry* during organogenesis of the testis is providing novel information about the links between the expression of a transcription factor and mechanistic processes that control structural morphogenesis and its relation to cell differentiation. Available indirect evidence suggests that pre-Sertoli cells express *Sry* and serve as an organizing center in the male gonad. We have discovered that *Sry* induces a biphasic, male-specific proliferation of coelomic epithelial cells, beginning just prior to the peak of *Sry* expression. By using a stable fluorescent lipophilic dye to lineage trace coelomic epithelial cells, we have shown that Sertoli cells arise from the coelomic epithelium during the earliest phase of proliferation. A second mechanism of testis organogenesis shown to depend on *Sry* is the male-specific migration of somatic cells from the mesonephros into the gonad. We have shown that migration of somatic cells from the mesonephros is required for testis cord formation in XY gonads in a stage-specific manner. Induction of mesonephric cell migration into bipotential XX gonads results in organization of XX cells into cord structures, upregulation of the male-specific marker *Sox9*, and downregulation of the female specific marker *Dax1*. When migration into XY gonads was blocked, expression of the male-specific marker *Sox9* declined. From these results we conclude that mesonephric cell migration plays a critical role in the formation of testis cords and the differentiation of Sertoli versus follicle cells in the gonad. These experiments defining mechanisms downstream of *Sry* are providing clear examples of how a regulatory transcription factor, *Sry*, initiates cellular processes, including proliferation and cell migration, which in turn influence architectural patterning, fate commitment, and differentiation of cells within an organ.

Acknowledgments. I would like to thank the members of my lab who have all contributed to these results: Jeannie Karl, Christopher Tilmann, Jeanna Schmahl, Jennifer Brennan, Dawn Franklin, and Kenny Ung. We are also grateful to Harold Erickson for antibodies against laminin-1, Ken-ichirou Morohashi for antibodies against SF1, Peter Koopman for an RNA probe against *Sox9*, and Robin Lovell-Badge for an RNA probe against *Dax1*. The work was supported by grants from the National Institutes of Health and the March of Dimes Research Foundation.

References

1. Jost A. Recherches sur la différentiation sexuelle de l'embryon de lapin. Archs Anat Microsc Morph Exp 1947;36:271–315.
2. Koopman P, Gubbay J, Vivian N, Goodfellow P, Lovell-Badge R. Male development of chromosomally female mice transgenic for *Sry*. Nature 1991;351:117–21.
3. Eicher EM, Shown EP, Washburn LL. Sex reversal in C57BL/6J-Y[POS] mice corrected by a *Sry* transgene. Phil Trans R Soc B 1995;350:263–69.
4. Gubbay J, Collignon J, Koopman P, Capel B, Economou A, Münsterberg A, et al. A gene mapping to the sex-determining region of the mouse Y chromosome is a member of a novel family of embryonically expressed genes. Nature 1990;346: 245–50.
5. Lovell-Badge R, Robertson E. XY female mice resulting from a heritable mutation in the murine primary testis determining gene, *Tdy*. Development 1990;109: 635–46.
6. Koopman P, Münsterberg A, Capel B, Vivian N, Lovell-Badge R. Expression of a candidate sex-determining gene during mouse testis differentiation. Nature 1990;348:450–52.
7. Hacker A, Capel B, Goodfellow P, Lovell-Badge R. Expression of *Sry*, the mouse sex determining gene. Development 1995;121:1603–14.
8. Jeske YWA, Bowles J, Greenfield A, Koopman P. Expression of a linear *Sry* transcript in the mouse genital ridge. Nat Gen 1995;10:480–82.
9. Bianchi ME, Falciola L, Ferrari S, Lilley D. The DNA binding site of HMG1 protein is composed of two similar segments (HMG boxes), both of which have counterparts in other eukaryotic regulatory proteins. Embo J 1992;11:1055–63.
10. Harley VR, Jackson DI, Hextal PJ, Hawkins JR, Berkovitz GD, Sockanathan S, et al. DNA binding activity of recombinant *SRY* from normal males and XY females. Science 1992;225:453–56.

11. Pontiggia A, Rimini R, Harley V, Goodfellow P, Lovell-Badge R, Bianchi M. Sex-reversing mutations affect the architecture of SRY-DNA complexes. EMBO 1994;13:6115–24.

12. Behrens J, von Kries J, Kühl M, Bruhn L, Wedlich D, Grosschedl R, et al. Functional interaction of β-catenin with the transcription factor LEF-1. Nature 1996;382:638–42.

13. Giese K, Cox J, Grosschedl R. The HMG domain of lymphoid enhancer factor 1 bends DNA and facilitates assembly of functional nucleoprotein structures. Cell 1992;69:1–20.

14. Grosschedl R, Giese K, Pagel J. HMG domain proteins: architectural elements in the assembly of nucleoprotein structures. Trends Genet 1994;10:94–100.

15. Jenuwein T, Forrester W, Fernandezherrero L, Laible G, Dull M, Grosschedl R. Extension of chromatin accessibility by nuclear matrix attachment regions. Nature 1997;38:269–72.

16. Palmer SJ, Burgoyne PS. *In situ* analysis of fetal, prepubertal and adult XX–XY chimaeric mouse testes: Sertoli cells are predominantly, but not exclusively, XY. Development 1991;112:265–68.

17. Wartenberg H. Human testicular development and the role of the mesonephros in the origin of a dual Sertoli cell system. Andrologia 1978;10:1–21.

18. Upadhyay S, Luciani JM, Zamboni L. The role of the mesonephros in the development of indifferent gonads and ovaries of the mouse. Ann Biolanim Biochim Biophys 1979;19:1179–96.

19. Zamboni L, Upadhyay S. The contribution of the mesonephros to the development of the sheep fetal testis. Am J Anat 1982;165:339–56.

20. Byskov AG. Differentiation of mammalian embryonic gonad. Physiol Rev 1986;66:71–117.

21. Capel B, Lovell-Badge R. The *Sry* Gene and Sex Determination in Mammals. In: Wasserman, P, ed. Advances in developmental biology. Vol 2. Greenwich: JAI Press, 1993:1–35.

22. Martineau J, Nordqvist K, Tilmann C, Lovell-Badge R, Capel B. Male-specific cell migration into the developing gonad. Curr Biol 1997;7:958–68.

23. Karl J, Capel B. Sertoli cells of the mouse testis originate from the coelomic epithelium. Dev Biol 1998;203:323–33.

24. Eicher EM, Washburn LL, Whitney IJ, Morrow KE. *Mus poschiavinus* Y chromosome in the C57BL/6J murine genome causes sex reversal. Science 1982;217: 535–37.

25. Friedrich G, Soriano P. Promoter trap in embryonic stem cells: a genetic screen to identify and mutate developmental genes in mice. Genes Dev 1991;5:1513–23.

26. Buehr M, Gu S, McLaren A. Mesonephric contribution to testis differentiation in the fetal mouse. Development 1993;117:273–81.

4

MIS Actions in the Developing Testis

Mary Min-chin Lee

Introduction

Müllerian inhibiting substance (MIS), a gonadal glycoprotein in the TGF-β family of growth and differentiation factors, is recognized primarily for its role in promoting involution of the Müllerian ducts during normal male sexual differentiation. Continued synthesis of MIS by Sertoli cells and expression of its cognate type II receptor in the postnatal testis, however, raised the possibility of additional functions for MIS. We hypothesized that MIS plays an important role in the regulation of Leydig-cell proliferation and maturation during postnatal testicular development. This chapter will summarize the expression and binding characteristics of the MIS receptor in the postnatal testis and elucidate the actions of MIS in Leydig cells at different stages of maturation using a primary rat Leydig-cell culture model. These data suggest that this fetal growth inhibitor affects androgen production by downregulating steroidogenic enzymes and helps to maintain a normal complement of Leydig cells by constraining their proliferation, thus supporting a direct role for MIS in the developing testis.

Background

The necessity for a distinct factor other than testosterone to achieve normal male sexual differentiation was first validated by Alfred Jost in the 1940s when he demonstrated that a testosterone crystal implanted next to a fetal rabbit urogenital ridge stimulated wolffian duct development but was unable to cause Müllerian duct regression (1). This substance was later named *Müllerian inhibiting substance* by Patricia Donahoe, and *anti-Müllerian hormone* by Nathalie Josso, the two investigators primarily responsible for the biochemical analysis and purification of MIS (2,3). In 1986, the gene (4), followed by the cDNA sequence (5) for MIS, was reported. MIS is a 140 kDa glycoprotein produced by Sertoli cells and postnatal granulosa cells that shares carboxy terminal homology with the TGF-β superfamily. MIS is produced as a dimeric prohormone precursor that undergoes proteolytic processing to generate a bioactive 25 kDa C-terminal dimer and an inactive N-terminal fragment (6). Like other proteins in the TGF-β family, MIS signals through a heterotetrameric receptor complex composed of structurally related serine threonine kinase receptors (7–9). After ligand-specific binding by the type II receptors, the type I receptors are recruited into the receptor complex and cross-phosphorylated on serine and threonine residues in the juxtamembrane domain. The type I receptor then phosphorylates downstream mediators of signaling, the best characterized of which are the SMAD family of proteins, for TGF-β signaling (10).

Although the Müllerian ducts are only sensitive to the regressive effects of MIS for a short period during midgestation, Sertoli-cell secretion of MIS persists postnatally. In rodents, both MIS mRNA and protein levels decline markedly after birth, but transiently rise at puberty and remain detectable in the adult (11,12). The MIS type II receptor is expressed in the fetal testis and downregulated at birth, then induced again by 2 weeks of age and remains abundant in the pubertal and adult testis (7,13). The expression of both MIS and its type II receptor in Sertoli cells is highest at stage VII of the spermatogenic cycle (13). The phenotypes of mice transgenic for MIS and those with null deletions of the MIS gene and its receptor subsequently provided clues for a potential role of MIS in the postnatal testis.

Although the majority of male transgenic mice overexpressing MIS had no discernible phenotype, males with high serum levels of MIS had feminized external genitalia with vaginal openings, undescended testes devoid of germ cells, and underdeveloped Wolffian ducts, which is consistent with inadequate androgenization during sexual differentiation (14,15). In fact, serum testosterone concentrations were lower and steroidogenic enzyme mRNA transcripts were less abundant in transgenic mice than they were in control mice (16). Although the total testicular volume was unchanged, the Leydig cell volume in adult transgenic mice was one third that of controls. This was attributed to a 50–80% decrease in the numbers of immature and mature Leydig cells, with a corresponding increase in mesenchymal precursor cells, which suggests that MIS may have induced a maturational block. Male mice with targeted deletions of the MIS gene or its receptor had conversely retained Müllerian ducts as expected, but they also developed Leydig-cell hyperplasia and neoplasia (14,15,17,18). Despite the increased Leydig-cell numbers, serum testosterone concentrations were not elevated, although P450c17 mRNA was more abundant (16).

These data indicated that perturbations in MIS expression could alter the number and/or function of Leydig cells in the testis. This led us to hypothesize that MIS is one of the critical hormones that balances the proliferative actions of known Leydig-cell mitogens and modulates steroidogenic capacity in the developing testis. The focus of these studies is to elucidate the actions of MIS in developing Leydig cells at different stages of maturation using a primary rat Leydig-cell culture model.

Expression of the MIS Receptors in Leydig Cells

Initial studies localized the MIS type II receptor to Sertoli cells of the fetal and postnatal testis (7,13). To determine if MIS acts directly or indirectly on Leydig cells, cell-specific expression of the MIS type II receptor was characterized (19). Primary rat Leydig-cell cultures were prepared by collagenase/DNase/Dispase digestion followed by elutriation and Percoll gradient centrifugation (20). Postnatal Leydig cells pass through three discrete maturational stages (21,22). Progenitor Leydig cells (PLCs), harvested from 21-day-old prepubertal rats, retain an elongated, mesenchymallike shape, but are recognizable as Leydig cells by their expression of the LH receptor and the steroidogenic enzymes. PLCs transform from a spindle to a round shape and acquire the abundant lipid inclusions that are characteristic of the immature or pubertal Leydig cells (ILC). ILCs, isolated from 35-day pubertal rats, express both steroidogenic and androgen-metabolizing enzymes. Further differentiation of the ILCs to adult Leydig cells (ALCs) is characterized by loss of lipid inclusions and increased steroidogenic capacity, which is typical of Leydig cells isolated from 90-day rats. Leydig-cell proliferative capacity decreases with increasing maturational stage in that PLCs actively divide, whereas ILCs only undergo one to two rounds of cell division and ALCs do not proliferate.

Sertoli cell–enriched cultures were obtained by subjecting the seminiferous tubule fraction to glycine treatment, followed by sequential collagenase/hyaluronidase digestion and filtration (23).

To ascertain the purity of the cellular preparations, the cells were stained for 3bHSD activity and analyzed for expression of cell-type–specific genes (19,24). The Leydig-cell preparations consistently contained fewer than 1 germ cell per high power field (<1%) and appeared homogeneous microscopically. Greater than 95% of the cells were positive for Leydig cell–specific 3β-hydroxysteroid dehydrogenase (3βHSD) (19). The Sertoli cell–enriched fractions and COS cells used for a negative control line did not stain for 3bHSD. Northern analysis confirmed that the Sertoli-cell genes, androgen-binding protein (ABP), MIS, and FSH receptor were expressed in the Sertoli, but not the Leydig-cell preps, whereas the LH receptor was only expressed in Leydig cells (Table 4.1) (19).

Cellular distribution of the MIS type II receptor mRNA was examined by northern analysis in total testis, primary Leydig cells at all three maturational ages and primary Sertoli cells from day 21 and day 35 rats (19). These studies showed that specific expression of the MIS type II receptor in primary Leydig cells at all three ages as well as in day 21 and day 35 Sertoli cells (Fig. 4.1, ALCs are not shown). ABP was not expressed in any of the

TABLE 4.1. Relative mRNA expression of cell-type specific genes.

	Postnatal day 21			Postnatal day 35		
	Testis	Leydig cells	Sertoli cells	Testis	Leydig cells	Sertoli cells
Sertoli cell genes						
MIS	103	0	490	211	0	75
FSH receptor	678	0	124	570	0	11
ABP	1892	0	404	931	5	49
Leydig cell genes						
LH receptor	61	765	0	221	883	0

ABP (gift of Dr. David Joseph, Biotechnology Development Institute at the University of Florida, Alachua, FL) (25), MIS (26), and the FSH receptor (Dr. Michael Griswold, Washington State University, Pullman, WA) (27) were selected as genes specific to Sertoli cells and the LH receptor (Dr. Deborah Segaloff, University of Iowa College of Medicine, Iowa City, IA) (28) as a Leydig cell–specific gene. The relative abundance of the signals were quantitated by densitometric analysis using NIH Image software. Reprinted with permission from Lee MM, et al. Mullerian inhibiting substance type II receptor expression and function in purified rat Leydig cells. Endocrinology 1999;140:2819–27. © The Endocrine Society.

Leydig-cell preparations, confirming the lack of Sertoli cell contamination. When normalized for GAPDH expression, MIS receptor mRNA levels declined in Sertoli cells from day 21 to day 35 but remained unchanged in Leydig cells.

Expression of the MIS types I and II receptors was also characterized by immunohistochemical staining, using chick antipeptide antibodies that had been demonstrated to detect the receptor on urogenital ridge sections and COS cells transfected with the receptor. This confirmed expression of both types I and II receptors for MIS in PLCs, ILCs, and ALCs (data not shown).

MIS Binding to Leydig Cells

To determine if primary Leydig cells express functional MIS receptors, binding was characterized by flow cytometry. Analysis of endogenous forward and side-angle scatter revealed that preparations of isolated Leydig cells differ in size and light scatter as they mature. PLCs were the smallest and ALCs the largest cells, whereas the ILCs were heterogeneous with three different-sized subpopulations of cells. For analysis of MIS binding, freshly isolated Leydig cells were incubated with biotinylated MIS and binding was visualized with avidin-phycoerythrin. The MIS was recombinantly produced and immunoaffinity purified in the laboratory of Patricia Donahoe and David MacLaughlin (25). It was then quantitated by ELISA (26) as well as by a rat urogenital ridge bioassay (27,28), verifying cross-species bioactivity. All three maturational stages of primary Leydig cells bound MIS specifically as contrasted with primary Sertoli cells from day 21 rats and COS cells (an

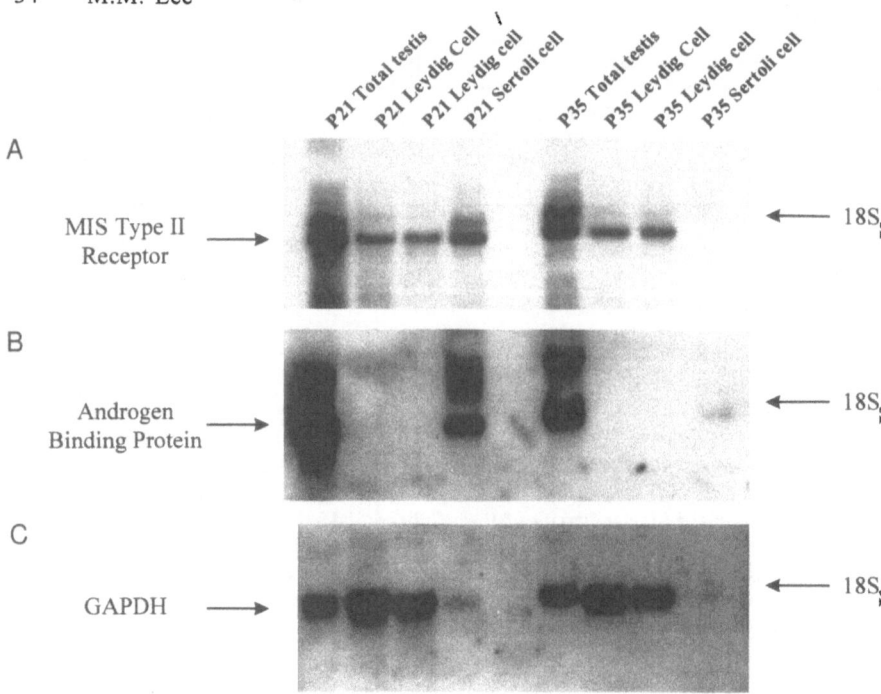

FIGURE 4.1. Northern analysis of the MIS type II receptor and androgen binding protein. Northern membranes were probed with a full-length rat MIS type II receptor riboprobe (7), and ABP (38) and GAPDH (39) random primed probes. (A) The MIS type II receptor was expressed abundantly in highly purified Leydig cells and Sertoli cells. The steady-state mRNA levels of the MIS type II receptor in Sertoli cells were more abundant on day 21 than day 35, when normalized for GAPDH expression, using NIH Image software for densitometric analysis. In contrast, the abundance of the receptor transcripts in Leydig cells was similar on days 21 (PLCs) and 35 (ILCs) (ALC data not shown). (B) ABP is present in total testis and Sertoli cells, but not in Leydig cells, even on an overexposed autoradiogram (not shown). To verify lack of Sertoli cell contamination in the Leydig-cell fractions, less Sertoli cell RNA (1–2 μg) was loaded to enable a prolonged exposure to be obtained without obscuring the Leydig cell lanes. (C) Rehybridization with a GAPDH probe confirmed that all lanes contained comparable amounts of RNA (less than twofold variation), except for the two Sertoli cell lanes that were initially loaded with only 2 μg (day 21) and 1 μg (day 35) total RNA. Reprinted with permission from Lee MM, et al. Mullerian inhibiting substance type II receptor expression and function in purified rat Leydig cells. Endocrinology 1999;140:2819–27. © The Endocrine Society.

MIS type II receptor negative cell line) (Fig. 4.2A). Mean fluorescence shifted back toward the baseline when the cells were preincubated with 10-fold excess nonbiotinylated MIS. With increasing concentrations of MIS, the PLCs, ILCs, and ALCs exhibited a progressive increase in the mean fluorescence per cell in contrast to primary Sertoli cells and COS cells.

The binding visualized by flow cytometry in the PLCs was concentration dependent from 10 to 150 nM and saturable (Fig. 4.2B) (19). The concentration of MIS required to reach half saturation was approximately 15 nM, a measure

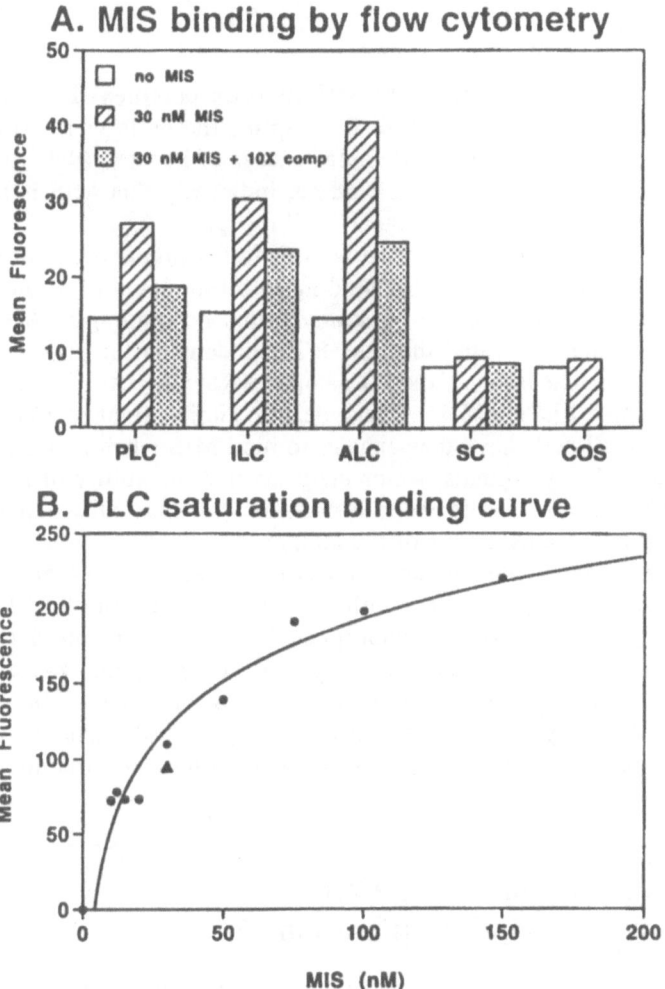

A. MIS binding by flow cytometry

no MIS

30 nM MIS

30 nM MIS + 10X comp

B. PLC saturation binding curve

FIGURE 4.2. MIS binding by flow cytometry. Freshly isolated Leydig or Sertoli cells were resuspended at 1×10^6 cells/ml in Leydig cell media, then incubated with biotinylated MIS or buffer for 1 hour. The cells were then washed and incubated with avidin-phycoerythrin conjugate (Molecular Probes, Eugene, OR) for 30 minutes in the dark. For competition experiments, either nonbiotinylated MIS (10-fold excess) or TGF-β1 (Promega; up to 40 nM) were co-incubated with biotinylated MIS. The cells were analyzed in a Becton Dickenson FACSCAN using LYSIS II acquisition and analysis software, with 10,000–20,000 events collected in list mode and analyzed per sample. Forward versus side-angle scatter gating and propidium iodide exclusion were used to distinguish viable cells from dead cells and debris. (A) Mean fluorescence per cell of PLCs, ILCs, and ALCs, but not Sertoli cells or COS cells, increased with 30 nM MIS and decreased when binding was competed with 10-fold excess nonbiotinylated MIS. (B) Mean and median fluorescence per cell were plotted against the MIS concentration to generate a saturation binding curve for PLCs, which was fitted by a polynomial regression algorithm. The binding of biotinylated MIS to PLCs was concentration dependent (from 0 to 150 nM) and saturable with a dissociation constant of 15 nM. In the presence of excess TGF-β(Δ), mean fluorescence per cell did not change significantly. Adapted with permission from Lee MM, et al. Mullerian inhibiting substance type II receptor expression and function in purified rat Leydig cells. Endocrinology 1999;140:2819–27. © The Endocrine Society.

of the dissociation constant of the MIS-receptor complex. To ascertain that MIS was not binding to the TGF-β receptor, the cells were co-incubated with TGF-β at 1000–10,000-fold molar excess of its ED_{50} (0.4–40 nM). Excess TGF-β did not compete for binding, indicating that MIS is binding to its own receptor rather than to the TGF-β receptor (Fig. 4.2B).

Multiple flow studies conducted with different preparations of PLCs and ALCS consistently demonstrated binding of biotinylated MIS, whereas ILC results were more variable. We initially found no binding with ILCs (19), but recent studies indicated that this is dependent on the subpopulation of cells examined. The larger-sized ILCs bound MIS, whereas the smallest cells, which resemble PLCs, did not. Thus, despite similar light scatter characteristics, the small cells have the capacity to bind MIS when isolated from 21-day, but not 35-day animals, which suggests that the ability of Leydig cells to bind MIS is not merely stage dependent, but may also depend on the overall pubertal status or age of the animal.

To further analyze the characteristics of the ILC fraction that bound MIS, we performed double labeling with biotinylated MIS and an LH-receptor antibody, using two different fluorogens. These experiments demonstrated that the majority of ILCs expressed the LH receptor, and that a subset of these LH receptor positive cells bound MIS. In ongoing studies, the ILCs are being sorted by their MIS binding capacity to further characterize these discrete subpopulations of cells and identify biological variables unique to each fraction.

Effects of MIS on Leydig Cell Steroidogenesis and Proliferation

With this evidence that primary Leydig cells bind MIS, functional studies were designed to examine the direct effects of MIS on Leydig-cell proliferation and steroidogenesis. To study steroidogenesis, Leydig cells were plated in triplicate overnight with 1 ng/ml LH, then treated with 30 nM MIS for 48 hours. Conditioned media were collected at three time points for testosterone RIA (29,30), with 22R-hydroxycholesterol added for the final 6-hour media collection. Mean basal production of testosterone by the PLCs was low (1.4–3.9 ng/million cells/24 hours). At all time points, PLC testosterone secretion decreased with MIS, and this effect was greater with a longer duration of exposure to MIS (88% of basal at 24 hours, $p < 0.05$; 78% at 48 hours, $p < 0.01$; and 69% at 54 hours, $p < 0.0001$) (Fig. 4.3A). The effect of MIS on testosterone secretion by ILCs varied from experiment to experiment, resulting in no significant mean difference (Fig. 4.3B). MIS treated ALCs consistently produced less testosterone, but this did not reach statistical significance (Fig. 4.3C). The differing actions of MIS at the three maturational ages may reflect the effect of MIS on the expression of both steroidogenic and metabolizing enzymes that contribute to net androgen production. To address this possibility, androstenediol, androsterone, and androstenedione are currently being assayed.

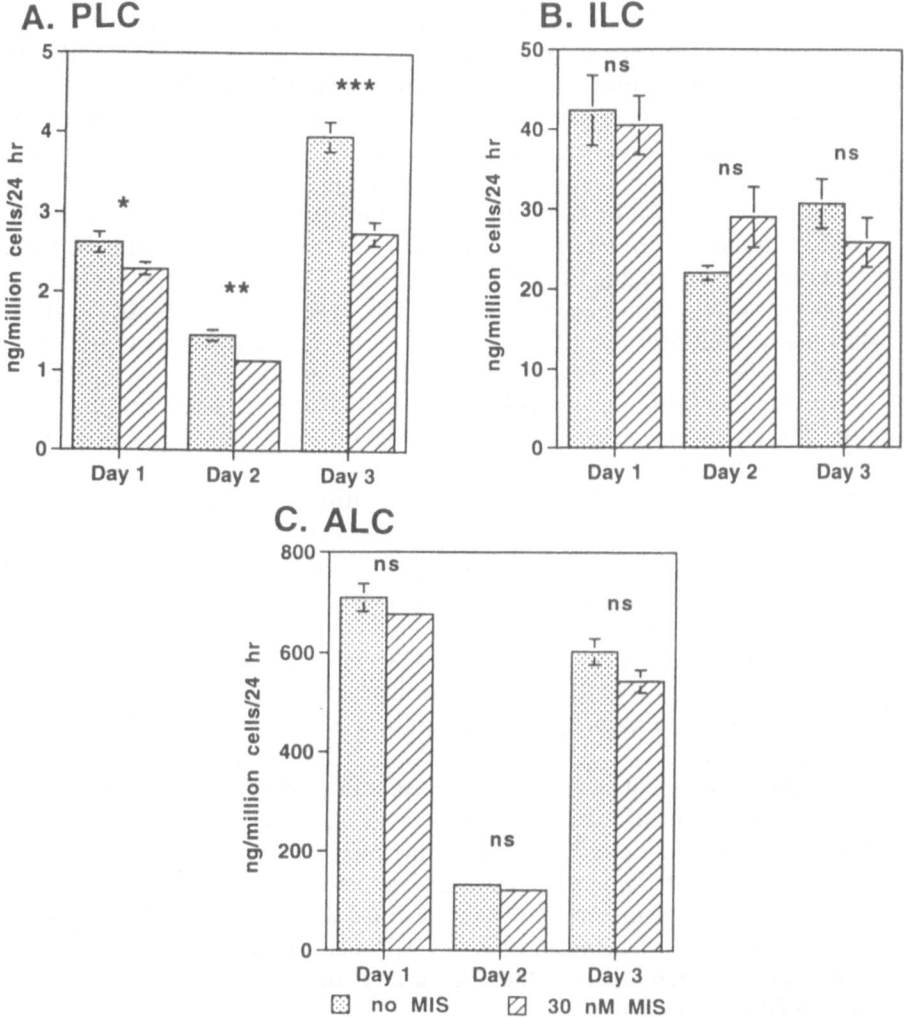

FIGURE 4.3. Effects of MIS on Leydig cell steroidogenesis. Primary Leydig cells were cultured overnight in serum-free DMEM/F12 (1:1) supplemented with 15 mM Hepes, 26 mM sodium bicarbonate, 0.1% BSA, 100 mg/ml bovine lipoprotein (Sigma), 12 µg/ml gentamycin, and 1 ng/ml LH (NIDDK-oLH-26, National Hormone and Pituitary Program) in a reduced oxygen incubator ($5\% CO_2/5\% O_2$) (Nuaire TS Autoflow Co_2/O_2 incubator) (20,40). The cells were treated with 30 nM MIS or buffer for 48 hours. Conditioned media were collected every 24 hours for steroid analysis. On the third day, 22R-hydroxycholesterol was added as a testosterone substrate for the last 6 hours. (A) Basal production of testosterone by PLCs in the absence of MIS was low (1.4–3.9 ng/million cells/24 hours), as had been reported previously. At all time points, testosterone production by PLCs decreased with MIS. A longer duration of exposure to MIS caused greater inhibition of testosterone production (88% of basal at 24 hours, $p < 0.05$; 78% at 48 hours, $p < 0.01$; and 69% at 54 hours, $p < 0.0001$). (B) In the ILCs, the results varied among experiments, resulting in no significant differences. (C) MIS-treated ALCs consistently produced less testosterone, but this did not reach statistical significance.

The effects of MIS on Leydig cell steroidogenesis in the MA-10 Leydig cell line have also been examined (Teixeira JT, Payne A, Donahoe PK, unpublished data). Treatment of MA-10 cells with 105 nM MIS for 48 hours decreased progesterone production by 30% and decreased testosterone production 10-fold. Moreover, MIS decreased P450c17 mRNA levels in both cAMP stimulated and unstimulated MA-10 cells. To determine whether MIS downregulates P450c17 transcription, a transgene containing 1 kb of the P450c17 promoter driving firefly luciferase was transfected into MA-10 cells. At concentrations ranging from 35 to 105 nM, MIS decreased luciferase activity of the transgene, confirming that MIS inhibits transcription of P450c17. These data proved that MIS directly regulates steroidogenic enzyme transcription in Leydig cells.

To elucidate the role of MIS in the regulation of Leydig-cell proliferation, the effect of exogenously added MIS on thymidine incorporation of PLCs and ILCs was examined. ALCs were not studied because they do not undergo cell division either in vivo or in vitro. For these studies, freshly isolated Leydig cells were cultured overnight in serum-free media, then treated with increasing concentrations of MIS in the presence or absence of low-dose LH (1 ng/ml) for 24–96 hours. The cells were labeled with tritiated thymidine for 4 hrs before harvesting.

Treatment of cultured PLCs with MIS caused a decrease in thymidine incorporation (Fig. 4.4A,B) (19). In the absence of LH, this effect was only significant at the highest MIS concentration of 43 nM (818–433 cpm/million cells; $p < 0.05$, $n = 4$) (Fig. 4.4A). Addition of low-dose LH (1 ng/ml) to the culture media enhanced basal incorporation of thymidine and potentiated the effects of MIS on DNA synthesis (Fig. 4.4B). At concentrations of 3.5–43 nM, MIS inhibited PLC thymidine incorporation (up to 64% of control, $p < 0.001$, $n = 7$), with no dose effects detectable by Tukey analysis. In contrast, thymidine incorporation in the ILCs was unaffected by MIS treatment regardless of the concentration of MIS used, up to 171 nM ($n = 5$, Fig. 4.4C). The addition of LH to the ILC cultures did not confer responsiveness to MIS (Fig. 4.4D).

Conclusions

These studies have proved conclusively that postnatal Leydig cells express functional MIS type I and type II receptors and that MIS inhibits proliferation and steroidogenesis of primary Leydig cells, confirming that the Leydig cell phenotypes in the mice models of MIS null and overexpression are mediated directly through cell–surface receptors on Leydig cells. Leydig-cell proliferation and steroidogenesis are regulated by diverse hormones and growth factors (e.g., androgens, insulinlike-growth factor-I, thyroid hormone, LH, and Sertoli cell paracrine factors) (31–37). MIS appears to be a previously unrecognized player in the regulation of Leydig-cell maturation and differentiation. The ability of MIS to decrease testosterone production, especially in the

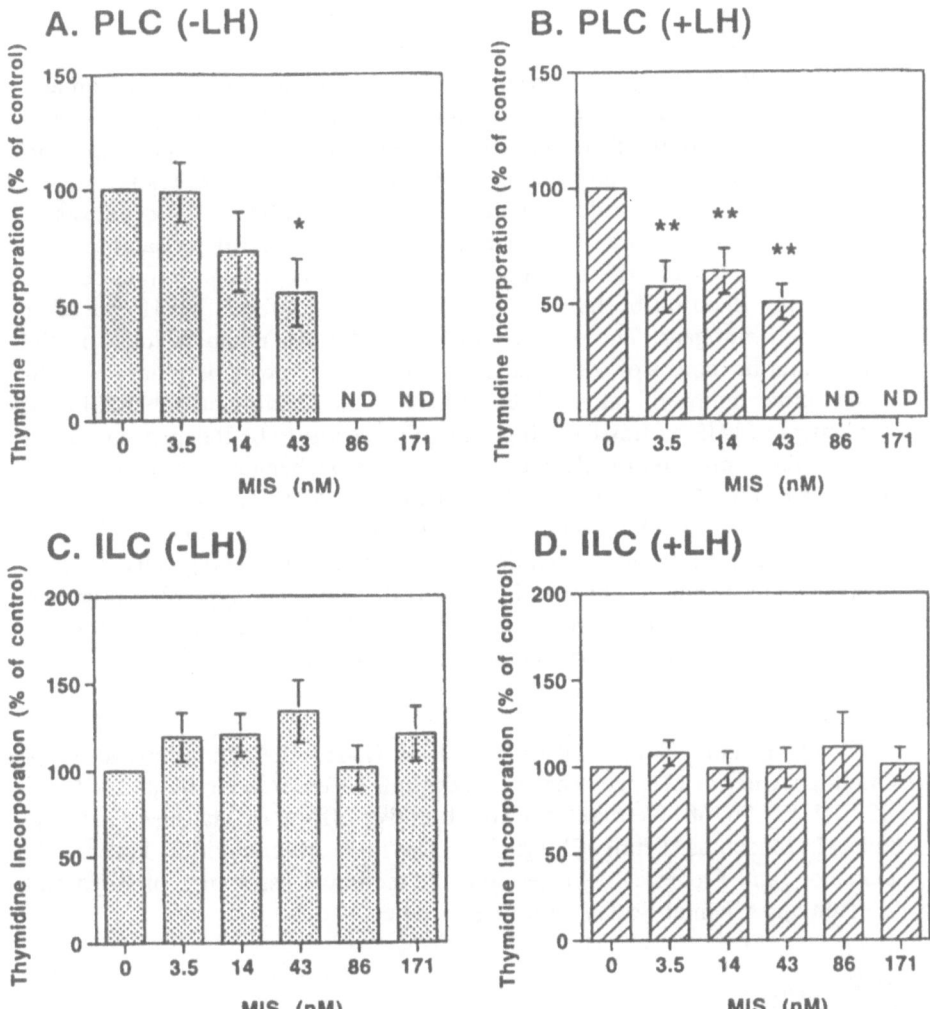

FIGURE 4.4. Effects of MIS on Leydig cell DNA synthesis. Primary Leydig cells were treated with buffer or MIS (3.5 to 172 nM) for 24–48 hours, in the presence and absence of low doses of LH (1 ng/ml) in triplicate. The cultures were labeled with 1 mCi/well [³H]thymidine (DuPont-New England Nuclear, Boston, MA) during the last 4 hours of hormonal treatment, then lysed in 0.5 ml hyamine hydroxide (ICN Radiochemicals, Irvine, CA), and counted in a liquid scintillation counter. The results for each MIS dose were expressed as thymidine incorporation as a percentage of mean uptake in the buffer-treated controls. The data were normalized and analyzed using one-way ANOVA to determine the overall effect of MIS treatment on thymidine incorporation. Tukey's test was then used to evaluate all pair-wise comparisons, with unequal ns adjusted using a Tukey-Kramer adjustment. (A) In the absence of LH, 43 nM MIS was needed to significantly decrease thymidine incorporation of PLCs (* $p < 0.05$). (B) Addition of LH (1 ng/ml) enhanced basal thymidine incorporation and potentiated the effects of MIS at all doses (** $p < 0.001$). In the absence (C) or presence of LH (D), MIS did not alter thymidine uptake in ILCs. Adapted with permission from Lee MM, et al. Mullerian inhibiting substance type II receptor expression and function in purified rat Leydig cells. Endocrinology 1999;140:2819–27. © The Endocrine Society.

prepubertal PLCs, may serve to prevent excessive androgen production and thereby restrict premature differentiation of the testis. Moreover, these studies and the work in the R2C cell, suggest that MIS might also participate in the modulation of androgen secretion by the sexually mature testis.

These data provide evidence that MIS directly inhibits DNA synthesis in PLCs, which is a measure of cellular proliferation, and LH potentiates this action. Thus, one role of MIS in the postnatal testis may be to help restrain Leydig-cell overproliferation by balancing the stimulatory effects of LH and other Leydig-cell mitogens. The perturbation of Leydig-cell numbers found in the genetic murine models of MIS excess or null expression can therefore be attributed to direct antiproliferative effects of MIS on the dividing prepubertal PLCs. This effect of MIS on Leydig-cell proliferation seems to be independent of LH because the expression of LH and its receptor is unchanged in mice with null deletions of the MIS gene (16). Future studies will focus on clarifying the molecular basis of this inhibition to determine whether MIS is causing cell cycle arrest or increasing apoptotic cell death of the progenitor Leydig cells. A better understanding of the mechanism by which MIS prevents hyperplastic growth and neoplastic transformation of Leydig cells will offer additional insights into the regulation of testicular development and tumorigenesis.

Acknowledgments. Supported by a Charles H. Hood Foundation Research Grant, an American Cancer Society Institutional Research Grant, and NICHD R29-HD/CA36768. We thank the collaborative efforts of Matthew P. Hardy, Peter T. Masiakos, Ching Ching Seah, David T. MacLaughlin, Patricia K. Donahoe, and Frederic I. Preffer, and the technical assistance of Raymond D. Tien and Chantal Sottas with these studies.

References

1. Jost A. Recherches sur la differentiation sexuelle de l'embryon de lapin. Arch Anat Microsc Morphol Exp 1947;36:271–315.
2. Donahoe PK, Cate RL, MacLaughlin DT, Epstein J, Fuller AF, Takahashi M, et al. Mullerian inhibiting substance: gene structure and mechanism of action of a fetal regressor. Rec Prog Horm Res 1987;43:431–67.
3. Josso N, Picard JY. Anti-Mullerian hormone. Physiol Rev 1986;66(4):1038–90.
4. Cate RL, Mattaliano RJ, Hession C, Tizard R, Farber NM, Cheung A, et al. Isolation of the bovine and human genes for Mullerian inhibiting substance and expression of the human gene in animal cells. Cell 1986;45(5):685–98.
5. Picard JY, Benarous R, Guerrier D, Josso N, Kahn A. Cloning and expression of cDNA for anti-Mullerian hormone. Proc Natl Acad Sci USA 1986;83(15): 5464–68.
6. MacLaughlin DT, Hudson PL, Graciano AL, Kenneally MK, Ragin RC, Manganaro TF, et al. Mullerian duct regression and anti-proliferative bioactivities of Mullerian inhibiting substance reside in its carboxy-terminal domain. Endocrinology 1992;131(1):291–96.

7. Teixeira J, He WW, Shah PC, Morikawa N, Lee MM, Catlin EA, et al. Developmental expression of a candidate Mullerian inhibiting substance type II receptor. Endocrinology 1996;137(1):160–65.
8. di Clemente N, Wilson C, Faure E, Boussin L, Carmillo P, Tizard R, et al. Cloning, expression, and alternative splicing of the receptor for anti-Mullerian hormone. Mol Endocrinol 1994;8(8):1006–20.
9. Baarends WM, van Helmond MJ, Post M, van der Schoot P, Hoogerbrugge JW, de Winter J, et al. A novel member of the transmembrane serine/threonine kinase receptor family is specifically expressed in the gonads and in mesenchymal cells adjacent to the mullerian duct. Development 1994;120(1):189–97.
10. Massague J. Receptors for the TGF-β family. Cell 1992;69:1067–70.
11. Kuroda T, Lee MM, Haqq CM, Powell DM, Manganaro TF, Donahoe PK. Mullerian inhibiting substance ontogeny and its modulation by follicle-stimulating hormone in the rat testes. Endocrinology 1990;127(4):1825–32.
12. Lee MM, Cate RL, Donahoe PK, Waneck GL. Developmentally regulated polyadenylation of two discrete messenger ribonucleic acids for Mullerian inhibiting substance. Endocrinology 1992;130(2):847–53.
13. Baarends WM, Hoogerbrugge JW, Post M, Visser JA, De Rooij D, Parvinen M, et al. Anti-Mullerian hormone and anti-Mullerian hormone type II receptor messenger ribonucleic acid expression during postnatal testis development and in the adult testis of the rat. Endocrinology 1995;136(12):5614–22.
14. Lyet L, Louis F, Forest MG, Josso N, Behringer RR, Vigier B. Ontogeny of reproductive abnormalities induced by deregulation of anti-mullerian hormone expression in transgenic mice. Biol Reprod 1995;52(2):444–54.
15. Behringer RR, Cate RL, Froelick GJ, Palmiter RD, Brinster RL. Abnormal sexual development in transgenic mice chronically expressing mullerian inhibiting substance. Nature 1990;345(6271):167–70.
16. Racine C, Rey R, Forest M, Louis F, Ferre A, Huhtaniemi I, et al. Receptors for anti-Mullerian hormone on Leydig cells are responsible for its effects on steroidogenesis and cell differentiation. Proc Natl Acad Sci USA 1998;95:594–99.
17. Mishina Y, Rey R, Finegold MJ, Matzuk MM, Josso N, Cate RL, et al. Genetic analysis of the Mullerian-inhibiting substance signal transduction pathway in mammalian sexual differentiation. Genes Dev 1996;10:2577–87.
18. Behringer RR, Finegold MJ, Cate RL. Mullerian inhibiting substance function during mammalian sexual development. Cell 1994;79(3):415–25.
19. Lee MM, Seah CC, Masiakos PT, Sottas CM, Preffer FI, Donahoe PK, et al. Mullerian inhibiting substance type II receptor expression and function in purified rat Leydig cells. Endocrinology 1999;140:2819–27.
20. Klinefelter GR, Kelce WR, Hardy MP. Isolation and culture of Leydig cells from adult rats. Meth Toxicol 1993;3:166–81.
21. Ge RS, Shan LX, Hardy MP. Pubertal development of Leydig cells. In: Payne AH, Hardy MP, Russell LD, eds. The Leydig cell. Vienna, VA: Cache River Press, 1996: 159–74.
22. Benton L, Shan LX, Hardy MP. Differentiation of adult Leydig cells. J Steroid Biochem Mol Biol 1995;53(1–6):61–68.
23. Mather J, Phillips DM. Primary culture of testicular somatic cells. In: Methods for serum-free culture of cells of the endocrine system. New York: Alan R. Liss, 1984:29–45.
24. Payne AH, Downing JR, Wong KL. Luteinizing hormone receptors and testoste-

rone synthesis in two distinct populations of Leydig cells. Endocrinology 1980;106:1424–29.

25. MacLaughlin DT, Epstein J, Donahoe PK. Bioassay, purification, cloning, and expression of Mullerian inhibiting substance. Meth Enzymol 1991;198:358–69.

26. Hudson PL, Dougas I, Donahoe PK, Cate RL, Epstein J, Pepinsky RB, et al. An immunoassay to detect human Mullerian inhibiting substance in males and females during normal development. J Clin Endocrinol Metab 1990;70(1):16–22.

27. Picon R. Action du testicule foetal sur le developpement in vitro des canaux de Muller chez le rat. Arch Anat Microsc Morphol Exp 1969;58(1):1–19.

28. Donahoe PK, Ito Y, Hendren WH. A graded organ culture assay for the detection of Müllerian inhibiting substance. J Surg Res 1977;23(2):141–48.

29. Cochran R, Ewing L, Niswender G. Serum levels of follicle stimulating hormone, luteinizing hormone, prolactin, testosterone, 5α-dihydrotestosterone, 5α-androstane-3α, 17β-diol, 5α-androstane-3β-, 17β-diol, and 17β-estradiol from male beagles with spontaneous or induced benign prostatic hyperplasia. Invest Urol. 1981;19:142–47.

30. Shan LX, Phillips DM, Bardin CW, Hardy MP. Differential regulation of steroidogenic enzymes during differentiation optimizes testosterone production by adult rat Leydig cells. Endocrinology. 1993;133(5):2277–83.

31. Ackland JF, Schwartz NB, Mayo KE, Dodson RE. Nonsteroidal signals originating in the gonads. Physiol Rev 1992;72:731–87.

32. Skinner MK. Cell-cell interactions in the testis. Endocrine Rev 1991;12:45–77.

33. Vergouwen R, Jacobs S, Huiskamp R, Davids J, de Rooj D. Proliferative activity of gonocytes, Sertoli cells and interstitial cells during testicular development in mice. J Reprod Fertil 1991;93:233–43.

34. Hardy MP, Gelber SJ, Zhou ZF, Penning TM, Ricigliano JW, Ganjam VK, et al. Hormonal control of Leydig cell differentiation. Ann NY Acad Sci 1991;637(152): 152–63.

35. Ewing LL, Keeney DS. Leydig cells: structure and function. In: Desjardins C, Ewing LL, eds. Cell and molecular biology of the testis. New York: Oxford University Press, 1993:137–65.

36. Payne AH, Youngblood GL. Regulation of expression of steroidogenic enzymes in Leydig cells. Biol Reprod 1995;52:217–25.

37. Shan L, Hardy DO, Catterall JF, Hardy MP. Effects of luteinizing hormone (LH) and androgen on steady state levels of messenger ribonucleic acid for LH receptors, androgen receptors, and steroidogenic enzymes in rat Leydig cell progenitors in vivo. Endocrinology 1995;136(4):1686–93.

38. Joseph D, Hall S, French F. Rat androgen-binding protein: evidence for identical subunits and amino acid sequence homology with human sex hormone-binding globulin. Proc Natl Acad Sci USA 1987;84:339–43.

39. Ercolani L, Florence B, Denaro M, Alexander-Bridges M. Isolation and complete sequence of a functional human glyceraldehyde-3-phosphate dehydrogenase gene. J Biol Chem 1988;263:15335–41.

40. Shan L, Hardy M. Developmental changes in levels of luteinizing hormone receptor and androgen receptor in rat Leydig cells. Endocrinology 1992;131(3): 1107–14.

5

Regulation of the Differentiation of the Undifferentiated Spermatogonia

Dirk G. de Rooij, Bianca H.G.J. Schrans-Stassen,
Ans M.M. van Pelt, Gladis A. Shuttlesworth,
Marvin L. Meistrich, Masaru Okabe, and Yoshitake Nishimune

Introduction

In the seminiferous epithelium of adult nonprimate mammals, so-called A-single (A_s) spermatogonia are the stem cells of spermatogenesis (1–3). Upon division of the A_s spermatogonia, the daughter cells either migrate away from each other and become two new stem cells, or the cells stay together becoming A-paired (A_{pr}) spermatogonia connected by an intercellular bridge. About half of the stem-cell population normally divides to form A_{pr} spermatogonia, whereas the other half goes through self-renewing divisions, thereby maintaining stem-cell numbers (Fig. 5.1).

The A_{pr} spermatogonia are the first cells in the spermatogenic lineage that are destined to the differentiation pathway and develop further to form chains of 4, 8, or 16 A-aligned (A_{al}) spermatogonia. The A_s, A_{pr}, and A_{al} spermatogonia together are called *undifferentiated spermatogonia* (1,2). The A_{al} spermatogonia differentiate into A_1 spermatogonia, which are the first generation of the differentiating-type spermatogonia (Fig. 5.1). The differentiating spermatogonia carry out a series of six divisions, resulting in A_2, A_3, A_4, Intermediate (In), and finally B spermatogonia, which give rise to primary spermatocytes through the last mitotic division.

Spermatogenesis is a cyclic process that can be subdivided in stages (4). In late-stage VIII of the cycle of the seminiferous epithelium, the spermatogonial population consists of A_1 spermatogonia that are about to divide into A_2 spermatogonia during the next epithelial stage, and A_s, A_{pr}, and a few A_{al} spermatogonia that are largely quiescent (5). During subsequent stages, the proliferative activity of the undifferentiated spermatogonia is stimulated by as yet unknown factors. During proliferation, the numbers of A_s and A_{pr} sper-

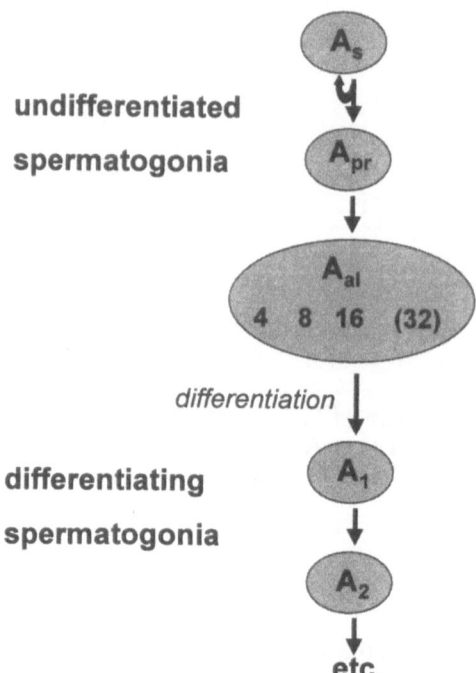

undifferentiated

spermatogonia

differentiating

spermatogonia

FIGURE 5.1. Scheme of spermatogonial multiplication and stem-cell renewal in rodents.

matogonia remain relatively constant, but increasing amounts of A_{al} spermatogonia are formed (6,7). The proliferative activity of the undifferentiated spermatogonia continues until about stages II/III, at which time these cells become largely quiescent again (6,7). At some time before epithelial stage VIII virtually all A_{al} spermatogonia that were formed during the preceding period of proliferative activity differentiate into A_1 spermatogonia.

The present knowledge on the regulation of the differentiation of undifferentiated spermatogonia will be discussed, especially findings indicating that this differentiation represents a rather vulnerable step in the spermatogenic process. Furthermore, the role of the c-kit/stem-cell factor system in spermatogonial differentiation will be reviewed.

Regulation of Stem-Cell Renewal

In the normal situation the probability of self-renewal of stem cells at each division will have to be close to 50% (8). When stem cells have been lost because of the cell killing effects of irradiation or administration of cytotoxic drugs, however, this percentage should be higher to enable recovery of stem-cell numbers. Indeed, detailed studies of the composition of repopulating colonies formed by surviving stem cells, 6–10 days after irradiation, revealed that virtually no A_{pr} spermatogonia were formed during the first five divisions after irradiation, and that the percentage of self-renewing divisions remained considerably higher than 50% for at least divisions six and seven (9). There are as yet no clues about the nature of the factors that determine the ratio between stem-cell renewal and formation of A_{pr} spermatogonia. It is also as yet unknown whether there is a functional differentiation (i.e., irreversible change in gene expression) when intercellular bridges are formed between the daughter cells of stem cells. A_{pr} and also A_{al} spermatogonia still possibly have stem-cell properties when the intercellular bridges break up, as occurs after irradiation (10), and they become single cells.

Differentiation of A_{al} Spermatogonia

Differentiation occurs in the compartment of undifferentiated spermatogonia when A_{al} spermatogonia differentiate into A_1 spermatogonia. This differentiation step marks the transition from the randomly cycling population of undifferentiated spermatogonia to the rigidly controlled series of six synchronous divisions of differentiating spermatogonia (8). It has become clear that this differentiation step is rather vulnerable to many kinds of disturbing factors.

It has been established that the differentiation of the A_{al} spermatogonia becomes blocked in case of vitamin A deficiency (VAD) (11,12). In VAD mice and rats, only undifferentiated spermatogonia remain except for a few residual preleptotene spermatocytes in rats. Vitamin A metabolites, directly or indirectly via Sertoli cells, apparently control undifferentiated spermatogonial differentiation. This differentiation step might be the only moment during the development of spermatogonia at which vitamin A is required. Almost immediately after the onset of the VAD situation, the formation of A_1 spermatogonia is arrested but the A_1 spermatogonia formed just before the onset of the deficiency develop normally and become preleptotene spermatocytes (13). The vitamin A–sensitive step is apparently at a very specific point in spermatogonial development.

Several other situations have been detected in which mouse and rat spermatogenesis becomes arrested at the spermatogonial level. In mice, this arrest is seen in C57Bl mice experimentally made cryptorchid 2 months before (14,15) and in *jsd/jsd* (16–18) and *Sl17H/Sl17H* mutant mice (19). In rats, spermatogonial arrest can be induced by administration of 2,5-hexanedione, which damages Sertoli cell function (20–22). In irradiated LBNF1 rats after an initial recovery, spermatogenesis deteriorates again until only A spermatogonia remain (23). In 2,5-hexanedione-treated rats results of modeling spermatogonial multiplication suggested spermatogonial cell death at the level of A_3 spermatogonia (22). The precise point at which spermatogonial development became arrested has been determined in the other four of these five models.

Spermatogonial Arrest in *jsd/jsd*, *Sl17H/Sl17H*, and Cryptorchild Mice and in Irradiated LBNF1 Rats

Germ Cells Remaining

In whole mounts of seminiferous tubules of *jsd/jsd*, *Sl17H/Sl17H* and cryptorchid mice and of irradiated LBNF1 rats, the population of spermatogonia remaining in the testis was studied (24,25). The great majority of the germ cells present in the tubules were found to be A spermatogonia with sporadic clones of more differentiated cells in all but the *Sl17H/Sl17H* mice, where no differentiating clones of germ cells were encountered (Fig. 5.2A). The size of the clones of A spermatogonia (i.e., the number of cells composing the clones) was studied and was found to vary from 1 to 16 cells and rarely more. This distribution of clonal sizes is similar to that of the undifferentiated spermatogonia in the normal epithelium in which clones of 1 (A_s), 2 (A_{pr}), and 4, 8, or 16 (A_{al}) undifferentiated spermatogonia are the most common (6,7). From both the morphology and the topographical arrangement of the remaining A spermatogonia it can be concluded that in all four models spermatogonial development stops at the moment at which the A_{al} spermatogonia should differentiate into A_1 spermatogonia.

Apoptotic Germ Cells

In all four models, the remaining A spermatogonia were actively proliferating, mitotic clones being common (Fig. 5.2B) (24,25). Nevertheless, no excessive numbers of spermatogonia were encountered because apoptotic spermatogonial clones were also found. Clones of all sizes were seen in apoptosis (Fig. 5.2C). When clonal sizes of viable and apoptotic clones were compared it appeared that the apoptotic clones on average consisted of more cells. The clones apparently become more vulnerable to apoptosis when they become larger. One reason for this could be that the cells composing a clone are connected to each other by intercellular bridges, and when one cell becomes apoptotic the other cells might have to follow because apoptosis regulatory molecules reach them via the bridges. The notion that when one cell of a clone degenerates they all do has already been proposed by Huckins (26). In the four models studied, the apoptosis of the undifferentiated spermatogonia does not appear to be related to the failure of the attempt of these cells to differentiate into A_1 spermatogonia. This is because many A_s and A_{pr} spermatogonia also become apoptotic, whereas these cells do not or only rarely attempt to differentiate in the normal epithelium (6,7).

Clumped Clones and Odd-Numbered Clones

Another phenomenon that was often seen in all four models was the occurrence of clumped clones (i.e., the presence of more than one nucleus in the same cytoplasm) (Fig. 5.2D). Clumps most often contained two nuclei, but clumps with eight nuclei also occurred. It is interesting that these clumps were also seen

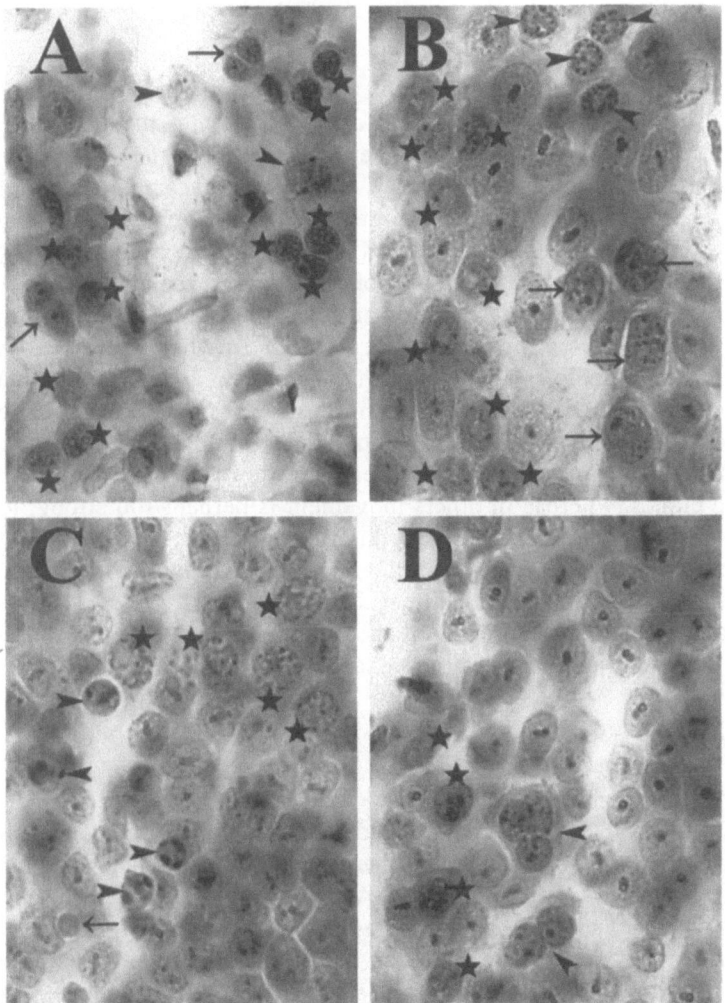

FIGURE 5.2. Photographs of cells on the basal membrane of whole mounts of seminiferous tubules of rats and mice in which a spermatogonial arrest is present. In general, the
same phenomena were seen in all four models. 850×. (A) LBNF1 rat 15 weeks after 6
Gy of X-irradiation. Only undifferentiated A spermatogonia (asterisks) and Sertoli cells
(two of which are indicated by arrowheads) are present. Undifferentiated spermatogonia are sometimes seen in clumps (i.e., one or more nuclei in the same cytoplasm,
arrows). (B) Cryptorchid C57Bl mouse. Tubular area with a high density of undifferentiated spermatogonia (asterisks), four of the cells are in telophase, which indicates that
they were just formed from a division of A$_{pr}$ spermatogonia (arrowheads) and a chain of
4 A$_{al}$ spermatogonia synchronously is in prophase (arrows). (C) *Sl17H/Sl17H* mutant
mouse. Like the other models the remaining A spermatogonia are actively proliferating,
as evidenced here by the prophasic A$_{al}$ spermatogonia (asterisks). Still no accumulation
of spermatogonia occurs because clones also become apoptotic (arrowheads and arrow). The morphology of the apoptotic cells may vary considerably within a clone
(compare arrowhead indicated cells with the one indicated by arrow). (D) *jsd/jsd* mutant mouse. The formation of clumps of undifferentiated spermatogonia was common
in all four models. The undifferentiated spermatogonia indicated by asterisks and arrowheads probably belong to the same clone, but groups of three and of two have formed
clumps (arrowheads).

in two other situations in which the cell density on the basal membrane of the seminiferous tubules is low (i.e., shortly after irradiation in the mouse) (10) and in the vitamin A–deficient rat, where they were called *clusters* (11).

Even though clones consisting of 1, 2, 4, 8, or 16, and sometimes 32 undifferentiated spermatogonia were found in the normal epithelium exclusively (6,27), odd-numbered clones were also observed in the present four models. These odd-numbered clones were also previously observed after irradiation (10,28,29).

It can be concluded that clumped and odd-numbered clones arise under all the widely different circumstances described earlier, with the common feature in all being the disappearance of the differentiating-type spermatogonia from the basal membrane. It is tempting to speculate that in this condition the movement of the cells required at mitotic divisions becomes disorganized. In some clones, movement does not take place, giving rise to clumped clones, whereas in others movement is perhaps too strong, leading to breaking up of some of the intercellular bridges and the formation of odd-numbered clones. As discussed earlier, when the formation of intercellular bridges does not involve a functional differentiation of the cells, the breaking up of clones of undifferentiated spermatogonia in such a way that single cells arise, could also be a way to enhance stem-cell renewal.

Conclusions

In cryptorchid, and *jsd/jsd* and *Sl17H/Sl17H* mutant mice (24), as well as in irradiated LBNF1 (25) and vitamin A–deficient rats (11,12), spermatogenesis was found to be arrested at the moment at which the A_{al} spermatogonia differentiate into A_1 spermatogonia (Fig. 5.3). A similar arrest has been speculated to occur in rats that underwent an experimental spinal cord injury (30). The arrest, however, may be somewhat earlier than it is in the 2,5-hexanedione rat model, in which the arrest was suggested to be at the level of A_3 spermatogonia (22).

The nature of the defect in the *jsd* mutation is not known, but the Sertoli cells do not produce a functional stem cell factor (SCF) in *Sl17H/Sl17H* mice (19). A functional c-kit receptor/SCF ligand system is apparently required for undifferentiated spermatogonial differentiation. Furthermore, the results in the vitamin A–deficient rat indicate that there is a retinoid-dependent step in the differentiation process of A_{al} spermatogonia either direct or indirect via Sertoli cells. Both spermatogonia and Sertoli cells possess nuclear receptors for retinoids (31–33). In the cryptorchid mice and the irradiated LBNF1 rats the underlying cause for the spermatogonial arrest is even more difficult to pinpoint. It is possible in both that Sertoli cell function is damaged, but the function(s) that fail that are crucial to spermatogonial differentiation are not yet known.

In both the irradiation and 2,5-hexanedione rat models, the spermatogonial differentiation arrest can be relieved by treatment with a gonadotropin-releasing hormone (GnRH) agonist or antagonist that cause a sustained suppression of luteinizing hormone (LH) and follicle stimulating hormone (FSH) levels, and consequently also an inhibition of testicular testosterone production (25,34–

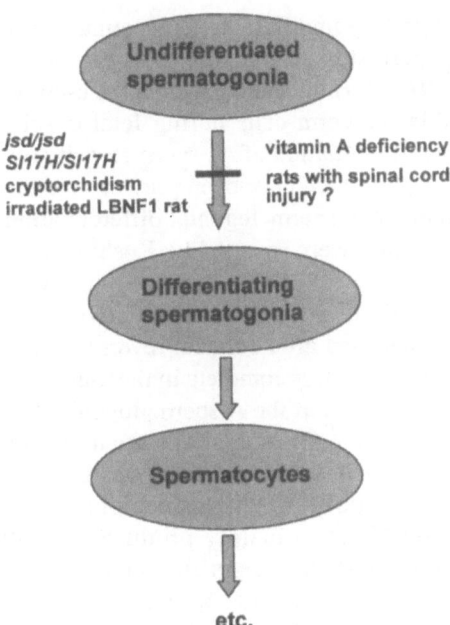

FIGURE 5.3. Rodent models presently available in which the differentiation step from undifferentiated into differentiating type spermatogonia has become blocked.

37). It is suggested that the decrease in hormone levels improves Sertoli cell function in such a way that some spermatogonial differentiation is again sustained. The hormone important in these models has been suggested to be testosterone or a metabolite (25,36). Even though serum levels of testosterone in these models do not change, the intratesticular testosterone concentration will be much higher than it is in the normal testis because the same amount of testosterone is produced in a testis that is much smaller due to the extensive germ cell loss. Levels of testosterone that are too high may negatively influence Sertoli cell function (25,36). It is interesting that it was found that in LBNF1 rats a spermatogonial arrest can also be induced by administration of procarbazine and in this case, too, suppression of GnRH stimulated recovery (38).

The Role of the C-Kit Receptor and SCF Ligand in Spermatogonial Differentiation

The c-kit receptor and its ligand, SCF, are encoded at the White spotting (W) and Steel (Sl) loci, respectively. Many mutations of these genes are known and most homozygous mutant mice are sterile because of a lack of germ cells (39). In these mutants the migration and/or proliferation of the primordial germ cells is impaired (40–42). In some, however, the effects are less severe, as they are in W^f/W^f mice, which are fully fertile (43) and in *Sl17H/Sl17H* mice, in which there are many proliferating undifferentiated spermatogonia that are unable to differentiate into A_1 spermatogonia, as discussed earlier (24).

The results in *Sl17H/Sl17H* mice indicate that the c-kit receptor and its ligand SCF are indispensable for germ cells during fetal development and have an important role in the differentiation of A_{al} spermatogonia in the adult. Although less well defined, however, there have been previous indications for such a role for c-kit/SCF. Problems with spermatogonial differentiation (i.e., the formation of In and B spermatogonia) were reported by Koshimizu et al. (44) and Tajima et al. (45) after surgical reversal of cryptorchidism in several fertile *White spotting* mutant and *Steel Dickie* mice, respectively. Even though recovery to full spermatogenesis was observed after surgical reversal of cryptorchidism in normal mice, recovery was much less complete in the mutants and it was concluded that there was a (partial) arrest at the A spermatogonial level.

It is interesting that in 2,5-hexanedione-treated rats, proliferation and survival of the remaining A spermatogonia was stimulated by administration of SCF (46). In addition, in 2,5-hexanedione-treated rats with a spermatogonial arrest, Sertoli cells mainly produce the soluble form of SCF, whereas the treatment with GnRH agonist, which stimulates spermatogonial differentiation again, is accompanied by an increase in the production of membrane-bound SCF (37). In the normal mouse at the start of spermatogenesis, shortly after birth, there is a dramatic shift in the production by Sertoli cells from soluble to membrane-bound SCF (37,47), which suggests that the membrane-bound SCF is most important in spermatogenesis.

In the testis, SCF was found to be produced by Sertoli cells (48,49) and the c-kit mRNA was localized to at least A_2–B spermatogonia (47). Morena et al. (50), studying spermatogonia isolated from young rats, reported the c-kit receptor protein to be present on all types of spermatogonia. Injection of the c-kit antibody ACK2 into adult mice, however, caused a depletion of differentiating spermatogonia even though the undifferentiated spermatogonia were unaffected (51), which suggests that at least some undifferentiated spermatogonia may not possess c-kit receptors. Immunohistochemical studies of c-kit expression in the normal adult testis revealed about 15% of the undifferentiated spermatogonia in epithelial stage VI to be weakly staining for c-kit, which is a percentage that increased in stage VII and reached about 80% in stage IX (52). This indicates that immunohistochemically detectable amounts of c-kit start to appear in undifferentiated spermatogonia just before or during differentiation. These results suggest that increasing c-kit expression marks the differentiation of A_{al} spermatogonia into A_1 spermatogonia.

Conclusions

During each epithelial cycle, the undifferentiated spermatogonia proliferate and produce many A_{al} spermatogonia. After a period of quiescence these A_{al} spermatogonia, without division, differentiate into the first generation of differentiating-type spermatogonia, the A_1 spermatogonia. This differentiation step has now been shown to be rather vulnerable because it can become blocked in a number of, at least seemingly, widely different situations: vitamin A deficiency, irradiation, homozygous *jsd* and *Sl17H* mutations, cryptorchidism, and probably also Sertoli cell intoxication by 2,5-hexanedione administration (Fig. 5.3). Further studies will have to make clear whether or not the important factors in these situations are all active in the same regulatory pathway. In at least two of the situations of spermatogonial arrest, the c-kit/SCF system seems to be involved and this regulatory system clearly has an important role in undifferentiated spermatogonial differentiation. The expression of the c-kit receptor in undifferentiated spermatogonia may be used to monitor the differentiation of A_{al} spermatogonia into A_1 spermatogonia.

Acknowledgment. The authors wish to thank Mr. R. Scriwanek for preparing Figure 5.2.

References

1. Huckins C. The spermatogonial stem cell population in adult rats. I. Their morphology, proliferation and maturation. Anat Rec 1971;169:533–57.
2. Oakberg EF. Spermatogonial stem-cell renewal in the mouse. Anat Rec 1971; 169:515–31.
3. de Rooij DG. Proliferation and differentiation of undifferentiated spermatogonia in the mammalian testis. In: Potten CS, ed. Stem cells. Their identification and characterization. Edinburgh: Churchill Livingstone, 1983.89–117.
4. Russell LD, Ettlin RA, Hikim APS, Clegg ED. Histological and histopathological evaluation of the testis. Clearwater, FL: Cache River Press, 1990.
5. Lok D, de Rooij DG. Spermatogonial multiplication in the Chinese hamster. III. Labelling indices of undifferentiated spermatogonia throughout the cycle of the seminiferous epithelium. Cell Tissue Kinet 1983;16:31–40.
6. Lok D, Weenk D, de Rooij DG. Morphology, proliferation, and differentiation of undifferentiated spermatogonia in the Chinese hamster and the ram. Anat Rec 1982;203:83–99.
7. Tegelenbosch RA, de Rooij DG. A quantitative study of spermatogonial multiplication and stem cell renewal in the C3H/101 F1 hybrid mouse. Mutat Res 1993;290:193–200.
8. de Rooij DG. Stem cells in the testis. Int J Exp Pathol 1998;79:67–80.
9. van Beek ME, Meistrich ML, de Rooij DG. Probability of self-renewing divisions of spermatogonial stem cells in colonies, formed after fission neutron irradiation. Cell Tissue Kinet 1990;23:1–16.
10. van Beek ME, Davids JA, van de Kant HJ, de Rooij DG. Response to fission neutron irradiation of spermatogonial stem cells in different stages of the cycle of the seminiferous epithelium. Radiat Res 1984;97:556–69.
11. van Pelt AM, de Rooij DG. The origin of the synchronization of the seminiferous epithelium in vitamin A-deficient rats after vitamin A replacement. Biol Reprod 1990;42:677–82.

12. van Pelt AM, van Dissel-Emiliani FM, Gaemers IC, van der Burg MJ, Tanke HJ, de Rooij DG. Characteristics of A spermatogonia and preleptotene spermatocytes in the vitamin A-deficient rat testis. Biol Reprod 1995;53:570–78.

13. de Rooij DG, van Pelt AMM, van de Kant HJG, van der Saag PT, Peters AHFM, Heyting C, et al. Role of retinoids in spermatogonial proliferation and differentiation and the meiotic prophase. In: Bartke A, ed. Function of somatic cells in the testis. New York: Springer Verlag, 1994:345–61.

14. Nishimune Y, Haneji T. Testicular DNA synthesis in vivo: comparison between unilaterally cryptorchid testis and contralateral intact testis in mouse. Arch Androl 1981;6:61–65.

15. Nishimune Y, Haneji T, Aizawa S. Testicular DNA synthesis in vivo: changes in DNA synthetic activity following artificial cryptorchidism and its surgical reversal. Fertil Steril 1981;35:359–62.

16. Mizunuma M, Dohmae K, Tajima Y, Koshimizu U, Watanabe D, Nishimune Y. Loss of sperm in juvenile spermatogonial depletion (jsd) mutant mice is ascribed to a defect of intratubular environment to support germ cell differentiation. J Cell Physiol 1992;150:188–93.

17. Kojima Y, Kominami K, Dohmae K, Nonomura N, Miki T, Okuyama A, et al. Cessation of spermatogenesis in juvenile spermatogonial depletion (jsd/jsd) mice. Int J Urol 1997;4:500–7.

18. Beamer WG, Cunliffe-Beamer TL, Shultz KL, Langley SH, Roderick TH. Juvenile spermatogonial depletion (jsd): a genetic defect of germ cell proliferation of male mice. Biol Reprod 1988;38:899–908.

19. Brannan CI, Bedell MA, Resnick JL, Eppig JJ, Handel MA, Williams DE, et al. Developmental abnormalities in Steel17H mice result from a splicing defect in the steel factor cytoplasmic tail. Genes Dev 1992;6:1832–42.

20. Boekelheide K. Rat testis during 2,5-hexanedione intoxication and recovery. II. Dynamics of pyrrole reactivity, tubulin content, and microtubule assembly. Toxicol Appl Pharmacol 1988;92:28–33.

21. Allard EK, Hall SJ, Boekelheide K. Stem cell kinetics in rat testis after irreversible injury induced by 2,5-hexanedione. Biol Reprod 1995;53:186–92.

22. Allard EK, Boekelheide K. Fate of germ cells in 2,5-hexanedione-induced testicular injury. II. Atrophy persists due to a reduced stem cell mass and ongoing apoptosis. Toxicol Appl Pharmacol 1996;137:149–56.

23. Kangasniemi M, Huhtaniemi I, Meistrich ML. Failure of spermatogenesis to recover despite the presence of a spermatogonia in the irradiated LBNF1 rat. Biol Reprod 1996;54:1200–8.

24. de Rooij DG, Okabe M, Nishimune M. Arrest of spermatogonial differentiation in jsd/jsd, Sl17H/Sl17H and cryptorchid mice. Biol Reprod 1999;61:842–47.

25. Shuttlesworth GA, de Rooij DG, Huhtaniemi I, Reissmann T, Russell LD, Shetty G, et al. Enhancement of A spermatogonial proliferation and differentiation in irradiated rats by GnRH antagonist administration. Endocrinology 2000;141:37–49.

26. Huckins C. The morphology and kinetics of spermatogonial degeneration in normal adult rats: an analysis using a simplified classification of the germinal epithelium. Anat Rec 1978;190:905–26.

27. de Rooij DG. Spermatogonial stem cell renewal in the mouse. I. Normal situation. Cell Tissue Kinet 1973;6:281–87.

28. Erickson BH. Survival and renewal of murine stem spermatogonia following 60Co gamma radiation. Radiat Res 1981;86:34–51.
29. Erickson BH, Hall GG. Comparison of stem-spermatogonial renewal and mitotic activity in the gamma-irradiated mouse and rat. Mutat Res 1983;108:317–35.
30. Huang HFS, Li MT, Anesetti R, Giglio W, Ottenweller JE, Pogach LM. Effects of spinal cord injury on spermatogenesis and the expression of messenger ribonucleic acid for Sertoli cell proteins in rat Sertoli cell-enriched testes. Biol Reprod 1999;60:635–41.
31. van Pelt AM, van den Brink CE, de Rooij DG, van der Saag PT. Changes in retinoic acid receptor messenger ribonucleic acid levels in the vitamin A-deficient rat testis after administration of retinoids. Endocrinology 1992;131:344–40.
32. Gaemers IC, van Pelt AM, van der Saag PT, Hoogerbrugge JW, Themmen AP, de Rooij DG. Effect of retinoid status on the messenger ribonucleic acid expression of nuclear retinoid receptors alpha, beta, and gamma, and retinoid X receptors alpha, beta, and gamma in the mouse testis. Endocrinology 1997;138:1544–51.
33. Gaemers IC, van Pelt AM, van der Saag PT, Hoogerbrugge JW, Themmen AP, de Rooij DG. Differential expression pattern of retinoid X receptors in adult murine testicular cells implies varying roles for these receptors in spermatogenesis. Biol Reprod 1998;58:1351–56.
34. Meistrich ML, Wilson G, Zhang Y, Kurdoglu B, Terry NH. Protection from procarbazine-induced testicular damage by hormonal pretreatment does not involve arrest of spermatogonial proliferation. Cancer Res 1997;57:1091–97.
35. Meistrich ML, Kangasniemi M. Hormone treatment after irradiation stimulates recovery of rat spermatogenesis from surviving spermatogonia. J Androl 1997;18:80–87.
36. Meistrich ML. Hormonal stimulation of the recovery of spermatogenesis following chemo- or radiotherapy. Review article. Apmis 1998;106:37–45.
37. Blanchard KT, Lee J, Boekelheide K. Leuprolide, a gonadotropin-releasing hormone agonist, reestablishes spermatogenesis after 2,5-hexanedione-induced irreversible testicular injury in the rat, resulting in normalized stem cell factor expression. Endocrinology 1998;139:236–44.
38. Meistrich ML, Wilson G, Huhtaniemi I. Hormonal treatment after cytotoxic therapy stimulates recovery of spermatogenesis. Cancer Res 1999;59:3557–60.
39. Nishimune Y, Okabe M. Mammalian male gametogenesis: growth, differentiation and maturation of germ cells. Develop Growth Differ 1993;35:479–86.
40. Mintz B. Embryological development of primordial germ cells in the mouse: influence of a new mutation, W^J. J. Embryol Exp Morphol 1957;5:396–403.
41. Mintz B, Russell ES. Gene-induced embryological modifications of primordial germ cells in the mouse. J Exp Zool 1957;134:207–37.
42. McCoshen JA, McCallion DJ. A study of the primordial germ cells during their migratory phase in Steel mutant mice. Experientia 1975;31:589–90.
43. Guenet JL, Marchal G, Milon G, Tambourin P, Wendling F. Fertile dominant spotting in the house mouse. A new allele at the W locus. J Hered 1979;70:9–12.
44. Koshimizu U, Sawada K, Tajima Y, Watanabe D, Nishimune Y. White-spotting mutations affect the regenerative differentiation of testicular germ cells: demonstration by experimental cryptorchidism and its surgical reversal. Biol Reprod 1991;45:642–48.
45. Tajima Y, Sakamaki K, Watanabe D, Koshimizu U, Matsuzawa T, Nishimune Y.

Steel-Dickie (Sld) mutation affects both maintenance and differentiation of testicular germ cells in mice. J Reprod Fertil 1991;91:441–49.

46. Allard EK, Blanchard KT, Boekelheide K. Exogenous stem cell factor (SCF) compensates for altered endogenous SCF expression in 2,5-hexanedione-induced testicular atrophy in rats. Biol Reprod 1996;55:185–93.

47. Manova K, Nocka K, Besmer P, Bachvarova RF. Gonadal expression of c-kit encoded at the W locus of the mouse. Development 1990;110:1057–69.

48. Rossi P, Albanesi C, Grimaldi P, Geremia R. Expression of the mRNA for the ligand of c-kit in mouse Sertoli cells. Biochem Biophys Res Commun 1991;176: 910–14.

49. Mauduit C, Chatelain G, Magre S, Brun G, Benahmed M, Michel D. Regulation by pH of the alternative splicing of the stem cell factor pre-mRNA in the testis. J Biol Chem 1999;274:770–75.

50. Morena AR, Boitani C, Pesce M, De Felici M, Stefanini M. Isolation of highly purified type A spermatogonia from prepubertal rat testis. J Androl 1996;17: 708–17.

51. Yoshinaga K, Nishikawa S, Ogawa M, Hayashi S, Kunisada T, Fujimoto T. Role of c-kit in mouse spermatogenesis: identification of spermatogonia as a specific site of c-kit expression and function. Development 1991;113:689–99.

52. Schrans-Stassen BHGJ, van de Kant HJG, de Rooij DG, van Pelt AMM. Differential expression of c-kit in mouse undifferentiated and differentiating type A spermatogonia. Endocrinology 1999;140:5894–900.

6

Regulation of Growth and Survival in the Mammalian Germline

MARIA P. DE MIGUEL, MARK J. FEDERSPIEL, AND PETER J. DONOVAN

From PGCs to B Spermatogonia

Correct testicular function requires that a full complement of testicular germ cells be present in the adult testis. The germ-cell compartment of the testis is established early in embryonic development from the germline progenitor cells, termed *primordial germ cells* (PGCs). In mammals, the embryonic history of the germline has been well established. PGCs can be traced in the embryo by staining embryo sections for tissue nonspecific alkaline phosphatase (TNAP) and by antigenic markers recognized by rabbit polyclonal and mouse monoclonal antibodies (1–5). That these TNAP+ cells are indeed PGCs is confirmed by the fact that these cells are deficient or absent in mouse mutants that are sterile (6–9). PGCs arise outside of the gonad anlagen, and colonization of the gonad is brought about partly through the morphogenetic movements of the embryo and partly through active directed migration (2). During this period of gonad colonization the numbers of germ cells increases.

In the mouse embryo the earliest identifiable population of PGCs is small (8–10 cells) (4,5,10,11). By the time the embryonic gonad is fully colonized by PGCs (approximately 12.5 days postcoitum in the mouse) the population of PGCs is greatly increased and is estimated to be about 25,000–30,000 cells (2,12). It is this population that will give rise to the spermatogonial stem cell of the adult testis. It seems obvious, therefore, that failure of PGCs to survive or proliferate on their way to, or in, the embryonic gonad can result in reduced fertility or, in some cases, complete sterility. In male embryos, once the PGCs have reached the embryonic gonad they cease proliferation and enter a quiescent period, where they are referred to as gonocytes (2). This occurs at about the same time as sexual differentiation is detected by the formation of testis cords in the gonad anlagen. In rodents, these germ cells, now termed *gonocytes*, will remain in this quiescent state until a few days after birth, at which time they will resume mitosis to form the mitotic stem cell of the testis, the *spermatogonium* (see 13,14 for reviews).

The transition from gonocytes to spermatogonia is still not well characterized. It has been hypothesized that, at the start of spermatogenesis, gonocytes give rise to either A stem spermatogonia (A_s) or directly to A_2 spermatogonia (15). In the adult, the A_s cell will divide to give rise to A paired (A_{pr}) and A aligned (A_{al}) undifferentiated spermatogonia, which remain connected by intercellular bridges. Then A_{al} spermatogonia will differentiate into A_1 spermatogonia, which are the first generation of differentiating type A spermatogonia. These differentiating spermatogonia go through a series of six divisions via A_2, A_3, A_4, In, and B spermatogonia, which will give rise to spermatocytes (for review see 16). The preceding description provides some information on how the various stages of germ-cell development in a male mammal are linked, but provide little information about the mechanisms regulating growth and differentiation. Defining the timing and extent of germ-cell proliferation are important because this information is vital to any meaningful understanding of how and when germ-cell proliferation is controlled in mammals.

In Vivo Proliferation

Mouse PGCs proliferate actively in vivo (17). In mice, fate mapping studies have identified the PGCs progenitors as early as 6.5 days postcoitum (dpc) (4,5,10). At this time the PGCs represent a small population of approximately 8–10 cells. During the next several days of embryonic development the PGCs will move toward the forming embryonic gonad. By 10.5 dpc approximately 1000 PGCs are identified in the embryo by alkaline phosphatase staining (6). In the fully colonized gonad at 12.5 dpc there are estimated to be 25,000 PGCs present (see Ref. 2 for review). The population doubling time of PGCs has been estimated to be between 14 and 16 hours (12). When PGCs are isolated into culture during the time period in which they are migrating to the gonad (8.5–11.5 dpc) they continue to proliferate and incorporate ^{3}H-thymidine or BrdU (3,18,19). PGCs isolated from 12.5 dpc or older embryonic gonads show a decreased ability to proliferate (3). Thus, their in vitro proliferation seems to mirror their in vivo proliferation.

The proliferation rate of embryonic mouse gonocytes decreases dramatically after they reach the embryonic testicular cord as described earlier. At 14 dpc, 7.7% of the mouse gonocytes are estimated to be proliferating, whereas this number drops to 0.2% at 16 dpc.[1] From 16 dpc until birth the gonocytes are arrested at G_1 phase of the cell cycle (20). In the rat (21), 5%

---

[1] For the purposes of this chapter, to make the numbers derived from various studies comparable, we have adjusted the proliferation rates to the percentage of cells labeled after 1 hour of either ^{3}H-thymidine or BrdU exposure.

of the gonocytes are proliferating at 16 dpc, 5.5% at 17dpc, and 1% at 18 dpc. As described earlier, mouse gonocytes resume mitosis after birth. At 1 day postpartum (dpp) their labeling index is 10.4%, 20.1% at 2 dpp, and 24.1% at 3 dpp (20), at which time the first A spermatogonia are identified. By contrast, in the rat, resumption of proliferation takes place around the third day of life and is strain dependent. In the U:WU Wistar rat, proliferation rates are zero during the first 3 days of life, 1.1% at 4 dpp, and 5.5% at 5 dpp (21). In a separate study, spermatogonial proliferation rates were examined over a longer timecourse and similar numbers were observed. For the first 3 days of life no spermatogonia incorporated BrdU. At 4 dpp, 0.5% incorporated BrdU, at 5 dpp 5% and a maximum of 19% at 6 dpp. At 7 dpp, 15% of the spermatogonia incorporated BrdU (22). In parallel, in the Chinese hamster the onset of spermatogenesis occurs at 5 dpp (15), while in humans the first B spermatogonia are seen at 4 years of age (23).

In the adult, A spermatogonial proliferation indexes depend on the testicular epithelial stage. In the mouse they have been described to be 58.3% and 50.6% in stages I and II, then decrease to 7.7% and 3.7% in stages III and IV. No spermatogonia are proliferating in stages V to VIII, but around 2% are proliferating in stages IX to XI, with a further increase to 52.4% in stage XII (24). In a more recent study, which did not take into account the testicular epithelial stage, the spermatogonial proliferation indexes are described to be 13.7% for type A and 14.3% for intermediate-B spermatogonia (25). It is important that defining the temporal and spatial windows during which germ cells proliferate allows the factors that act at these times and places to be identified and characterized. Over the past 5 years much progress has been made toward understanding the molecular mechanisms controlling germ-cell growth and differentiation during embryonic and postnatal development. Some of this information has come from the analysis of mouse mutants or knockout mice, and some has come from cell culture studies in which the actions of purified growth factors can be analyzed.

Factors That Affect Germ Cell Proliferation

PGC Growth

PGC growth has been studied extensively in vitro and many of the factors that have been found to affect PGC numbers in vitro have physiological relevance. The factors that are necessary for PGC survival are not completely understood. Nevertheless, it has been possible to culture these cells for extended periods of time over feeder-cell layers with the addition of several growth factors. Among the factors that act on PGCs, the most studied is stem cell factor (SCF), encoded by the Steel (Sl) locus. This factor has been shown to increase PGC survival in vitro (3,18,19,26–28). Several mutants have been found to affect either the factor or its receptor, c-kit, encoded by the W locus

(29–31). Mice homozygous for many of these mutations are sterile, which demonstrates the critical role for SCF in PGC survival.

The interleukin-6 (IL-6) family of growth factors most likely also plays an important role in PGC survival: Leukemia inhibitory factor (LIF) has been shown to increase PGC survival in vitro; in combination with SCF, it induces proliferation (3,18,26–28,32,33). Other members of this family—ciliary neurotrophic factor (CNTF) and oncostatin m (OSM)—have also been shown to increase mouse PGCs survival (34), whereas IL-6 does not affect PGC growth in vitro (32). It is of note that mice lacking the common signaling component of the receptor for all members of this cytokine family, termed *gp130*, show PGC depletion (Taga unpublished, cited in 35–37). These data unequivocally demonstrate that signaling via gp130 is required for PGC growth.

Other growth factors such as tumor necrosis factor-α (TNF-α) (38), interleukin-4 (IL-4) (39), and epidermal growth factor (EGF) (Cooke unpublished, cited in Ref. 40) have all been demonstrated to increase PGC survival in vitro, but their role in regulating PGC numbers in vivo remains unclear. On the other hand, insulinlike growth factor I (IGF-I), interleukins 1 and 3 (IL-1&3), platelet-derived growth factor (PDGF) (32), activin, bone morphogenetic protein 4 (bmp-4), and β-nerve growth factor (β-NGF) (41) have been found to have no effect on PGC survival in culture. Finally, other factors have been described to inhibit PGC proliferation in vitro, and include tumor necrosis factor-β (TNF-β) and transforming growth factor-β1 (TGF-β1) (42). Once again the role of these negative regulators in controlling PGC growth in vivo remains unclear.

Gonocyte Proliferation

The factors that affect gonocyte proliferation and differentiation are still poorly understood. So far it has not been possible to culture these cells in the absence of the accompanying Sertoli cells, which gives an indication that the factors controlling gonocyte survival involve both soluble as well as membrane-anchored factors and matrix proteins. In vitro, gonocytes isolated from 2-day-old mice and cultured in serum-supplemented medium have been shown to proliferate actively, but for a very short period (1 day) before disappearing from the culture (43). In contrast to the situation in mice, newborn rat gonocytes, which resume mitosis 3 days after birth, do not proliferate for the first 2 days of culture in accordance with the in vivo situation. In fact, when rat gonocytes are cultured in serum-free medium over Matrigel, their labeling indexes are 0.2% on day 3, 5% on day 4 and 6.1% on day 5 of culture, and they can be cultured for up to 10 days (44,45).

It is surprising that the main hormones controlling spermatogenesis in vivo, follicle stimulating hormone (FSH) and testosterone (T), do not affect newborn rat gonocytes when co-cultured with Sertoli cells (46). Other hormones, such as 17-β-estradiol, which is produced locally by Sertoli cells (47) and the so-called thymuline from thymus extracts (48), increase the proliferation rate of cultured gonocytes. On the other hand, anti-Müllerian hormone (AMH, MIS) has been reported to induce mouse gonocyte differentiation in vitro (49).

In contrast to the relatively little information about the endocrine control of gonocyte fate, a wide variety of growth factors have been reported to affect gonocyte survival, proliferation or differentiation in vitro. For example, basic fibroblast growth factor (bFGF) (50), increases both survival and proliferation of newborn rat gonocytes in co-culture with rat Sertoli cells. PDGF has similarly been shown to stimulate proliferation of newborn rat gonocytes in vitro (47). LIF (45) and OSM (22) have been demonstrated to increase both survival and proliferation of rat gonocytes and at least survival of mouse gonocytes (35). CNTF affects only the in vitro survival of these cells (45). It is interesting to note that other members of the OSM family of cytokines [e.g., IL-6 and granulocyte-colony stimulating factor (G-CSF)] do not affect gonocyte survival in culture (51). This most likely reflects the type of cytokine receptor expressed by gonocytes.

The major difference between PGCs and gonocytes seems to be in the expression of the c-kit receptor and, therefore, in the dependence on SCF. Gonocyte proliferation and differentiation are not regulated by SCF, whereas PGC survival and proliferation are. In vitro, SCF has no effect on rat gonocytes (45), and injection of an anti–c-kit antibody into 2-day-old mice does not affect spermatogenesis (52). It is interesting that SCF seems to play an important role later on in the control of the spermatogonial population and reflects the fact that c-kit levels are upregulated in type A spermatogonia (see later).

Undifferentiated Spermatogonia Kinetics

There are very few studies concerning the endocrine/paracrine control of the undifferentiated spermatogonia kinetics, which is mostly due to the difficulty in distinguishing these cells morphologically from both gonocytes and differentiating spermatogonia. In vivo injection of inhibin to Chinese hamsters does not affect proliferation and differentiation of undifferentiated spermatogonia (53). Only one mutation, *juvenile spermatogonial depletion* (*jsd*), has been described to affect the population of undifferentiated spermatogonia specifically (54). In these mice, one wave of spermatogenesis takes place, but spermatogonia then fail to divide further. It is interesting that transplantation of seminiferous tubules of cryptorchid B6+/+ mice, in which the only germ cells remaining are presumably undifferentiated spermatogonia (55), into B6-*jsd/jsd* testis leads to the differentiation of A spermatogonia into spermatids. In contrast, when B6-*jsd/jsd* tubules are transplanted into WBB6F1-W/Wv testes, type A spermatogonia are stimulated to proliferate mitotically, but they do not differentiate (56). The authors concluded that the *jsd* mutation causes a defect in the intratubular environment that supports germ-cell differentiation. The differentiation of undifferentiated spermatogonia into differentiating spermatogonia has been reported to be vitamin A-dependent because in vitamin-A deficient animals (57) only undifferentiated A spermatogonia remain (58). These cells are unable to differentiate unless vitamin A/retinoic acid is replaced in the diet (13,59,60). In vitro, addition of retinol to cultures of cryptorchid mouse testes leads to the differentiation of undifferentiated spermatogonia (61).

Growth of Differentiating Spermatogonia

In most of the studies carried out to date a mixture of undifferentiated and differentiating spermatogonia are cultured together. In these conditions, addition of activins A and B promotes both survival and proliferation of pubertal rat spermatogonia (62). In vivo injection of inhibin to Chinese hamsters provokes cell loss (53). FSH has been described to induce the differentiation of differentiating spermatogonia in organ culture (63), and to increase ^{3}H-thymidine incorporation of A and intermediate spermatogonia of adult rats (64).

As described earlier, differentiating spermatogonia, like PGCs, are dependent on the SCF/c-kit signaling pathway. Intravenous injection of an anti–c-kit monoclonal antibody into adult mice caused depletion of differentiating A spermatogonia. Intraperitoneal injection of this antibody into prepubertal mice similarly completely blocked mitosis of differentiating A spermatogonia, without affecting the mitosis of the undifferentiated cells (65). The cell loss caused by anti–c-kit injection has been determined to be by apoptosis (66). In vitro, addition of SCF to 13 dpp mouse cultures induces the proliferation of spermatogonia (67), as has also been described for adult rat spermatogonial stage-defined seminiferous tubules in culture (68).

Other factors, such as IL-1 (69,70), IGF-II (71), and TGF-β (72) have been described to induce proliferation of differentiating spermatogonia in vitro. IGF-I (73) induces both proliferation and differentiation of the spermatogonial population of cryptorchid adult mice. EGF can induce or inhibit differentiation in vitro, depending on the concentration (74). Finally, TGF-α has been demonstrated to induce the differentiation of spermatogonia from cryptorchid mice (73).

In addition, other still-unidentified growth factors (e.g., the so-called seminiferous growth factor) promote A spermatogonia proliferation (75). This factor could be a polypeptide growth factor that induces intracellular protein phosphorylation, like all the factors described earlier. On the other hand, this factor could utilize the other main signal transduction pathway, which involves G-coupled receptors that increase intracellular cAMP, which will activate protein kinases. The effects of such factors have been less extensively studied; however, both PACAPs (76) and molecules known to increase intracellular cAMP [e.g., Forskolin (33)] have been demonstrated to increase the proliferation rate of mouse PGCs. The identification of the factors regulating the growth of germ cells at any stage of development is important because of the implications for fertility. In addition, knowledge of germ-cell growth regulators will be vital to attempts to establish long-term cultures of germ cells.

In Vitro Culture of Germ Cells

In vitro culture systems have been used extensively both to identify and to study the factors that regulate PGC growth. Isolation and culture of PGCs has been described extensively elsewhere (3,77). In brief, the most successful and most commonly used method involves culturing PGCs on a confluent feeder layer. In this system, the PGCs can be identified using classic germ-cell markers such as TNAP and SSEA-1 (3). Many of the factors that have been identified using this system have subsequently been shown to be relevant to PGC growth in vivo. Moreover, culture systems have also been useful for studying other aspects of PGC development in addition to growth regulation, especially PGC differentiation and migration (3,42,78–80). The application of such culture techniques to the analysis of spermatogonial development would provide a powerful means of analyzing spermatogonial differentiation. We have begun to examine the effects of a variety of growth factors on the survival, growth, and differentiation of spermatogonia in vitro. In brief, mouse Sertoli cells and germ cells are isolated enzymatically from 1–3-day-old animals (see Ref. 31) and cultured essentially as described in detail elsewhere for their rat counterparts (22). For culturing mouse gonocytes and undifferentiated spermatogonia, we made minor modifications to the growth factor combinations that gave the highest proliferation rate. Using a combination of Forskolin, LIF, EGF, and OSM, we could achieve a proliferation rate of the germ cells of 35–40% after 7 days in culture. Improved culture methods for spermatogonia could allow many aspects of their basic physiology to be examined in addition to having many practical applications.

Manipulating Gene Expression in the Mammalian Germline

In most of the examples described earlier, several cell types are cultured together. This makes it difficult and sometimes impossible to determine if the effects of a specific factor on a specific cell type are direct or indirect. This led us to try to create a system in which questions about the factors that control germ-cell development can be asked in a more defined manner by introducing genes into specific cells (i.e., somatic or germ cells). It has been demonstrated that adenoviruses can infect germ cells in vivo, but only for a short period of time; after 30 days, transgene expression is lost (82). In this regard, the use of retroviral vectors has been demonstrated to lead to long-term in vivo infection of several cell types. Tissue-specific targeting of experimental gene delivery and expression in mouse tissues had been demonstrated previously with the RCAS family of avian leukosis virus (ALV)–based retroviral vectors (83). The use of this avian retroviral vector system in mammalian cells has several unique advantages. First, this system includes retroviral vectors that are replication-competent in avian cells and grow to high titers (>10^7 IFU/ml). Second, ALVs are naturally replication-defective in mammalian cells; consequently, the vectors cannot spread to other cells. The defect(s) results in little or no viral protein expression, but does not affect experimental gene expression. Third, mammalian cells are not susceptible to efficient infection by ALVs because they lack the appropriate receptors. The cloning of the receptor for subgroup A ALVs, tv-a, (84, 85), however, made possible the generation of mammalian cell lines and transgenic mouse lines that express the tv-a receptor.

The utility of the ALV retroviral vector system in mice was initially demonstrated with two different types of transgenic mice: α-AKE lines in which the susceptibility to ALV infection was made specific for skeletal muscle by expressing the tv-a gene under the control of the tissue-specific chicken α-sk-actin promoter (86), and β-AKE lines in which the tv-a receptor is expressed in most if not all tissues and in the early embryo by expressing the tv-a gene under the control of the constitutive chicken β-actin promoter (87). Most tissues in the β-AKE mice were susceptible to ALV infection, including germ cells because the integrated ALV proviruses were transmitted as a transgene. Tissue-specific gene expression was also obtained with the β-AKE lines by expressing the experimental gene under the control of an internal promoter, β-sk-actin (86,87). This experimental approach to tissue-specific gene delivery and expression was used to develop a transgenic mouse line in which the susceptibility to ALV infection was specific for astrocytes (88–90). In summary, tissue-specific gene targeting can be achieved with the RCAS family of ALV retroviral vectors by expressing the receptor under the control of a tissue-specific promoter, thereby targeting the expression of the experimental gene to the appropriate tissue. It should be possible to restrict the expression of the exogenous gene further by including an internal tissue-specific promoter in the vector.

We have completed a series of preliminary experiments to test if cultured mouse germ cells are susceptible to ALV-based retroviral vector infection. Germ cells were isolated from β-AKE mice at different stages of embryonic and postnatal development and infected with RCASBP(A)GFP (91), which is the highest-titer subgroup RCASBP vector that contains the enhanced green fluorescent protein (GFP) under the control of the viral promoter. PGCs were cultured as described previously on STO cell monolayers (3,19), and infection followed by GFP expression and co-expression of PGC markers (e.g., anti-SSEA-1) (Fig. 6.1A,B). In these cultures, up to 20% of the dividing PGCs isolated from β-AKE mice became infected as judged by expression of GFP. This represents 15% of all the PGCs in culture because in these cultures 80% of the PGCs are dividing on day 7 of culture in the presence of Forskolin, LIF, and SCF. Simple retroviruses (e.g., ALV, murine leukemia virus) require dividing cells for efficient gene delivery and expression. We also noted that embryonic somatic cells (but not the STO cells) were also infected in this system (Fig. 6.1A). In cultures of gonocytes and Sertoli cells, GFP expression could also be identified in RCASBP(A)GFP-infected cells

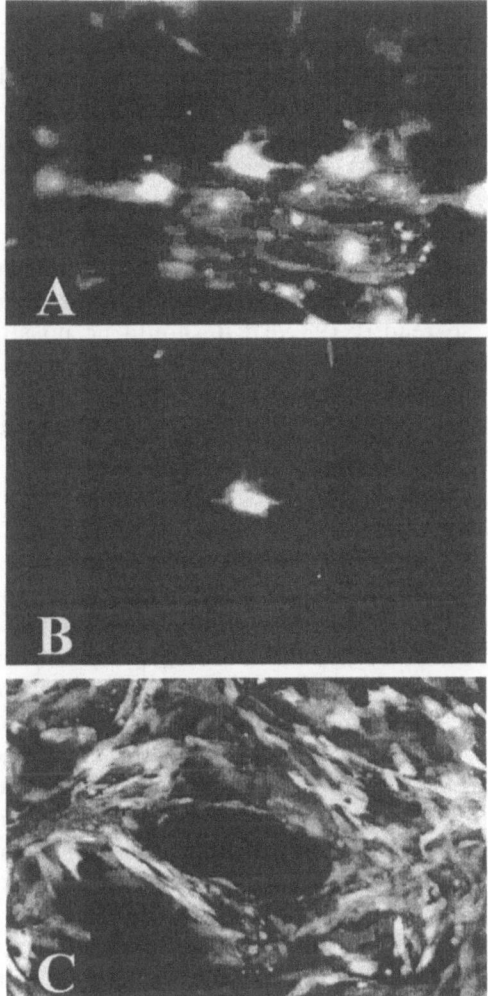

FIGURE 6.1. (A) Fluorescence photomicrograph of GFP expression in retrovirally infected cultures of PGCs and embryonic somatic cells. PGCs and accompanying somatic cells were isolated from 8.5 dpc β-AKE mouse embryos and the cells cultured over irradiated STO feeder cell layer. Twenty-four hours later the cultures were infected with an avian retrovirus expressing GFP from the retroviral LTR. Infected cells expressing GFP are recognized under fluorescence light using GFP excitation and emission filters. Magnification = 1200×. (B) Expression of GFP in PGCs. The same field as (A), in which a PGC can be recognized by staining for the SSEA-1 antigen with a mouse anti-SSEA-1 monoclonal antibody and a rabbit antimouse immunoglobulin antiserum coupled to Rhodamine isothiocyanite. Magnification = 1200×. (C) Expression of GFP in cultures of newborn spermatogonia and Sertoli cells. Spermatogonia and accompanying Sertoli cells were isolated from 3-day-old β-AKE mice and placed into culture. Twenty-four hours later they were infected with an avian retrovirus expressing GFP from the retroviral LTR. Infected cells expressing GFP are recognized under fluorescence light using GFP excitation and emission filters. Note the large numbers of cells expressing GFP. Magnification = 1200×.

(Fig. 6.1C). Great sophistication clearly can be built into this system simply by expression of the avian retroviral receptor in different lineages or cell types. For example, introduction of the tv-a cDNA into the Oct-4 locus would allow expression of the receptor in PGCs, but not in embryonic somatic cells (92). The application of this ALV-based retroviral vector gene transfer to the analysis of postnatal germ-cell development could provide a rapid and facile mechanism by which to address questions about spermatogonial growth, development, and differentiation. Furthermore, because spermatogonial transplantation works so readily (93,94), it should be possible to introduce retroviruses into spermatogonia in culture and then return them to a host testis. The results presented earlier suggest that retroviral-mediated gene expression is a viable system for investigating growth control of the mammalian germline.

Conclusions

The molecular mechanisms regulating germ-cell growth and differentiation are slowly being determined, but there still remains much to be learned about these processes. The use of existing mouse mutants and mice carrying targeted gene mutations has allowed the characterization of some of the genes involved in germline development in mammals. Cell culture systems have similarly been used to study some of the factors that control germ-cell growth, survival, and differentiation. The identification of genes expressed in the mammalian germline is straightforward, but a major problem facing the field is how to determine the function of such genes in controlling germ-cell growth. Targeted expression of genes to specific stages of germline development is still problematical because the promoters that could be used for such experiments also direct gene expression to other cell types present in the early embryo. A similar problem exists for carrying out cell- and stage-specific gene targeting in the germline. The use of retroviruses to accomplish gene delivery would overcome some, but not all, of these problems. Many of the questions that one would want to ask about the function of a specific gene could be addressed using retroviral-mediated gene expression. Moreover, because the testis is so accessible in the adult animal, viral delivery to the testis is likely to be straightforward. In addition, the ability to isolate and culture spermatogonial stem cells and then transplant them back into the testis may allow retroviral-mediated manipulation of the mammalian germline. These types of studies should allow many of the questions regarding germline growth control to be addressed.

References

1. Fox N, Damjanov I, Martinez-Hernandez A, Knowles BB, Solter D. Immunohistochemical localization of the early embryonic antigen (SSEA-1) in postimplantation

mouse embryos and fetal and adult tissues. Dev Biol (Orlando) 1981;83(2): 391–98.

2. McLaren A. Germ cells and soma: a new look at an old problem. New Haven: Yale University Press, 1981.

3. Donovan PJ, Stott D, Cairns LA, Heasman J, Wylie CC. Migratory and postmigratory mouse primordial germ cells behave differently in culture. Cell 1986;44(6): 831–38.

4. MacGregor GR, Zambrowicz BP, Soriano P. Tissue non-specific alkaline phosphatase is expressed in both embryonic and extraembryonic lineages during mouse embryogenesis but is not required for migration of primordial germ cells. Development 1995;121(5):1487–96.

5. Ginsburg M, Snow MH, McLaren A. Primordial germ cells in the mouse embryo during gastrulation. Development 1990;110(2):521–28.

6. McCoshen JA, McCallion DJ. A study of the primordial germ cells during their migratory phase in Steel mutant mice. Experientia 1975;31(5):589–90.

7. Mintz B, Russell ES. Gene-induced embryological modifications of primordial germ cells in the mouse. J Exp Morphol 1957;134:207–37.

8. Mintz B. Embryological development of primordial germ cells in the mouse: influence of a new mutation, Wj. J Embryol Exp Morphol 1957;5:396–406.

9. Buehr M, McLaren A, Bartley A, Darling S. Proliferation and migration of primordial germ cells in We/We mouse embryos. Dev Dynam 1993;198(3):182–89.

10. Lawson KA, Hage WJ. Clonal analysis of the origin of primordial germ cells in the mouse. Ciba Foundation Symposium 1994;182:68–84; discussion 84–91.

11. Lawson KA, Pedersen RA. Clonal analysis of cell fate during gastrulation and early neurulation in the mouse. Ciba Foundation Symposium 1992;165:3–21; discussion 21–26.

12. Tam PP, Snow MH. Proliferation and migration of primordial germ cells during compensatory growth in mouse embryos. J Embryol Exp Morphol 1981;64: 133–47.

13. De Rooij DG, van Dissel-Emiliani FM, van Pelt AM. Regulation of spermatogonial proliferation. Ann NY Acad Sci 1989;564:140–53.

14. De Rooij DG. Regulation of the proliferation of spermatogonial stem cells. J Cell Sci 1988;10(Suppl.)10:181–94.

15. Van Haaster LH, de Rooij DG. Spermatogenesis is accelerated in the immature Hjungarian and Chinese hamster and rat. Biol Reprod 1993;49(6):1229–35.

16. De Rooij DG. Stem cells in the testis. Int J Exp Pathol 1998;79(2):67–80.

17. Tam PP. The control of somitogenesis in mouse embryos. J Embryol Exp Morphol 1981;65(Suppl.):103–28.

18. Matsui Y, Toksoz D, Nishikawa S, Williams D, Zsebo K, Hogan BL. Effect of Steel factor and leukaemia inhibitory factor on murine primordial germ cells in culture. Nature 1991;353(6346):750–52.

19. Dolci S, Williams DE, Ernst MK, Resnick JL, Brannan CI, Lock LF, et al. Requirement for mast cell growth factor for primordial germ cell survival in culture. Nature 1991;352(6338):809–11.

20. Vergouwen RP, Jacobs SG, Huiskamp R, Davids JA, de Rooij DG. Proliferative activity of gonocytes, Sertoli cells and interstitial cells during testicular development in mice. J Reprod Fertil 1991;93(1):233–43.

21. Hilscher B, Hilscher W, Bulthoff-Ohnolz B, Kramer U, Birke A, Pelzer H, et al.

Kinetics of gametogenesis. I. Comparative histological and autoradiographic studies of oocytes and transitional prospermatogonia during oogenesis and prespermatogenesis. Cell Tiss Res 1974;154(4):443–70.

22. De Miguel MP, de Boer-Brouwer M, de Rooij DG, Paniagua R, van Dissel-Emiliani FM. Ontogeny and localization of an oncostatin M-like protein in the rat testis: its possible role at the start of spermatogenesis. Cell Growth Different 1997;8(5): 611–18.

23. Paniagua R, Nistal M. Morphological and histometric study of human spermatogonia from birth to the onset of puberty. J Anatomy 1984;139(Pt 3):535–52.

24. Oakberg EF. Spermatogonial stem-cell renewal in the mouse. Anat Rec 1971; 169(3):515–31.

25. Sawada K, Sakamaki K, Nishimune Y. Effect of the W mutation, for white belly spot, on testicular germ cell differentiation in mice. J Reprod Fertil 1991;93(2): 287–94.

26. Godin I, Deed R, Cooke J, Zsebo K, Dexter M, Wylie CC. Effects of the steel gene product on mouse primordial germ cells in culture. Nature 1991;352(6338):807–9.

27. Resnick JL, Bixler LS, Cheng L, Donovan PJ. Long-term proliferation of mouse primordial germ cells in culture [see comments]. Nature 1992;359(6395):550–51.

28. Stewart CL, Kaspar P, Brunet LJ, Bhatt H, Gadi I, Kontgen F, et al. Blastocyst implantation depends on maternal expression of leukaemia inhibitory factor [see comments]. Nature 1992;359(6390):76–79.

29. Russell ES. Hereditary anemias of the mouse: a review for geneticists. Adv Gen 1979;20:357–459.

30. Kitamura Y, Sonoda T, Nakano T, Hayashi C, Asai H. Differentiation processes of connective tissue mast cells in living mice. International Arch Aller Appl Immunol 1985;77(1–2):144–50.

31. Yarden Y, Kuang WJ, Yang-Feng T, Coussens L, Munemitsu S, Dull TJ, et al. Human proto-oncogene c-kit: a new cell surface receptor tyrosine kinase for an unidentified ligand. EMBO J 1987;6(11):3341–51.

32. De Felici M, Dolci S. Leukemia inhibitory factor sustains the survival of mouse primordial germ cells cultured on TM4 feeder layers. Dev Biol (Orlando) 1991; 147(1):281–84.

33. Dolci S, Pesce M, De Felici M. Combined action of stem cell factor, leukemia inhibitory factor, and cAMP on in vitro proliferation of mouse primordial germ cells. Molecular Reproduction & Development 1993;35(2):134–39.

34. Cheng L, Gearing DP, White LS, Compton DL, Schooley K, Donovan PJ. Role of leukemia inhibitory factor and its receptor in mouse primordial germ cell growth. Development 1994;120(11):3145–53.

35. Hara T, Tamura K, de Miguel MP, Mukouyama Y, Kim H, Kogo H, et al. Distinct roles of oncostatin M and leukemia inhibitory factor in the development of primordial germ cells and Sertoli cells in mice. Dev Biol (Orlando) 1998;201(2):144–53.

36. Koshimizu U, Taga T, Watanabe M, Saito M, Shirayoshi Y, Kishimoto T, et al. Functional requirement of gp130-mediated signaling for growth and survival of mouse primordial germ cells in vitro and derivation of embryonic germ (EG) cells. Development 1996;122(4):1235–42.

37. Yoshida K, Taga T, Saito M, Suematsu S, Kumanogoh A, Tanaka T, et al. Targeted disruption of gp130, a common signal transducer for the interleukin 6 family of cytokines, leads to myocardial and hematological disorders. Proc Nat Acad Sci USA 1996;93(1):407–11.

38. Kawase E, Yamamoto H, Hashimoto K, Nakatsuji N. Tumor necrosis factor-alpha (TNF-alpha) stimulates proliferation of mouse primordial germ cells in culture. Dev Biol (Orlando) 1994;161(1):91–5.
39. Cooke JE, Heasman J, Wylie CC. The role of interleukin-4 in the regulation of mouse primordial germ cell numbers. Dev Biol (Orlando) 1996;174(1):14–21.
40. Wylie C. Germ cells. Cell 1999;96(2):165–74.
41. Matsui Y, Zsebo K, Hogan BL. Derivation of pluripotential embryonic stem cells from murine primordial germ cells in culture. Cell 1992;70(5):841–47.
42. Godin I, Wylie CC. TGF beta 1 inhibits proliferation and has a chemotropic effect on mouse primordial germ cells in culture. Development 1991;113(4):1451–57.
43. Maekawa M, Nishimune Y. In-vitro proliferation of germ cells and supporting cells in the neonatal mouse testis. Cell Tiss Res 1991;265(3):551–54.
44. Orth JM, McGuinness MP. Neonatal gonocytes co-cultured with Sertoli cells on a laminin-containing matrix resume mitosis and elongate. Endocrinology 1991; 129(2):1119–21.
45. De Miguel MP, de Boer-Brouwer M, Paniagua R, van den Hurk R, de Rooij DG, van Dissel-Emiliani FM. Leukemia inhibitory factor and ciliary neurotrophic factor promote the survival of Sertoli cells and gonocytes in coculture system. Endocrinology 1996;137(5):1885–93.
46. Van Dissel-Emiliani FM, de Boer-Brouwer M, Spek ER, van der Donk JA, de Rooij DG. Survival and proliferation of rat gonocytes in vitro. Cell Tiss Res 1993; 273(1):141–47.
47. Li H, Papadopoulos V, Vidic B, Dym M, Culty M. Regulation of rat testis gonocyte proliferation by platelet-derived growth factor and estradiol: identification of signaling mechanisms involved. Endocrinology 1997;138(3):1289–98.
48. Prepin J, Le Vigouroux P, Dadoune JP. Effects of thymulin on in vitro incorporation of ^{3}H-thymidine into gonocytes of newborn rat testes. Reprod, Nutr, Dev 1994;34(4):289–94.
49. Zhou B, Watts LM, Hutson JM. Germ cell development in neonatal mouse testes in vitro requires mullerian inhibiting substance. J Urol 1993;150(2 Pt 2):613–16.
50. Van Dissel-Emiliani FM, De Boer-Brouwer M, de Rooij DG. Effect of fibroblast growth factor-2 on Sertoli cells and gonocytes in coculture during the perinatal period. Endocrinology 1996;137(2):647–54.
51. De Miguel MP, van Dissel-Emiliani MF. Paracrine regulation of the start of spermatogenesis: The Il-6 family. In: Martinez-Garcia F, Regadera J, eds. Male Reproduction: A multidisciplinary overview. Madrid, Spain: Churchill Communications, 1998:57–66.
52. Tajima Y, Sakamaki K, Watanabe D, Koshimizu U, Matsuzawa T, Nishimune Y. Steel-Dickie (Sld) mutation affects both maintenance and differentiation of testicular germ cells in mice. J Reprod Fertil 1991;91(2):441–49.
53. Van Dissel-Emiliani FM, Grootenhuis AJ, de Jong FH, de Rooij DG. Inhibin reduces spermatogonial numbers in testes of adult mice and Chinese hamsters. Endocrinology 1989;125(4):1899–903.
54. Beamer WG, Cunliffe-Beamer TL, Shultz KL, Langley SH, Roderick TH. Juvenile spermatogonial depletion (jsd): a genetic defect of germ cell proliferation of male mice. Biol Reprod 1988;38(4):899–908.
55. Nishimune Y, Aizawa S, Komatsu T. Testicular germ cell differentiation in vivo. Fertil Steril 1978;29(1):95–102.
56. Mizunuma M, Dohmae K, Tajima Y, Koshimizu U, Watanabe D, Nishimune Y.

Loss of sperm in juvenile spermatogonial depletion (jsd) mutant mice is ascribed to a defect of intratubular environment to support germ cell differentiation. J Cell Physiol 1992;150(1):188–93.

57. Mitranond V, Sobhon P, Tosukhowong P, Chindaduangrat W. Cytological changes in the testes of vitamin-A-deficient rats. I. Quantitation of germinal cells in the seminiferous tubules. Acta Anatomica 1979;103(2):159–68.

58. De Rooij DG, van Pelt AMM, de Kant HJG, van der Saag PT, Peters AHFM, Heyting C, et al. Role of retinoids in spermatogonial proliferation and differentiation and the meiotic prophase. In: Bartke A, ed. Function of somatic cells in the testis. New York: Springer Verlag, 1994:345–61.

59. Morales C, Griswold MD. Retinol-induced stage synchronization in seminiferous tubules of the rat. Endocrinology 1987;121(1):432–34.

60. Smith JE. Preparation of vitamin A-deficient rats and mice. Meth Enzymol 1990;190:229–36.

61. Haneji T, Koide SS, Nishimune Y, Oota Y. Dibutyryl adenosine cyclic monophosphate regulates differentiation of type A spermatogonia with vitamin A in adult mouse cryptorchid testis in vitro. Endocrinology 1986;119(6):2490–96.

62. Mather JP, Attie KM, Woodruff TK, Rice GC, Phillips DM. Activin stimulates spermatogonial proliferation in germ-Sertoli cell cocultures from immature rat testis. Endocrinology 1990;127(6):3206–14.

63. Boitani C, Politi MG, Menna T. Spermatogonial cell proliferation in organ culture of immature rat testis. Biol Reprod 1993;48(4):761–67.

64. Henriksen K, Kangasniemi M, Parvinen M, Kaipia A, Hakovirta H. In vitro, follicle-stimulating hormone prevents apoptosis and stimulates deoxyribonucleic acid synthesis in the rat seminiferous epithelium in a stage-specific fashion. Endocrinology 1996;137(5):2141–49.

65. Yoshinaga K, Nishikawa S, Ogawa M, Hayashi S, Kunisada T, Fujimoto T. Role of c-kit in mouse spermatogenesis: identification of spermatogonia as a specific site of c-kit expression and function. Development 1991;113(2):689–99.

66. Packer AI, Besmer P, Bachvarova RF. Kit ligand mediates survival of type A spermatogonia and dividing spermatocytes in postnatal mouse testes. Mol Reprod Dev 1995;42(3):303–10.

67. Rossi P, Dolci S, Albanesi C, Grimaldi P, Ricca R, Geremia R. Follicle-stimulating hormone induction of steel factor (SLF) mRNA in mouse Sertoli cells and stimulation of DNA synthesis in spermatogonia by soluble SLF. Dev Biol (Orlando) 1993;155(1):68–74.

68. Hakovirta H, Yan W, Kaleva M, Zhang F, Vanttinen K, Morris PL, et al. Function of stem cell factor as a survival factor of spermatogonia and localization of messenger ribonucleic acid in the rat seminiferous epithelium. Endocrinology 1999; 140(3):1492–98.

69. Pollanen P, Soder O, Parvinen M. Interleukin-1 alpha stimulation of spermatogonial proliferation in vivo. Reprod Fertil Dev 1989;1(1):85–87.

70. Parvinen M, Soder O, Mali P, Froysa B, Ritzen EM. In vitro stimulation of stage-specific deoxyribonucleic acid synthesis in rat seminiferous tubule segments by interleukin-1 alpha. Endocrinology 1991;129(3):1614–20.

71. Soder O, Bang P, Wahab A, Parvinen M. Insulin-like growth factors selectively stimulate spermatogonial, but not meiotic, deoxyribonucleic acid synthesis during rat spermatogenesis. Endocrinology 1992;131(5):2344–50.

72. Hakovirta H, Kaipia A, Soder O, Parvinen M. Effects of activin-A, inhibin-A, and

transforming growth factor-beta 1 on stage-specific deoxyribonucleic acid synthesis during rat seminiferous epithelial cycle. Endocrinology 1993;133(4): 1664–68.

73. Tajima Y, Watanabe D, Koshimizu U, Matsuzawa T, Nishimune Y. Insulin-like growth factor-I and transforming growth factor-alpha stimulate differentiation of type A spermatogonia in organ culture of adult mouse cryptorchid testes. Int J Androl 1995;18(1):8–12.

74. Haneji T, Koide SS, Tajima Y, Nishimune Y. Differential effects of epidermal growth factor on the differentiation of type A spermatogonia in adult mouse cryptorchid testes in vitro. J Endocrinol 1991;128(3):383–88.

75. Bellve AR, Zheng W. Growth factors as autocrine and paracrine modulators of male gonadal functions. J Reprod Fertil 1989;85(2):771–93.

76. De Felici M, Pesce M. Interactions between migratory primordial germ cells and cellular substrates in the mouse. Ciba Foundation Symposium 1994;182:140–50; discussion 150–53.

77. Donovan PJ. Growth factor regulation of mouse primordial germ cell development. Curr Topics Dev Biol 1994;29:189–225.

78. Stott D, Wylie CC. Invasive behaviour of mouse primordial germ cells in vitro. J Cell Sci 1986;86:133–44.

79. Godin I, Wylie C, Heasman J. Genital ridges exert long-range effects on mouse primordial germ cell numbers and direction of migration in culture. Development 1990;108(2):357–63.

80. De Felici M, Dolci S. Cellular interactions of mouse fetal germ cells in in vitro systems. Curr Topics Dev Biol 1987;23:147–62.

81. Bellve AR, Cavicchia JC, Millette CF, O'Brien DA, Bhatnagar YM, Dym M. Spermatogenic cells of the prepubertal mouse. Isolation and morphological characterization. J Cell Biol 1977;74(1):68–85.

82. Blanchard KT, Boekelheide K. Adenovirus-mediated gene transfer to rat testis in vivo. Biol Reprod 1997;56(2):495–500.

83. Federspiel MJ, Hughes SH. Retroviral gene delivery. Meth Cell Biol 1998;52: 179–214.

84. Young JA, Bates P, Varmus HE. Isolation of a chicken gene that confers susceptibility to infection by subgroup A avian leukosis and sarcoma viruses. J Virol 1993;67(4):1811–16.

85. Bates P, Young JA, Varmus HE. A receptor for subgroup A Rous sarcoma virus is related to the low density lipoprotein receptor. Cell 1993;74(6):1043–51.

86. Federspiel MJ, Bates P, Young JA, Varmus HE, Hughes SH. A system for tissue-specific gene targeting: transgenic mice susceptible to subgroup A avian leukosis virus-based retroviral vectors. Proc Nat Acad Sci USA 1994;91(23):11241–45.

87. Federspiel MJ, Swing DA, Eagleson B, Reid SW, Hughes SH. Expression of transduced genes in mice generated by infecting blastocysts with avian-leukosis virus-based retroviral vectors. Proc Nat Acad Sci USA 1994;93(10):4931–36.

88. Holland EC, Varmus HE. Basic fibroblast growth factor induces cell migration and proliferation after glia-specific gene transfer in mice. Proc Nat Acad Sci USA 1998;95(3):1218–23.

89. Holland EC, Hively WP, Gallo V, Varmus HE. Modeling mutations in the G1 arrest pathway in human gliomas: overexpression of CDK4 but not loss of INK4a-ARF induces hyperploidy in cultured mouse astrocytes. Genes Dev 1998; 12(23):3644–49.

90. Holland EC, Hively WP, DePinho RA, Varmus HE. A constitutively active epidermal growth factor receptor cooperates with disruption of G1 cell-cycle arrest pathways to induce glioma-like lesions in mice. Genes Dev 1998;12(23):3675–85.

91. Schaefer-Klein J, Givol I, Barsov EV, Whitcomb JM, Van Brocklin M, Foster DN, et al. The EV-O-derived cell line DF-1 supports the efficient replication of avian leukosis-sarcoma viruses and vectors. Virology 1998;248(2):305–11.

92. Yeom YI, Fuhrmann G, Ovitt CE, Brehm A, Ohbo K, Gross M, et al. Germline regulatory element of Oct-4 specific for the totipotent cycle of embryonal cells. Development 1996;122(3):881–94.

93. Brinster RL, Avarbock MR. Germline transmission of donor haplotype following spermatogonial transplantation [see comments]. Proc Nat Acad Sci USA 1994; 91(24):11303–7.

94. Brinster RL, Zimmermann JW. Spermatogenesis following male germ-cell transplantation [see comments]. Proc Nat Acad Sci USA 1994;91(24):11298–302.

Part II

Paracrine and Endocrine Interactions

Part III

Enzyme Immunoassays

7

Synthesis, Fate, and Proposed Function of Clusterin (SGP-2) in the Testis

Robert W. Bailey, Ann Clark, Elena Lymar, Walter A. Tribley, and Michael D. Griswold

History of Clusterin and Presence in the Male Reproductive System

Clusterin (SGP-2) is the major protein in the spent medium of rat Sertoli cell cultures (1,2). Rat clusterin is a glycoprotein of pI approximately 4.0 and is made up of two nonidentical disulfide-linked subunits of 34 kD and 47 kD with extensive charge heterogeneity (3,4). The highly negative charge and overall charge heterogeneity of the protein have been attributed to sulfation of the carbohydrate moieties and the presence of sialic acid (5). The cDNA sequence obtained after immunoprecipitation of polysomes and cloning of the mRNA contained an open reading frame sufficient in length to code for both monomers (4). It was shown that clusterin is made as a full-length precursor, undergoes posttranslational modifications, and is cleaved into two disulfide-linked subunits prior to secretion. Northern analysis of RNA from Sertoli cells with probes generated from the cDNA revealed a 2 kb message present in high abundance in testis, epididymis, and in Sertoli cells in culture (4). A similar-sized transcript was also observed in many other tissues. A search of nucleic acid and protein databases at the time revealed no identities with known sequences (see Fig. 7.1 for more structural information).

Normal Tissue Distribution and Proposed Functions

Since its discovery in the testis, clusterin has been described in many mammalian species and in birds. It was initially isolated in systems other than the testis as a complement inhibitor, an apolipoprotein J, and a component

73

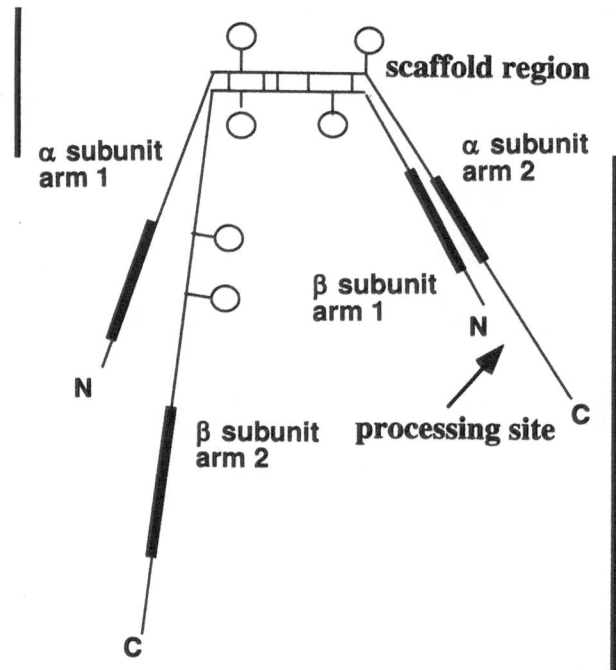

FIGURE 7.1. Diagrammatic representation of the structure of rat clusterin. The mature secreted form of clusterin is a dimer whose subunits are held together by five closely spaced disulfide bonds. The disulfide bonds and several oligosaccharide structures (circles) comprise a region designated as the scaffold region. The processing site is where a single proteolytic clip converts proclusterin to clusterin. There are four antiparallel arms that each have a region of amphipathic helixes (black bars). The arms form the putative hydrophobic binding domain of clusterin.

of secretory granules (for review see Ref. 6). Clusterin appears to be induced at the mRNA and protein level in regressing, involuting, or injured tissues. It is clearly induced in surviving cells in the process of apoptosis, and in polycystic kidney disease, renal ablation, and experimental hydronephrosis (7). Clusterin is a marker of neurodegeneration. Clusterin mRNA in the brain was shown to increase in the hippocampus of human Alzheimer patients, in human gliomas and epileptic foci, and in the hippocampus of castrated rats. In Alzheimer's disease, the amount of clusterin mRNA was doubled in the hippocampus and the entorhinal cortex (8).

Clusterin has been shown to bind with high affinity to several different proteins. Clusterin binds with high affinity to glycoprotein 330/megalin, which is a member of the low-density lipoprotein receptor family (9). Clusterin has also been shown to bind very tightly to the amyloid b peptide. It has been suggested that clusterin may act as a carrier of amyloid b and that it protects cells against amyloid b toxicity (10). Other studies have shown the binding of clusterin to apolipoprotein A (11), paraoxonase (12), the surface of *Staphylococcus aureus* (13), LRP-2 receptor (14), complement components (15), and transforming growth factor β receptor (16). Many of these interactions are characteristic of the general hydrophobic binding nature of clusterin.

Sertoli-Specific Regulation of the Clusterin Gene

The complete genomic organization and sequence of the rat, mouse, and human clusterin gene and the promoter region has been published (17,18). There is a high degree of conservation of amino acid sequence in the protein and nucleotide sequence in the coding regions and promoter of the gene. We used a number of promoter constructs with 5'-deleted clusterin promoter fragments linked to the luciferase reporter gene and transiently transfected primary Sertoli cells and MSC-1 mouse Sertoli cells, NIH3T3, mouse fibroblast, and COS7, monkey kidney cell lines. We found that a proximal 313 bp promoter was active in all cell types and was sufficient to drive maximal expression of the reporter gene in all cell lines. In contrast, an additional 120 bp region was also required for the maximal reporter activity in primary Sertoli cells. The addition of this 120 bp region increased the transcriptional activity 2.5 times only in Sertoli cells. This region, designated the sertoli-specific region (SSR) is apparently required only by Sertoli cells for maximal expression of the clusterin gene (Fig. 7.2).

We investigated DNA-protein interactions of this region in vitro by excising it from the plasmid as a 135 bp fragment. This fragment was then used as a probe in electrophoretic mobility shift assays (EMSA). We found that Sertoli cells contained a unique set of nuclear factors that interacted with this region of the promoter.

We have attempted to identify the exact sites within the SSR that are recognized by Sertoli cell nuclear proteins and, thus, may be involved in cell-specific regulation. Competition EMSA using wild-type (wt) and mutant oligonucleotide competitors derived from the different regions of the SSR identified a Sertoli-specific band. An element with similar sequence characteristics is known to be the major element in the 72 bp enhancer of the SV40 early gene promoter and is called the *core enhancer site*. The core enhancer site can be recognized by the core binding protein (CBF), which is also known as a critical factor for the cell-specific expression of some cellular genes in T-lymphocytes, myeloid cells, and osteoblasts. CBF is thought to be a transcriptional organizer mediating formation of the cell-specific complexes.

After we identified the sites of protein interactions within the SSR, we tested binding of the recombinant factors to these sites. EMSA using Sp1 and CBF-2 proteins demonstrated that they bind to these sites with good

```
                                              PurBP
-450   TCTTTTACTC TTCCATTAAA ATAGGAACAA AGAAAAGGAG TGCAGTAATG
                         Sp1        Sp1        Ets
-400   GGTTAATGTG AAAGATGAAC GTGGGCGTCG GGCGGTGAAA TCCTGAACCT
                         Ets/Pu-box core-enhancer(CBF)
-350   GTTTGGGGCT AGGAGCGGTC CAGAGTAGAG TGTGGATTCC TCTTCCCTTA
               Sp1
-300   AGGCTCTTCT GTTGGGGCCT GGCTGAGCCC TTAGGTACCT AGCAGAGAAT

-250   AGAACAGCCA TCAATCTAGC TAGGGGCCCT CAGGCAACCA GCGCGGTCAT
                    Sp1                        Sp1
-200   TTGTGATGCC CCTGCGCCCC CTGGTGCCCC CCGCTGGGTG CTGCGCCTCT
                                                      HSE
-150   CGTCCCCTCC CGACCCCCCC ACCAGGCTTC CAGAAAGCTC CTAGTGCATT
                    Sp1/ Ap1                       Sp1
-100   CCCCGGCATT CTCTGGGCGT GAGTCACGCA GGTTTGCAGC CAGCCCCAAA
                         TBP
 -50   GGGGGTGTAC TTGAGCAGAG CGCTATAAAT AGGGCGCTTC CCCGGTGCTC
```

FIGURE 7.2. The rat clusterin gene promoter region numbered upstream from the transcriptional start site. The Sertoli-specific region (SSR) is underlined. The core-enhancer (CBF)/Ets site in the SSR is proposed to regulate the high level of constitutive synthesis in Sertoli cells. The proximal elements (SP1 and heat shock element, HSE) are proposed to be important in the inductive processes during cellular damage.

affinity (the dissociation constant was estimated at $\sim10^{-8}$ M). The extent of the mobility shift and the effect of base substitutions in a probe were similar for recombinant CBF and for the Sertoli-specific band. This result suggested that the core enhancer site could be bound by CBF or a CBF family member. The putative Sp1 binding site in the SSR was bound by Sp1 and also by some of the nuclear extracts. We also found that SSR is able to bind recombinant Ets 1 (two sites in SSR) with good affinity (see Fig. 7.2).

Finally, in a search for the Sertoli cell-specific transcription factors we found a sequence-specific single-stranded DNA binding protein (PurBP) that binds to the oligopurine sequence within SSR and seems to be present only in Sertoli cells of all cells tested. A similar protein Pura has been shown to regulate clusterin expression in quail (19).

To determine whether certain of these elements are involved in the regulation, we undertook transient transfaction experiments using clusterin wt or mutant promoter constructs generated by PCR mutagenesis and linked to the luciferase reporter gene. The pWT promoter construct contained the clusterin gene fragment from −480 to +57. Transfection of the primary Sertoli cells demonstrated that deletion of the CBF site decreased promoter activity by 60% and was equivalent to the removal of the whole Sertoli-stimulatory region. From our results we concluded that core-enhancer and upstream Sp1 elements, presumably recognized by CBF and Sp1, respectively, may mediate cell-specific constitutive expression of clusterin in Sertoli cells. Conservation of these elements in all mammalian clusterin promoters lends further support to the idea of their functional importance in vivo. Several interesting features in the organization of the SSR are also characteristic of the enhancers of a large group of mammalian type C retroviruses (more than 100 representatives are known), papovaviruses, and polyoma virus. These features include the presence of the core-enhancer and the presence of an Ets binding site. This element is the most conserved of four conserved elements identified in the mammalian retroviral enhancers and is invariably flanked on its 3'-side by the core-enhancer. Finally, the amazing concentration of transcription-factor binding sites that have been shown to interact with Sertoli cell nuclear proteins, is another feature that relates the SSR to the viral enhancers. The high density of binding sites allows multiple cooperative interactions among different transcription factors.

Clusterin Accumulation by Dying Pachytene Spermatocytes: What Does This Tell Us About Function?

We treated adult rats with methoxyacetic acid (MAA), an alkylating agent that selectively destroys pachytene spermatocytes through apoptosis within 3 days of a single bolus application. The protein and mRNA for testicular clusterin were investigated at 6, 12, 24, 36, 48, and 72 hours posttreatment by removing one testis from each rat for extraction of RNA and fixing the remaining testis for histological examination (20).

Immunohistochemical labeling of clusterin in testes from control animals was localized to Sertoli cell cytoplasm, the surface of late elongated spermatids, and the cytoplasm of relatively few earlier germ cells. At 6 hours after MAA treatment, however, clusterin protein was also localized to the cytoplasm of pachytene spermatocytes. This staining occurred before any morphological changes in the spermatocytes were seen. Pyknosis of the degenerating spermatocytes was apparent by 12 hours after MAA treatment, and the cytoplasm of these cells still stained for clusterin at this and later time points. Complete degeneration of the spermatocytes had occurred by 72 hours after treatment with MAA.

To determine whether the degenerating germ cells were producing the clusterin that was immunolocalized to their cytoplasm, we performed in situ hybridization for localization of clusterin mRNA and saw that the distribution of silver grains was similar between sections from control and MAA-treated animals. Thus, we determined that the clusterin protein that was accumulating in the spermatocyte cytoplasm was probably secreted by Sertoli cells. Northern blot analysis of RNA from whole testis showed that steady-state amounts of clusterin mRNA was not affected by treatment with MAA, indicating that the Sertoli cell-derived clusterin in the degenerating germ cells was from the constitutively secreted pool. It is not known how the clusterin protein was taken into the degenerating germ cells.

Because clusterin is known to be involved in apoptosis of other cell and tissue types, we performed the TUNEL method on sections of testis from control and MAA-treated rats to label fragmented DNA in apoptotic cells. Fragmentation of DNA in nuclei of degenerating pachytene spermatocytes was seen at 12 hours post-MAA, and reached its maximum by 24 hours. This fragmentation coincided with the morphological changes and pyknosis of the degenerating germ cells. Thus, accumulation of clusterin protein in pachytene spermatocytes of MAA-treated rats was seen before any noticeable morphological degeneration of the germ cells or apoptotic fragmentation of their DNA had occurred.

Clusterin: Structure–Function Relationships

To understand clusterin structure and function better we reanalyzed the clusterin amino acid sequence to look for structural elements that may be important for function. Previous computer analysis had predicted the presence of potential amphipathic α-helixes in clusterin but these predictions varied depending on the species and the method used. We attempted specifically to define putative amphipathic α-helixes that are conserved among clusterins.

Secondary structure predictors ProteinPredict and NNPredict as well as amphipathic region predictors Amphi and MOM were used to find potential amphipathic α-helixes 15–20 amino acids long in the rat clusterin sequence. This process was repeated for several different clusterins from different species to look for conserved structural elements. We found six putative amphipathic α helices conserved across the different clusterin proteins. Although the sequence varied among the clusterins, the helixes display the same pattern of hydrophobic and hydrophilic residues on the respective two faces of the amphipathic α-helixes.

We believe that clusterin may function to maintain the solubility of otherwise insoluble molecules. This property was investigated by analyzing the ability of clusterin to solubilize bacteriorhodopsin, a protein from the purple membrane of *Halobacterium halobium*. Bacteriorhodopsin (BR) is insoluble in aqueous buffer and can only be solubilized with addition of detergent. If clusterin can act to solubilize proteins, then BR should become soluble in its presence. The idea for this experiment came out of the work of Schafmeister, where peptides with amphipathic properties were shown to be detergents by their ability to solubilize bacteriorhodopsin (21). Insoluble, delipidated ^{125}I-bacteriorhodopsin was added to clusterin purified from rat Sertoli cell cultures in variable molar ratios in Na acetate buffer. After an incubation of 24 hours, the mixture was analyzed for soluble bacteriorhodopsin. After centrifugation the soluble fraction was examined on SDS-PAGE gels followed by autoradiography. The result clearly showed that bacteriorhodopsin was solubilized in the presence of equal molar amounts of clusterin. We concluded that clusterin has definite detergentlike properties and may function to solubilize hydrophobic proteins and possibly lipids during spermatogenesis.

The ability of clusterin to associate with hydrophobic molecules was also assessed using the dye 1-anilinonapthalene-8-sulfonic acid (ANS). The fluorescence of ANS increases as it moves from polar to nonpolar environments (e.g., hydrophobic pockets, surfaces, and binding sites of proteins). The putative amphipathic helixes of clusterin should provide an environment for ANS binding. The fluorescence of ANS increased fivefold when in the presence of clusterin, which showed that hydrophobic interactions are occurring between clusterin and the fluorescent probe.

What Does Clusterin Do?

We believe that the appearance of clusterin in various tissues and its association with various processes has some common connection. The following lists the general properties of clusterin.

First, although clusterin is also induced in a wide variety of tissues in response to cellular injury and/or insult many tissues make a basal level of clusterin. During apoptosis clusterin is made primarily by the surviving cells or the cells next to the dying cells (20,22–24). Clusterin is induced by heat-shock in many cell types and has been shown to have a heat-shock element conserved in the promoter (25). Clusterin can be considered a secreted heat-shock or acute-phase protein.

Second, in many tissues, including the reproductive system, epithelial cells secrete clusterin into a lumen. Many cell types that secrete clusterin are highly secretory and consist of the cells surrounding tissue–fluid interfaces (26).

Third, the protein has amphipathic properties (i.e., it is soluble and has a pI of about 4.0 and yet it binds tightly to hydrophobic surfaces). Clusterin contains four to five amphipathic helixes associated with the distal arms (i.e., located away from the clustered cysteines). These amphipathic regions have a number of important properties including myosinlike rod structure (27), possible coiled–coiled structures (28), and a relative lack of defined structure.

Fourth, clusterin binds readily to some proteins, to hydrophobic membrane proteins, and to some lipids.

When these general properties are considered it is possible to speculate that clusterin may function to form molecular complexes during cellular death and injury and to prevent their accumulation and the subsequent blockage of the ducts or lumen. In this role clusterin functions as a biological detergent. Binding of clusterin to hydrophobic molecules and complexes may also promote their clearance by assisting their uptake into cells. Uptake into cells might be aided by the association of clusterin with a variety of cell-surface receptors including GP-330.

References

1. Griswold MD, Morales C, Sylvester SR. Molecular biology of the Sertoli cell. Oxf Rev Reprod Biol 1988;10(124):124–61.
2. Griswold MD. Protein secretions of Sertoli cells. Int Rev Cytol 1988;110(133): 133–56.
3. Kissinger C, Skinner MK, Griswold MD. Analysis of Sertoli cell-secreted proteins by two-dimensional gel electrophoresis. Biol Reprod 1982;27(1):233–40.
4. Collard MW, Griswold MD. Biosynthesis and molecular cloning of sulfated glyco-protein 2 secreted by rat Sertoli cells. Biochemistry 1987;26(12):3297–303.
5. Griswold MD, Roberts K, Bishop P. Purification and characterization of a sulfated glycoprotein secreted by Sertoli cells. Biochemistry 1986;25(23):7265–70.
6. Fritz IB. Introduction to clusterin: history and perspectives. In: Harmony JAK, ed. Clusterin: role in vertebrate development, function and adaptation. New York: Springer-Verlag, 1995:1–7.
7. Wilson M, Easterbrook-Smith SB, Lakins J, Tenniswood M. Mechanisms of in-duction and function of clusterin at sites of cell death. In: Harmony JAK, ed. Clusterin: role in vertebrate development, function and adaptation. New York: Springer-Verlag, 1995:75–91.
8. Finch CE, May PC. Recent findings on clusterin in neural tissues: neuroanatomy, cell sources, development and aging, Alzheimer disease and other brain lesions. In: Harmony JAK, ed. Clusterin: role in vertebrate development, function and ad-aptation. New York: Springer-Verlag, 1995:163–78.
9. Kounnas MZ, Loukinova EB, Stefansson S, Harmony JA, Brewer BH, Strickland DK, et al. Identification of glycoprotein 330 as an endocytic receptor for apolipoprotein J/clusterin [published erratum appears in J Biol Chem 1995 Sep 29;270(39):23234]. J Biol Chem 1995;270(22):13070–75.
10. Oda T, Wals P, Osterburg HH, Johnson SA, Pasinetti GM, Morgan TE, et al. Clusterin (apoJ) alters the aggregation of amyloid beta-peptide (A beta 1-42) and forms slowly sedimenting A beta complexes that cause oxidative stress. Exp Neurol 1995; 136(1):22–31.
11. Jenne DE, Lowin B, Peitsch MC, Bottcher A, Schmitz G, Tschopp J. Clusterin (complement lysis inhibitor) forms a high density lipoprotein complex with apolipoprotein A-I in human plasma. J Biol Chem 1991;266(17):11030–36.
12. Mackness B, Hunt R, Durrington PN, Mackness MI. Increased immunolocalization of paraoxonase, clusterin, and apolipoprotein A-I in the human artery wall with the progression of atherosclerosis. Arterioscler Thromb Vasc Biol 1997;17(7): 1233–38.
13. Partridge SR, Baker MS, Walker MJ, Wilson MR. Clusterin, a putative comple-ment regulator, binds to the cell surface of Staphylococcus aureus clinical isolates. Infect Immunol 1996;64(10):4324–29.
14. Hammad SM, Ranganathan S, Loukinova E, Twal WO, Argraves WS. Interaction of apolipoprotein J-amyloid beta-peptide complex with low density lipoprotein

receptor-related protein-2/megalin. A mechanism to prevent pathological accumulation of amyloid beta-peptide. J Biol Chem 1997;272(30):18644–49.

15. McDonald JF, Nelsestuen GL. Potent inhibition of terminal complement assembly by clusterin: characterization of its impact on C9 polymerization. Biochemistry 1997;36(24):7464–73.

16. Reddy KB, Karode MC, Harmony AK, Howe PH. Interaction of transforming growth factor beta receptors with apolipoprotein J/clusterin. Biochemistry 1996;35(1): 309–14.

17. Wong P, Taillefer D, Lakins J, Pinault J, Chader G, Tenniswood M. Molecular characterization of human TRPM-2/clusterin, a gene associated with sperm maturation, apoptosis and neurodegeneration. Eur J Biochem 1994;221917–25.

18. Wong P, Pineault JM, Lakins J, Taillefer D, Leger J, Wang C, et al. Genomic organization and expression of the rat TRPM-2 (clusterin) gene, a gene implicated in apoptosis. J Biol Chem 1993;268:5021–31.

19. Michel D, Chatelain G, Herault Y, Brun G. The expression of the avian clusterin gene can be driven by two alternative promoters with distinct regulatory elements. Eur J Biochem 1995;229(1):215–23.

20. Clark AM, Maguire SM, Griswold MD. Accumulation of clusterin/sulfated glycoprotein-2 in degenerating pachytene spermatocytes of adult rats treated with methoxyacetic acid. Biol Reprod 1997;57(4):837–46.

21. Schafmeister CE, Miercke LJ, Stroud RM. Structure at 2.5 A of a designed peptide that maintains solubility of membrane proteins. Science 1993;262(5134):734–38.

22. French LE, Soriano JV, Montesano R, Pepper MS. Modulation of clusterin gene expression in the rat mammary gland during pregnancy, lactation, and involution. Biol Reprod 1996;55(6):1213–20.

23. Clark AM, Griswold MD. Expression of clusterin/sulfated glycoprotein-2 under conditions of heat stress in rat Sertoli cells and a mouse Sertoli cell line. J Androl 1997;18(3):257–63.

24. Dragunow M, Preston K, Dodd J, Young D, Lawlor P, Christie D. Clusterin accumulates in dying neurons following status epilepticus. Brain Res Mol Brain Res 1995;32(2):279–90.

25. Michel D, Chatelain G, North S, Brun G. Stress-induced transcription of the clusterin/apo J gene. Biochemistry 1997;328: 45–50.

26. Aronow BJ, Lund SD, Brown TL, Harmony J, Witte DP. Apolipoprotein J expression at fluid-tissue interfaces: Potential role in barrier cytoprotection. Proc Natl Acad Sci 1993;90:725–29.

27. Tsuruta JK, Wong K, Fritz IB, Griswold MD. Structural analysis of sulphated glycoprotein 2 from amino acid sequence. Biochem J 1990;268:571–78.

28 Jenne DE, Tschopp J. Molecular structure and functional characterization of a human complement cytolysis inhibitor found in blood and seminal plasma: Identity to sulfated glycoprotein 2, a constituent of rat testis fluid. Proc Natl Acad Sci USA 1989;86:7123–27.

8

HRT for the Aging Male:
A Therapy That
Has Come of Age?

J. Lisa Tenover

Introduction

Although hormonal replacement therapy (HRT) for the postmenopausal woman has been studied and promoted for years, interest in the possibility of male HRT is a relatively new development. Reasons for growing enthusiasm in this area include an increasing body of data supporting an age-related decline in testosterone production and the increasing number of older adults who are eager to maintain robust health and avoid dysfunction and frailty.

Accompanying the decline in serum testosterone with age are a number of clinically detrimental physiologic changes in organs and functions that can be positively affected by testosterone therapy, at least in the younger adult hypogonadal man (Table 8.1). For the older man, the goals of HRT would be to prevent, stabilize, or reverse some of these detrimental target organ changes. Although interest in male HRT is strong at the current time, knowledge in this field is at least 20 years behind that of female HRT, and large-scale evaluations of the efficacy and risks of such therapy have yet to be done. Nonetheless, the lay media continues to emphasize the timeliness of male HRT and promote its potential, while at the same time the scientific community is expanding exploration of its clinical utility. It is the purpose of this chapter, therefore, to present the current state of clinical knowledge regarding male HRT.

Testosterone Levels in Aging Men

Although conflicting data existed in the early medical literature, both cross-sectional and longitudinal studies during the 1980s and 1990s have demonstrated an age-related decline in serum total testosterone, free testosterone, and/or testosterone not bound to sex hormone binding globulin (nonSHBG-

TABLE 8.1. Androgen target organ changes with aging and with testosterone replacement in hypogonadal young adult men.

Target organ/function	Change with	
	Aging	Testosterone
Muscle mass	⇓	⇑
Muscle strength	⇓	⇑
Fat mass	⇑	⇓
Bone mass	⇓	⇑
Libido	⇓	⇑
Erectile dysfunction	⇑	⇓
Mood	NC/⇓	⇑

⇑ = increase; ⇓ = decrease; NC = no change

bound testosterone; 1–3). Because levels of SHBG also tend to increase with age, levels of nonSHBG-bound testosterone (also referred to as "bioavailable testosterone") usually decrease more dramatically with age than do levels of total testosterone (4).

It is not known if the age-related decline in serum testosterone, which is due to decline in testosterone production by the testis, is universal in men; available data are from studies of predominantly Caucasian men of Western European descent. In addition, the rate of testosterone decline among men can vary greatly, can be affected by disease and medications, and does not inevitably result in clinically recognizable hypogonadism. In fact, it is difficult to determine the prevalence of "hypogonadism" among aging men because of the uncertainty of how to define this entity. Lacking a clear definition, most investigators in the area of male HRT have used some value at or below the lower limit of the normal range for serum total testosterone or bioavailable testosterone in young adult men to define the level below which an older man might be considered "testosterone deficient." Using this type of definition, the prevalence of testosterone deficiency has been reported to vary from 8% to more than 50% of men older than 60 years of age (5).

The possible benefits of male HRT are listed in Table 8.2. To date, studies of HRT in older men have been carried out in generally healthy individuals, with limited numbers of study participants; replacement therapy has been short term (24 months or less), and methods of evaluation of efficacy also have varied from study to study. Organizing outcome data by target organ system assists with analysis.

Benefits of Male HRT

Body Composition

In addition to several studies reported in abstract form only, there have been five published trials in which older men had testosterone replaced and body

TABLE 8.2. Potential benefits and risks of male HRT.

Benefits	Risks
Preserve or improve bone mass and prevent fractures	Fluid retention
Increase muscle mass	Precipitation or worsening of sleep apnea
Increase strength, stamina, and physical function	Development of gynecomastia
Improve libido	Induction of polycythemia
Improve well-being and mood	Hasten onset of clinically significant benign or malignant prostate disease
Decrease cardiovascular disease risk	Increase cardiovascular disease risk

composition evaluated (6–10). Three of these studies (6,7,9), as well as one other (11), have also evaluated strength changes with treatment. Changes in body composition with testosterone therapy have consistently demonstrated either a decline in total body fat, an increase in lean body mass (mostly muscle mass), or both. The magnitude of the fat mass changes in older men in response to testosterone therapy are similar to that seen with testosterone replacement in young hypogonadal men, whereas lean body mass changes are usually less dramatic in older men (3–6% increase) compared with younger men (9–19% increase). In terms of strength changes seen, most studies (7,9,11), but not all (6), have demonstrated a statistically significant increase in strength with testosterone treatment.

Most of these studies have been blinded and placebo controlled, but most have used only grip strength as the primary measure of strength. Only one published study evaluated the effect of testosterone therapy on lower extremity strength, and this study involved only six men treated for 1 month, and it was not placebo controlled (11). Although one of the goals of improving muscle strength in older men would be to maximize or preserve mobility and function, no study to date in older men has evaluated the effects of testosterone treatment on functional performance.

Bone

There have been at least five published studies (6–8,12,13), along with several in abstract form only, that have evaluated the effects of testosterone therapy on bone mineral density or biochemical parameters of bone turnover in older men. These studies have lasted from 3 to 36 months, with the shorter-term studies evaluating only bone turnover parameters. Some of these studies enrolled men who were osteoporotic at baseline, and one study evaluated the effect of testosterone in men on chronic glucocorticoid therapy (14). In general, testosterone therapy has resulted in a slowed rate of bone degradation and an increase in bone mineral density. Table 8.3 is a summary of the results from those published studies where bone mineral density was evaluated. Whether positive effects on bone mineral density can be main-

TABLE 8.3. Testosterone HRT effects on bone mineral density (BMD) in older men.

Treatment length (months)	Change in BMD[a]			Reference
	Study N	L-spine	Other site	
18	29	⇑	—	8
12	4	⇑	⇑	12
12	15	⇑	NC	14

[a] ⇑ = increase; NC = no change

tained over longer periods of time than have been studied to date with testosterone therapy, and what the optimal testosterone replacement dose to achieve maximal benefits for bone might be, are both unknown at this time.

Sexual Function and Mood

There are no clinical trials that have evaluated the effect of testosterone therapy on aspects of sexual function in healthy older "testosterone deficient" men; however, there are some studies that have evaluated the effects of raising serum testosterone levels in older men with various types of sexual dysfunction. In general, men with low libido have shown improvement (15–17), whereas erectile dysfunction is only occasionally improved by such therapy (18).

Several blinded, placebo-controlled testosterone replacement studies in older men have evaluated effects on "sense of well-being" or other aspects of mood (6,10). Although the studies are small, they have shown that older men on testosterone report an improved or higher sense of well-being compared with a group receiving placebo.

The Cardiovascular System

Most epidemiologic studies have shown that lower cardiovascular disease risk in men correlates with higher serum testosterone levels (19). Compared with premenopausal women, however, men have a higher incidence of cardiovascular disease and mortality. It is unknown whether or not androgens in men play any role in this sexual dichotomy. Cardiovascular disease risk factors that might be affected by sex steroids include serum lipoprotein levels, vascular tone, platelet and red blood cell clotting parameters, and direct atherogenesis. There are no data as yet on the effects of testosterone therapy in older men on most of these parameters. Several preliminary studies have suggested that testosterone therapy may decrease platelet aggregation or positively affect vasomotor tone, but these data need to be expanded. The effect on serum lipoprotein levels in older men is the one area where testosterone therapy has been more extensively evaluated. In general, parenteral testosterone therapy (i.e., by intramuscular injection or scrotal or transdermal patch) in older men has led to a decrease in total and low-density lipoprotein–cholesterol levels, with either no change or a small decrease in high-density lipoprotein–cholesterol levels (20). These lipoprotein level changes with testosterone therapy are modest, and the ultimate impact on cardiovascular disease is unknown.

Adverse Effects of Male HRT

The only absolute contraindications to male HRT are the presence of prostate carcinoma or breast cancer. Other potential risks of such therapy are listed in Table 8.2. Even though many of these adverse effects can be predicted by pretreatment medical history and examination, and others are easily manageable, several of the potential adverse effects (e.g., long-term effects on the prostate) are virtually unknown. Because of the uncertainty regarding the effect of male HRT on cardiovascular disease, as noted previously, this is also listed in the potential risk category.

Fluid retention is possible, especially within the first few months of treatment, but it is not as dramatic with testosterone as it is with the oral anabolic steroids such as oxandrolone. No studies of male HRT with testosterone have reported problems with peripheral edema or exacerbation of hypertension or congestive heart failure, but these studies have treated only relatively healthy men. In the chronically ill or more frail older man, fluid retention might pose a concern.

Sleep apnea has been reported to contribute to low serum testosterone levels, and testosterone therapy has been reported to exacerbate sleep apnea (21,22). Although the reports are limited, because sleep apnea is prevalent in the middle-aged and older man, screening for this condition by history prior to initiation of male HRT and throughout treatment seems prudent.

Tender breasts or development of gynecomastia occur in a small number of men on HRT. This may be due to the relatively greater increase in serum estradiol levels, as compared with serum testosterone levels, that result from such therapy in many older men. This side effect can often be overcome with a downward adjustment in HRT replacement dose.

Testosterone replacement therapy in older men can often result in a significant increase in red blood cell mass and hemoglobin levels. The increases reported are much larger than those usually seen when young hypogonadal men are given testosterone. In some cases, where polycythemia has developed, it has been necessary with the older man to either terminate therapy or to decrease the dose of testosterone used for replacement (9,20). Even though the coexistence of sleep apnea and elevated body mass index may contribute to the development of polycythemia in certain older men, this has not been the case for many of the men studied. The method of testosterone replacement may affect the magnitude of the change in red blood cell mass (20).

Both benign prostatic hyperplasia (BPH) and prostate cancer are diseases common to the older man and both are promoted by androgens. Androgen deprivation therapy has been used for the treatment of both of these processes, but whether male HRT places a man at increased risk of developing clinically significant prostate disease from preexisting, but subclinical disease, is unknown. A number of testosterone replacement studies in men aged 40–89 years have evaluated serum levels of prostate specific antigen (PSA), prostate size, or functional prostate parameters. The large majority of these studies have reported no significant change in PSA or other prostate parameters with testosterone therapy (20); however, because both prostate cancer and BPH are diseases with long natural histories, and the observation time to date with testosterone therapy in older men is limited to less than 800 man-years, the long-term effects of male HRT on the prostate of older men is still of concern.

Summary

During the 1990s much has been learned about the potential benefits and risks of male HRT. Although larger and longer-term studies are needed, data suggest that male HRT may have real potential benefit in terms of improving bone mineral density and increasing muscle mass and strength; however, whether these effects translate into decreased long-term fracture risk and functional improvement are uncertain. Male HRT also may positively influence mood and sexual function for some older men. In the short term (up to 3 years) the adverse effects of male HRT seem predictable and manageable, but the longer term effects on target organs such as the cardiovascular system and the prostate are yet to be determined. Thus, men interested in male HRT should be counseled that the risk–benefit ratio for such therapy is yet to be fully determined.

References

1. Vermeulen A. Clinical review 24: androgens in the aging male. J Clin Endocrinol Metab 1991;73:221–24.
2. Morley JE, Kaiser FE, Perry HM, Patrick P, Morley PMK, Stauber PM, et al. Longitudinal changes in testosterone, luteinizing hormone, and follicle-stimulating hormone in healthy older men. Metabolism 1997;46:410–13.
3. Gray A, Berlin JA, McKinlay JB, Longcope C. An examination of research design effects on the association of testosterone and male aging: results of a meta-analysis. J Clin Epidemiol 1991;44:671–84.
4. Nankin HR, Calkins JH. Decreased bioavailable testosterone in aging normal and impotent men. J Clin Endocrinol Metab 1986;63:1418–20.
5. Tenover JL. Trophic factors and male hormone replacement. In: Hazzard WR, Blass JP, Ettinger WH, Halter JB, Ouslander JG, ed. Principles of geriatric medicine and gerontology. Fourth ed. New York: McGraw-Hill, 1999:1029–40.

6. Tenover JS. Effects of testosterone supplementation in the aging male. J Clin Endocrinol Metab 1992;75:1092–98.

7. Morley JE, Perry HM, Kaiser FE, Kraenzle D, Jensen J, Houston K, et al. Effects of testosterone replacement therapy in old hypogonadal males: a preliminary study. J Am Geriatr Soc 1993;41:149–52.

8. Katznelson L, Finkelstein JS, Schoenfeld DA, Rosenthal DI, Anderson EJ, Klibanski A. Increase in bone density and lean body mass during testosterone administration in men with acquired hypogonadism. J Clin Endocrinol Metab 1996;81:4358–65.

9. Sih R, Morley JE, Kaiser FE, Perry HM, Patrick P, Ross C. Testosterone replacement in older hypogonadal men: a 12-month randomized controlled trial. J Clin Endocrinol Metab 1997;82:1661–67.

10. Marin P, Holmang S, Gustafsson C, Jonsson L, Kvist H, Elander A, et al. Androgen treatment of abdominally obese men. Obesity Res 1993;1:245–51.

11. Urban RJ, Bodenburg YH, Gilkison C, Foxworth J. Coggan AR, Wolfe RR, et al. Testosterone administration in elderly men increases skeletal muscle strength and protein synthesis. Am J Physiol 1995;269:E820–26.

12. Greenspan SL, Oppenheim DS, Klibanski A. Importance of gonadal steroids to bone mass in men with hyperprolactinemic hypogonadism. Ann Intern Med 1989;110:526–31.

13. Jackson JA, Kleerekoper M, Parfitt AM, Rao DS, Villanueva AR, Frame B. Bone histomorphometry in hypogonadal and eugonadal men with spinal osteoporosis. J Clin Endocrinol Metab 1967;65:53–58.

14. Reid IR, Wattie DJ, Evans MC, Stapleton JC. Testosterone therapy in gluco-corticoid treated men. Arch Intern Med 1996;156:1173–77.

15. Carani CM, Zini D, Baldini A. Effects of androgen treatment in impotent men with normal and low levels of free testosterone. Arch Sex Behav 1990;19:223–34.

16. Guay AT, Bansal S, Heatley GJ. Effect of raising endogenous testosterone levels in impotent men with secondary hypogonadism: double blind placebo-controlled trial with clomiphene citrate. J Clin Endocrinol Metab 1995;80:3546–52.

17. O'Carroll R, Bancroft J. Testosterone therapy for low sexual interest and erectile dysfunction in men: a controlled study. Br J Psychiatr 1984;145:146–51.

18. Bagatell CJ, Bremner WJ. Androgen and progestagen effects on plasma lipids. Prog Cardiovasc Dis 1995;38:255–71.

19. Tenover JL. The male climacteric: fact or fiction? In: Morales A, ed. Erectile dysfunction. London: Martin Dunitz, 1998:39–48.

20. Tenover JL. Effects of androgen supplementation in the aging male. In: Oddens BJ, Vermeulen A, eds. Androgens and the aging male. New York: Parthenon, 1996:91–204.

21. Sandblom RE, Matsumoto AM, Schoene RB, Lee KA, Giblin ED, Bremner WJ, et al. Obstructive sleep apnea syndrome induced by testosterone administration. N Engl J Med 1983;308:508–10.

22. Santamaria JD, Prior JC, Fleetham JA. Reversible reproductive dysfunction in men with obstructive sleep apnoea. Clin Endocrinol (Oxf) 1998;28:461–70.

9

Androgen Replacement in Young Men

FREDERICK C.W. WU

Introduction

Androgen replacement is one of the earliest forms of hormone replacement therapy, having been in continuous clinical use in since 1937. Since the 1940s, androgen treatment has been hardwired into the subconscious of routine clinical practice. The clinical use of androgens has previously been exclusively confined to the treatment of patients with specific pathologies in the pituitary–testicular axis (i.e., conditions causing classical hypogonadism). Most of these patients, however, have to be treated with unsatisfactory or even obsolete formulations of testosterone (T), with suboptimal pharmacokinetics, developed mostly in the 1950s. In the 1990s, however, we entered a new era in which the anabolic, growth-promoting, and contraceptive actions of testosterone were being exploited for legitimate clinical applications in healthy males and in patients without primary pathologies in the pituitary–testicular axis (Table 9.1). This chapter will discuss the use of T in young males using two clinical situtations: the management of delayed puberty and hormonal male contraception. These two applications highlight (1) the contrasting philosophies and requirements between physiological replacement and pharmacological treatment, (2) how application of basic knowledge on androgen action has influenced the approach to achieving therapeutic goals, and (3) the deficiencies of currently available testosterone preparations.

The use of T in delayed puberty is a prime example of physiological replacement aiming to replicate physiological tissue exposure by maintaining circulating levels as closely as possible within the normal range appropriate to the age and phase of sexual development. Provided pharmacokinetics of T preparations are capable of reproducing physiological concentrations, temporal patterns, and metabolic profiles of the natural hormone, it should be possible to expect efficacy and long-term safety of physiological replacement to be no different from that in healthy eugonadal men. Male contra-

TABLE 9.1. Indications for androgen replacement.

Classical
Hypogonadism
Delayed puberty

Nonclassical or extended
Male contraception
HIV infections
Osteoporosis
  Hypogonadal
  Eugonadal
  Glucocorticoid-induced
Rheumatoid arthritis
Chronic renal failure
COAD
Aplastic anemia
Tall stature
Angioneurotic edema

ception, on the other hand, is an example of pharmacological treatment that exploits the full biological potential of androgen actions to achieve maximal therapeutic effects within the boundaries of clinical safety. Supraphysiological to pharmacological doses of androgens employed are often operating in the log-linear portion of the dose–response curve such that therapeutic targets are often achieved at the expense of some unwanted effects. Rigorous evaluation of efficacy, safety, and cost-effectiveness similar to any new drug is therefore required.

Androgen Action

Androgens are required lifelong in man to fulfill diverse functions at different epochs of male reproductive life. Despite the diversity of biological action, there is only one well-defined species of androgen receptor, which is differentially responsive to T and dihydrotestosterone (DHT). Metabolism of T, which is the principal circulating androgen produced by the testis, to effector hormones by tissue 5 α and β reductases and aromatase (to estradiol) is the key mechanism for increasing diversity of biological actions without losing specificity (1). T itself is adequate for internal genitalia and skeletal muscle development as well as the activation of sexual behavior. DHT on the other hand is required for the development of external genitalia, prostate and seminal vesicles and secondary sexual hair. The increasing number of functions served by local aromatization of T to E2 has become apparent with the ERKO and aromataze-deficiency phenotypes (2). Aromatization of testosterone to estradiol is necessary for sexual differentiation of the brain, bone mass accretion, and fusion of the epiphyses during puberty. Increasing

levels of testosterone stimulate the development of secondary sexual characteristics and acquisition of fertility during puberty so that extragenital sexual di-
morphism and reproductive capacity become fully expressed. These functions
are maintained in adulthood until the gradual decline in senescence.

Puberty

Puberty is the stage of physiological transition from childhood to adulthood
during which dramatic physical as well as psychological changes occur. The
actions of T are particularly obvious and crucial during puberty, emphasized
by the fact that congenital hypogonadotrophic hypogonadism usually present
at this time as delayed puberty through lack of T-driven sexual development.
The dominant events are the development of secondary sexual characteristics and the pubertal growth spurt during which linear growth velocity increases from 4–6 to 10–15 cm per annum (contributing 15% of final adult
height) followed by a deceleration until epiphyseal closure is complete.

Gonadotrophin and T Secretion
During Pubertal Development

The proximate endocrine mechanism underlying these physical changes is
the gradual amplification of sleep-entrained gonadotrophin secretion that
produces a nightly rise and fall in T. The nightly rise in T through Puberty is
more clearly shown in the cross-sectional data from 129 boys with 8 P.M. and
8 A.M. differentials (Fig. 9.1). Steepest O/N rise in T correspond to PHV in
latter half of puberty at G4, testes volume 10 mL, and 8 A.M. T around 10
nmol/L during which time the overnight rise in T is the steepest. The gradual
rise of T, initially only at night, extended over a duration of 3–4 years, is
responsible for the well-defined *synchronized sequence* of developmental
changes (reflecting the differential tissue sensitivity to T). Even if wide individual variation in the onset and rate of progression of puberty is the rule,
the sequence of the developmental events remains unchanged.

Growth in Puberty

The slowly progressive increment and differential sensitivity of long bones
to T are the keys to optimizing total height gain during pubertal growth.
Thus, at the modest levels of T in the first half of puberty, long bone growth
and proliferation of chondrocytes at the growth plate are stimulated. Growth
velocity is accelerated without fusion of the epiphyses. In late puberty, increasing circulating levels of T and tissue levels of estradiol (from aromatization of T) stimulate the terminal differentiation of chondrocytes and
calcification of the epiphyses, which eventually leads to fusion of the long
bone growth plates and cessation of growth.

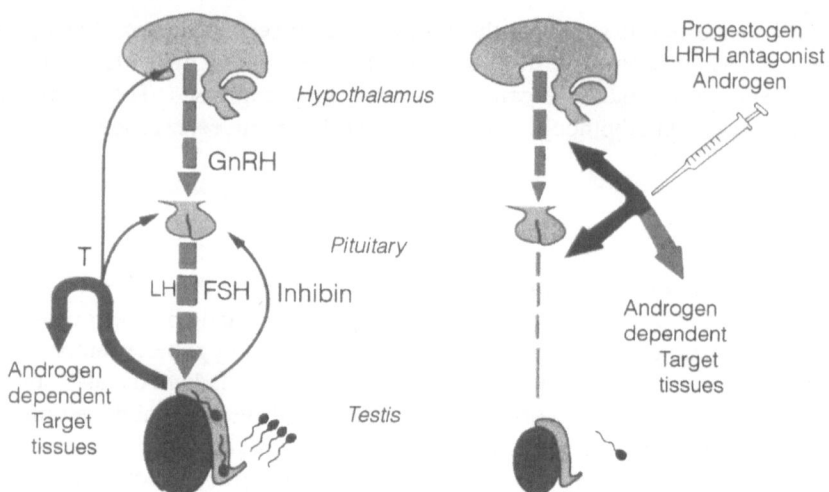

FIGURE 9.1. Suppression of spermatogenesis via inhibition of gonadotrophins by androgens, progestins, or GnRH analogs. Solid lines represent inhibitory actions; broken lines stimulatory actions. Androgens are required to maintain secondary sexual functions.

Both sex steroids and GH are required for maximal pubertal height gain. Sex steroids, GH/IGF-1, and growth velocity increase contemporaneously during puberty (3). The interaction between the gonadotrophic and somatotrophic axes are complicated and involve both independent and synergistic actions. T and DHT directly stimulate local growth factor (IGF-1 and FGF) production by epiphyseal chondrocytes and proliferation of osteoblasts and chondrocytes. GH and androgens act synergistically on the growth plates. Androgens (i.e., only aromatizable androgens) stimulate circulating GH pulse amplitude, which gives rise to a sexually dimorphic increase in GH. Estrogens, locally aromatized or circulating, are critical to epiphyseal closure. Males with inactivating mutations in the estrogen receptor α gene or the aromataze gene have open epiphyses, and growth continues into midadulthood, causing extreme tall stature (4,5).

Constitutional Delayed Growth and Puberty

Delayed puberty is a common (affecting 3% of otherwise healthy adolescent boys) clinical problem affecting boys who do not show any signs of pubertal onset at the age of 13.5–14 years (2 SD above the mean age of onset). In practice, this also includes those patients whose pubertal development is stalled or is progressing too slowly. Specific pathologies in the hypothalamic–pituitary–testicular (HPT) axis are rare (6); the vast majority of cases have constitutional delayed puberty, which is a temporary extension of the physiological prepubertal hypogonadotrophic hypogonadism. This is essentially self-limiting because spontaneous puberty is merely postponed but will eventually supervene, albeit at a later chronological age. Patients often have a family history of delayed puberty. Although a self-limiting condition, the prolongation of gonadotrophin and sex steroid deficiency beyond the midteens frequently causes inordinate distress, leading to psychosocial and/or educational sequelae, some of which persist in adulthood (Table 9.2).

Although the overwhelming majority of boys presenting with delayed puberty have constitutional or physiological delay, failure of pubertal development is frequently the presenting complaint in patients with congenital hypogonadism (6). Even though hypergonadotropic hypogonadism is readily diagnosed by documenting high levels of gonadotrophins, in the absence of clinical stigmata consistent with Kallmann's syndrome (e.g., anosmia, hyposmia, red–green color blindness), differentiation between permament isolated hypogonadotrophic hypogonadism (IHH) and constitutional delayed puberty (CDP) is difficult. Even with third-generation gonadotropin assays, it is not possible to distinguish normal prepubertal basal gonadotropin levels from those in hypogonadotrophic hypogonadism (7,8). There is also overlap in the response to bolus GnRH stimulation between the two conditions (7). It is not surprising that CDP, which is a variant of normal where the juvenile physiological hypogonadotrophic state is overextended, is functionally similar to permanent hypogonadotropic conditions (IHH) except by the former's self-limiting nature. Thus, the main distinguishing feature between the two is that CDP advances spontaneously to pubertal onset and progression, whereas IHH typically remains unchanged with time. Although no single

TABLE 9.2. Clinical features associated with delayed puberty.

Physical
Short stature (temporary)
Lack of sexual development (temporary)
Low peak bone mass (permanent)

Psychosocial
Low self-esteem/poor body image
Poor school performance/truancy
Social immaturity and isolation
Lower intellectual achievements
Psychosomatic complaints
Depression
Antisocial behavior

test at one time can indubitably differentiate between IHH and CDP (6), serial testing (e.g., morning plasma T or GnRH stimulation) combined with careful clinical monitoring (e.g., changes in testicular volume) can usually provide helpful information that permits clinical decision to be made at an earlier stage than before. In reaching the correct clinical decision (i.e., to induce "puberty" with androgens or to wait), it is prudent to emphasise the variable and diverse course of spontaneous pubertal development and the unfolding of permanent hypogonadotrophic hypogonadism (9,10). Partial gonadotrophin deficiency and arrest of pubertal development after normal onset are examples. Even the most informative tests are therefore limited by the nature of an evolving process, the pace and pattern of which is often unpredictable (9,10).

Androgen Treatment in Delayed Puberty

It is now a widely accepted management strategy in CDP to induce and maintain the patient's secondary sexual development in line with the peer group norm in order to prevent adverse psychosocial and physical sequelae of untreated delayed puberty. Boys showing no signs of pubertal development by the age of 14 years should be considered for induction or initiation of puberty. One of the most persuasive arguments for early treatment is the realization that males with a history of untreated delayed pubertal onset beyond 15 years have significantly lower peak bone mass in adulthood even though spontaneous development eventually supervened (11,12). There is no reason to withhold or delay treatment even if a definitive diagnosis has not been established. The overriding immediate priority should be to relieve symptoms and prevent long-term consequences of T deficiency. Decisions on the need to continue long-term treatment can be deferred when the correct diagnosis eventually emerges during followup.

After the age of 18, if there is no clinical sign of spontaneous pubertal development or increase in gonadotrophins and testosterone after withdrawal of treatment, the diagnosis of permanent IHH is probable. In the past, a major concern with early induction of puberty has been that androgens may cause a disproportionate advance in bone age and premature closure of epiphyses, leading to loss of growth potential and stunting of final adult height. However, cumulative data since 1980 have repeatedly confirmed that induction of secondary sexual characteristics and acceleration of growth can be safely accomplished by using low doses of parenteral testosterone (13,14), oral testosterone undecanoate (15,16), oral oxandrolone (16–20), and mesterolone (21) in boys with CDP without undue advance in skeletal age or compromising final height (22). This has been achieved by avoiding full adult doses and using low gradually incremental amounts of androgens that replicate the biological actions of progressively increasing levels of T in early and midpuberty.

Testosterone should be the androgen of choice because it can mimic the full spectrum of physiological sex steroid actions during puberty, including virilization, growth stimulation, and bone accretion via aromatization to estrogen. The pharmacokinetics of currently available T (and other androgen) preparations, however, are such that none can reproduce the pubertal physiological diurnal patterns of T accurately. Nonetheless, it would seem that these pharmacokinetically suboptimal preparations can be adapted successfully to induce pubertal development. The most commonly employed regimes are intramuscular T enanthate or mixtures of T esters 50 mg monthly or oral testosterone undecanoate 40 mg daily or alternate days for 6–12 months (Table 9.3). The orally active synthetic 17α-alkyl substituted anabolic steroid, oxandrolone (0.1mg/kg/day or 2.5mg daily), has enjoyed some popularity because it does not require injections. It is not aromatizable and may therefore also offer the theoretical advantage of stimulating growth velocity with a lower risk of premature epiphyseal closure, which is estrogen dependent. There is no difference, however, between oral oxandrolone and either oral or parenteral testosterone in terms of growth stimulation or bone age advance (16). The lack of virilization (20), the potential risk of cholestatic jaundice, the implications of using an anabolic steroid in an adolescent population, and the increasing (favorable) experience of using testosterone are factors that have restricted the wider use of oxandrolone in the treatment of delayed puberty in boys.

Because CDP is a self-limiting condition, some clinicians prefer to treat intermittently for 3–6 months only, followed by a similar period of observation to allow spontaneous puberty to progress. The induced growth acceleration is usually sustained for 6 months or more after the end of treatment. If there is no sign of spontaneous pubertal progression, a further course of treatment is given. This cautious stop–start regime permits earlier cessation of treatment, but it is disruptive and requires frequent monitoring. It is my practice to give patients the more assured clinical benefits of a longer period of treatment, T enanthate 50 mg IM monthly or equivalent for up to 12 months without interruption, before reassessing endogenous activity of the HPT axis. Since IM preparations of T have durations of action of only two weeks, the monthly dosing regime effectively provides intermittent rather than continuous treatment. Thus, during treatment, increases in testicular volume and predose plasma T levels can be monitored as evidence of endogenous pro-

TABLE 9.3. Choices for androgen treatment in delayed puberty.

T enanthate 50mg IM/month
T esters mixture (Sustanon) 50 mg IM/month
T undecanoate 40 mg p.o./day
Oxandrolone 2.5 mg p.o./day
HCG 1500–2000 U s.c. twice weekly
Transdermal T

gression to signal the redundancy of continued therapy. If continued treatment is required, however, the dose of T enanthate can be increased to 100 mg monthly in the second year and 200 mg monthly in the third. Bone age can be monitored, although experience has shown that excessive stimulation of skeletal development is unlikely with this regime. Because of their long duration of action and need for a surgical implantation, T pellets have no place in the induction of puberty. Newer formulations of T delivered transdermally (body patches or gels) would seem ideal for induction of puberty because of the physiological pharmacokinetic profiles, greater flexibility for dosing, and the painless administration. Current licensed indications for these new formulations, however, prohibit their use in the adolescent patient and there is no published data on their efficacy or safety in induction of puberty.

There is no evidence that exogenous testosterone treatment accelerates the endogenous maturation of the GnRH pulse generator or the Leydig cells (10,23). The complexity, low acceptability, and higher costs of hCG, menopausal gonadotrophins, or pulsatile GnRH in the induction of puberty negates any perceived advantage of increasing testicular size and early induction of spermatogenesis. Therapeutic stimulation of the testes should be deferred until fertility is actively sought. Testosterone treatment in adolescence does not impair adult gonadal functions (24).

Conclusions

In conclusion, the use of androgen for induction of puberty in boys with delayed puberty is effective, safe, and should be started without undue deferral. The dose of T, the androgen of choice, should be low initially and increased gradually over 3 years to replicate endogenous pubertal progression. T can be discontinued when signs of spontaneous development become apparent during treatment.

Hormonal Suppression of Spermatogenesis for Male Contraception

The synergistic actions of T and FSH are required for normal spermatogenesis (25,26). Hormonal male contraception is effected via the endocrine suppression of pituitary gonadotrophic drive to the testis, thereby simultaneously abrogating Leydig cell steroidogenesis and nullifying FSH (Figure 9.1). The consequent depletion of intratesticular testosterone and loss of FSH action result in a collapse of spermatogenesis characterized by a block in spermatogonial maturation and disruption of premeiotic stages of spermatogenesis without affecting stem cells (27,28). Maintenance of spermatogonial stem cell population ensures that hormonal suppression of spermatogenesis is reversible. The need to induce maximal inhibition of T production from the testis (29), however, invariably creates a systemic hypoandrogenic state. This dictates the need for exogenous T replacement to maintain extratesticular secondary sexual functions (e.g., sex drive and androgen-dependent metabolic functions on bone, muscle, and haemopoiesis). Exogenous T administered systemically is unable to raise *intratesticular* testosterone to an extent that will fully maintain spermatogenesis in the presence of gonadotrophin suppression.

Male Contraceptives Based on Androgens Alone

The androgen-only approach has been a popular prototype for further study because of its economy as a dual-acting single agent as well as familiarity with its use in many years of clinical practice. The contraceptive efficacy of T enanthate 200 mg IM weekly was investigated in two World Health Organization (WHO) clinical trials (30,31). The risk of pregnancy was directly correlated with sperm concentrations. One pregnancy occurred during 352 coupleyears of exposure giving a Pearl rate (pregnancy per 100 couples using method for 1 year) of 0.003. With sperm densities between 0.1 and 3.0 million /ml, four pregnancies occurred during 49.5 coupleyears of exposure, yielding a Pearl rate of 8.1 (2.2–20.70 per 100 coupleyears). The Pearl rate of the method as a whole, including all men with sperm densities below 3 million/ml (i.e., azoospermia to 3 million/ml), was 1.4 (0.4–3.7) per 100 coupleyears. This is comparable to the typical first-year failure rate of modern female reversible contraceptives (e.g., OCP, injectables, medicated IUDs) and is superior to the condom (12 per 100 personyears), withdrawal (18 per 100 personyears) and periodic abstinence (20 per 100 personyears). Ninety-eight percent of Asian and 95% of Caucasian men were suppressed to 3 million/ml, indicating that the vast majority of men are able to achieve this oligozoospermic threshold of contraceptive efficacy. These two trials established the important principle that hormonal suppression of spermatogenesis can provide effective reversible contraception for men. The incidence of side effects (e.g., acne, weight gain, changes in sex drive, and mood) was low apart from acne (29.3%) and the cumulative annual medical discontinuation rate was 9.7% (32). HDL-cholesterol and total cholesterol decreased by 18% and 6%, respectively, although haematocrit increased by 6%. These reflect the high peak and markedly fluctuating levels of T produced by weekly IM injections of the supraphysiological dose (200 mg T enanthate weekly is equivalent to 22 mg of T daily) rather than an inherent feature of androgen–only hormonal male contraception.

Surgical implantation of T pellets at a supraphysiological dose of 1200 mg to normal men produced azoospermia with apparently fewer side effects than weekly IM TE (32). This confirmed that a relatively high dose of T (9 mg daily) is required for effective suppression of spermatogenesis by the androgen–only approach. The feasibility of maintaining spermatogenesis suppression by and the acceptability of repeated T implantation at least every 6 months are currently unknown.

T-17α-trans-4-*n*-butyl-cyclohexylcarboxylate (T buciclate) is formulated as an aqueous suspension of finely milled crystals and administered as a depot intramuscular injection. A single dose of 1200 mg of T buciclate produced azoospermia in only three out of eight eugonadal men whose plasma T remained within the physiological range (34). This again confirmed that higher levels of T are required for spermatogenesis suppression.

T undecanoate was originally formulated in oleic oil for orally administered androgen replacement; however, it has been reformulated in castor oil for IM injections. A single dose of T undecanoate 1000 mg achieved a prolonged half–life of 33.9 days in hypogonadal men compared with 4.5 days for 250 mg of T enanthate (35). A multicenter contraceptive efficacy study using IM T undecanoate (in tea seed oil) 500–1000 mg four to six times per week is currently in progress in China.

19-Nortestosterone (19-NT) or nandrolone is an anabolic steroid with both a higher affinity for the androgen receptor than T as well as a potent progestogen. 19-NT hexoxyphenylproprionate injected every 3 weeks for 3 months induced suppression of gonadotrophins and testosterone, and achieved azoospermia in 6 out of 12 volunteers without any symptoms of androgen-deficiency (36). If 19NT can maintain essential androgen dependent functions without producing undesirable metabolic, prostatic, and behavioral effects with more prolonged exposure, a 19-NT ester can be further investigated as a potential single-agent antifertility formulation.

Chemical manipulation of the steroid ring structure can alter the biopotency and tissue selectivity of androgens. 7α-methyl-19-nortestosterone (MENT) is a potent synthetic androgen that is not 5α-reduced, but is instead aromatized to 7α-methyl-estradiol. In the castrated rat and monkey, MENT is four times more potent than T in maintaining ventral prostate and seminal vesicle weights, but 10–12 times more potent in maintaining muscle mass and in suppressing gonadotrophins (37,38). The favorable therapeutic index gives MENT the potential of being used at lower doses (one tenth that of T) to suppress gonadotrophins and maintain adult sexual functions and muscle mass without stimulating the prostate (39). This and other selective androgen receptor modulators (SARM) are currently being investigated as a potential agent for androgen replacement and male contraception.

Combined Hormonal Male Contraceptives

Because supraphysiological levels of testosterone are required to produce maximal suppression of spermatogenesis, dose-dependent androgen-related side effects are a concern. An alternative approach in which the primary antigonadotrophic agent is nonandrogenic allows testosterone to be deployed in lower physiological replacement doses.

Progestogen and Androgen Combination

Progestogens are potent inhibitors of gonadotrophin secretion in men. They can act synergistically or additively with androgens, thus permitting lower doses of each steroid to be combined with possibly greater efficacy than when either compound is used alone. A single administration of 300 mg of DMPA combined with 800 mg of T implants induced azoospermia in 9 out of 10 Caucasian men (40). DMPA (200 or 100 mg) and T enanthatae (250 or 100 mg) at monthly intervals for 4 months suppressed spermatogenesis to azoospermia in 19 out of 20 Indonesian men (41). These studies showed that combination regimens of progestogen and androgen can be highly effective. Oral levonorgestrel 500 µg combined with IM T enanthate 100 mg/week induced azoospermia in 12 of 18 (67%) men (42). Reducing the dose of levonorgestrel to 250 and 125 µg daily produced similar results. Oral desogestrel 150–300 µg daily ombined with IM T enanthate 50–100 mg IM per week suppressed 18 of 24 (75%) men to azoospermia (43). There is some indication that an optimized combination (e.g., desogestrel 300 µg per day with T enanthate 50 mg weekly) can induce azoospermia in all men. Oral cyproterone acetate is highly effective in suppressing spermatogenesis to azoospermia in nearly all subjects in a dose-dependent manner (12.5–100 mg daily) when supplemented by intramuscular T enanthate (44) but not oral T undecanoate (45). There were no changes observed in lipids; however, a small decrease in hematocrit was recorded. The antiandrogenic properties of cyproterone acetate may account for the superior results of this combination compared with other combinations or androgens alone.

GnRH Analogs and Androgen Combinations

Abolition of gonadotrophin secretion can be achieved via blockade of GnRH action on the GnRH receptors, which are virtually exclusively expressed in the anterior pituitary gonadotrophs. This unique specificity of action confined to the pituitary–gonadal axis offers the prospect of hormonal male contraception with freedom from nonreproductive side effects. Continuous administration of superactive agonistic analogues of the natural GnRH decapeptide initially stimulates gonadotrophins followed by downregulation of the GnRH receptors. The potential of GnRH agonists (with T replacement) to reduce sperm production has been explored in 12 clinical studies (see Ref. 46 for review). Only 23% of subjects achieved azoospermia, and there was evidence that this modest efficacy can be further blunted by the simultaneous use of exogenous androgen replacement. Inadequate doses of the agonists and persistence of FSH are two possible reasons for their relative ineffectiveness. GnRH agonists have virtually been abandoned as a potential candidate for male contraception due to the availability of GnRH antagonists.

GnRH antagonists are capable of reversibly suppressing gonadotrophins more completely and rapidly than agonists (47). GnRH antagonists, with either simultaneous or delayed introduction of T replacement, suppressed spermatogenesis to azoospermia in 35 out of 40 (88%) men within 6–8 weeks (48–50); local histamine reaction has been reported with some antagonists. Compared with most sex steroid–based regimens, GnRH antagonists produce more rapid and complete suppression of spermatogenesis. Because of the low biopotency, however, milligram amounts of these peptides are required to be administered daily to achieve adequate gonadotrophin suppression in man. They are complex compounds containing several synthetic amino acids, and they are expensive to produce (51). For these reasons, current GnRH antagonists are unlikely to be developed as practical and economic contraceptive agents. In the future, nonpeptide, orally active GnRH antagonists may be available to revive further investigations.

Heterogeneity of Response to Hormonal Suppression of Spermatogenesis

A striking finding from the studies described is the marked individual difference within and between population groups in the extent of spermatogenesis arrest in response to uniform gonadotrophin suppression.

Heterogeneity Within Population Groups

Within Caucasian populations, sex steroids induce rates of azoospermia (responders) ranging from 40 to 70%, with the remainder becoming oligozoospermic (partial responders). No major difference in physical or hormonal characteristics or pharmacokinetics and pharmacodynamics between the responders and partial responders have been identified. One possibility is the extent of residual androgenic stimulation in the seminiferous tubules, which is supported by evidence that partial responders exhibit higher 5α-reductase activity during treatment (52). Data in rats showed that Leydig cells continue to secrete small amounts of T after hypophysectomy (26). Elimination of this persistent intratesticular androgen action is important in achieving maximal spermatogenesis blockade (29).

Heterogeneity Between Population Groups

One of the surprising findings from the WHO trials was that Asian (i.e., Chinese, Indonesian, and Thai) men showed a consistently higher rate of spermatogenic suppression (90%) when compared with European or American (74%) men (53). Baseline anthropometric characteristics, biochemical, endocrine, and semen parameters, or the levels of T and gonadotrophins during treatment do not explain the interethnic heterogeneity in spermatogenic (and other tissue metabolism, e.g., liver enzymes and lipid) response to sex steroids. Caucasians and Chinese men residing in the United States have higher levels of androgenic steroid precursors, which serve as substrates for 5α-reduced metabolites compared to Chinese in China (54); however, there is no interethnic difference in 5α-reductase activity. This raises the interesting possibility of an environmental or dietary origin to these population differences. Greater sensitivity of LH to exogenous T infusion (55) and lower daily sperm production rates (56) in Asians compared with Caucasians have been reported. It is currently unclear whether or not these differences are responsible for the heterogeneity in suppression of spermatogenesis.

Conclusions

Androgens are integral to hormonal male contraception as fulfilling the dual role of replacement and inhibition of spermatogenesis. Differences (i.e., interindividual and interethnic) in response to the metabolism of testosterone may underlie the heterogeneity in suppression of spermatogenesis. Androgen-only regimes are most effective and safe in Asian men. Androgen/progestin or GnRH antagonist combinations may be more suitable for Caucasians. Pharmaceutical companies are currently developing new androgens and improved formulations aimed specifically for male contraception. The long-term safety of contraceptive androgen use in men needs to be documented.

Androgen Treatment in Young Males—A New Dawn

Sixty five years after testosterone was first introduced into clinical practice, we are witnessing a new dawn in androgen replacement. Testosterone is being increasingly considered as a growth-promoting, contraceptive and legitimate anabolic (e.g., muscle and bone) agent in wasting or debilitating conditions (e.g., AIDS or rheumatoid arthritis). Careful placebo-controlled studies using state-of-the art techniques are currently in progress to accumulate data on efficacy, quality of life, and safety to usher in the extended therapeutic roles of androgens.

Current preparations of testosterone do not meet the goals for physiological replacement and will be of historic interest only before long. The search for SARM has begun. As new and improved androgen preparations become available for the much wider market of nonclassical indications, management of the relatively small number of patients with classic hypogonadism will also be improved.

References

1. Quigley CA, de Bellis A, Marschke KB, et al. Androgen receptor defects: historical, clinical and molecular perspective. Endocrinol Rev 1995;16:271–95.
2. Bulun SE. Aromatase deficiency in women and men: would you have predicted the phenotypes? J Clin Endocrinol Metab 1996;81:867–71.

3. Metzger MD, Kerrigan JR, Rogol AD. Gonadal steroid hormone regulation of the somatotropic axis during puberty in humans: mechanisms of androgen and estrogen action. Trends Endocrinol Metab 1994;5:290–96.

4. Smith EP, Boyd J, Frank GR, et al. Estrogen resistance caused by a mutation in the estrogen-receptor gene in a man. N Engl J Med 1994;331:1056–61.

5. Morishima A, Grumbach MM, Simpson ER, Fisher C, Kenan Q. Aromatase deficiency in male and female siblings caused by a novel mutation and the physiological role of estrogen. J Clin Endocrinol Metab 1995;80:3689–98.

6. Wu FCW. Male puberty and its disorders. In: Wang C, ed. Male reproductive function. Norwell, MA: Kluwer Academic Publishers, 1999:85–118.

7. Wu FCW, Butler GE, Kelnar CJH, Stirling HF, Huhtaniemi I. Patterns of pulsatile luteinizing and follicle stimulating hormone secretion in prepubertal (midchildhood) boys and girls and patients with idiopathic hypogonadotrophic hypogonadism (Kallmann's syndrome): a study using an ultrasensitive time-resolved immunofluorometric assay. J Clin Endocrinol Metab 1991;72:1229–37.

8. Brown DC, Stirling HF, Butler GE, Kelnar CJH, Wu FCW. Use of the ultrasensitive time-resolved immunofluorometric assay of LH in the differential diagnosis of normal male prepuberty and hypogonadotrophic hypogonadism. Horm Res 1996;46:83–87.

9. Kulin HE. Extensive personal experience. Delayed puberty. J Clin Endocrinol Metab 1996;81:3460–64

10. Kulin HE, Finkelstein JW, D'Arcangelo R, et al. Diversity of pubertal testosterone changes in boys with constitutional delay in growth and/or adolescence. J Pediatr Endocrinol Metab 1997;10:395–400.

11. Finkelstein JS, Neer RM, Biller BMK, Crawford JD, Klibanski A. Osteopenia in adult men with histories of delayed puberty. N Engl J Med 1992;326:600–4.

12. Finkelstein JS, Klibanski A, Neer RM. A longitudinal evaluation of bone mineral density in adult men with histories of delayed puberty. J Clin Endocrinol Metab 1996;81:1152–55.

13. Zachman M, Studer S, Prader A. Short-term testosterone treatment at bone age 12 to 13 years does not reduce adult height in boys with constitutional delay of growth and adolescence. Helv Paediatr Acta 1987;42:21–28.

14. Richman RA, Kirsch LR. Testosterone treatment in adolesent boys with constitutional delay in growth and development. N Engl J Med 1988;319:1563–67.

15. Butler GE, Walker RF, Kelnar CJH and Wu FCW. Oral testosterone undecanoate in puberty: pharmacodynamics and effects on growth and sexual maturation. J Clin Endocrinol Metab 1992;75:37–44.

16. Albanese A, Kewley GD, Long A, et al. Oral treatment for constitutional delay of growth and puberty in boys: a randomised trial of an anabolic steroid or testosterone undecanoate. Arch Dis Child 1994;71:315–17.

17. Stanhope R, Buchanan CR, Fenn GC, Preece MA. Double blind placebo controlled trial of low dose oxandrolone in the treatment of boys with constitutional delay of growth and puberty. Arch Dis Child 1988;63:501–5.

18. Papadimitriou A, Wacharasindhu S, Pearl K, et al. Treatment of constitutional growth delay in prepubertal boys with a prolonged course of low-dose oxandrolone. Arch Dis Child 1991;66:841–43.

19. Bassi F, Neri AS, Gheri RG, et al. Oxandrolone in constitutional delay of growth: analysis of the growth patterns up to final stature. J Endocrinol Invest 1993;16:133–37.

20. Wilson DM, McCauley E, Brown DR et al. Oxandrolone therapy in constitutional delayed growth and puberty. Pediatrics 1995;96:1095–100.
21. Strickland AL. Long-term results of treatment with low-dose fluoxymesterone in constitutional delay of growth and puberty and in generic short stature. Pediatrics 1993;91:716–20.
22. Uruena M, Pantsiotou S, Preece MA, et al. Is testosterone therapy for boys with constitutional delay of growth and puberty associated with impaired final height and suppression of the hypothalamic-pituitary gonadal axis? Eur J Pediatr 1992;151:15–18.
23. Brown DC, Butler GE, Kelnar CJH, Wu FCW. A double blind placebo controlled study of the effects of low dose testosterone undecanoate on the growth of small for age, prepubertal boys. Arch Dis Child 1995;73:131–35.
24. Lemcke B, Zentgraf J, Behre HM, Kliesch S, Bramswig JH, Nieschlag E. Long-term effects on testicular function of high-dose testosterone treatment for excessive tall stature. J Clin Endocrinol Metab 1996;81:296–301.
25. Sharpe RM. Regulation of spermatogenesis. In: Knobil E, Neill JD, eds. The Physiology of Reproduction. New York: Raven Press, 1994:1363–434.
26. Weinbauer GF, Gromoll J, Simoni M, Nieschlag E. In: Nieschlag E, Behre HM, eds. Andrology, male reproductive health and dysfunction. Berlin: Springer. 1997:25–57.
27. El Shannawy A, Gates R, Russel L. Hormonal regulation of spermatogenesis in the hypophysectomized rat: cell viability after hormonal replacement in adults after intermediate periods of hypophysectomy. J Androl 1998;19:320–34.
28. Yang ZW, Wreford NG, Royce P, de Krester DM, McLachlan RI. Stereological evaluation of human spermatogenesis after suppression by testosterone treatment: heterogeneous pattern of spermatogenic impairment. J Clin Endocrinol Metab 1998;83(4):1284–91.
29. Franca LR, Parreira GG, Gates RJ, Russel LD. Hormonal regulation of spermatogenesis in the hypophysectomised rat: quantitation of germ-cell population and effect of elimination of residual testosterone after long-term hypophysectomy. J Androl. 1998;19(3):335–40.
30. World Health Organization Task Force on Methods for the Regulation of Male Fertility. Contraceptive efficacy of testosterone-induced azoospermia in normal men. Lancet 1990;335:955.
31. World Health Organization Task Force on Methods for the Regulation of Male Fertility. Contraceptive efficacy of testosterone-induced oligozoospermia in normal men. Fertil Steril 1996;65:821–29.
32. Wu FCW, Farley TMM, Peregoudov A, Waites GMH, World Health Organization Task Force on Methods for the Regulation of Male Fertility. Effects of exogenous testosterone in normal men: experience from a multicentre contraceptive efficacy study using testosterone enanthate. Fertil Steril 1996;65:626–36.
33. Handelsman DJ, Conway AJ, Boylan LM. Suppression of human spermatogenesis by testosterone implants. J Clin Endocrinol Metab 1992;75:1326.
34. Behre HM, Baus S, Kliesch S et al. Potential of testosterone buciclate for male contraception: endocrine differences between responders and non-responders. J Clin Endocrinol Metab 1995;80: 2394–403.
35. Behre HM, Abshagen K, Oettel M, Hubler D, Nieschlag E. Intramuscular injection of testosterone undecanoate for the treatment of male hypopgonadism: phase I studies. Eur J Endocrinol 1999:140(5):414–19.

36. Knuth UA, et al. Clinical trial of 19-nortestosterone-hexoxyphenyl-propionate (Anadur) for male fertility regulation. Fertil Steril 1985;44:814.
37. Cummings DE, Kumar N, Bardin CW, Sundaram K, Bremner WJ. Prostate sparing effects of the potent androgen 7α-methyl-19-nortestosterone: a potential alternative to testosterone for androgen replacement and male contraception. J Clin Endocrinol Metab 1998;83:4212–19.
38. Sundaram K, Kumar N, Bardin CW. 7α-methyl-19-nortestosterone (MENT); the optimal androgen for male contraception. Ann Med 1993;25:199–205.
39. Suvisaari J, et al. Pharmacokinetics and pharmacodynamics of 7α-methyl-19-nortestosterone after intramuscular administration in healthy men. Hum Reprod. 1997;12:967–73.
40. Handelsman DJ, Conway AJ, Howe CJ, Turner L, Mackey MA. Establishing the minimum effective dose and additive effects of depot progestin in suppression of human spermatogenesis by a testosterone depot. J Clin Endocrinol Metab 1996;81:4113–21.
41. Pangkahila W. Reversible azoospermia induced by an androgen-progestin combination regimen in Indonesian men. Int J Androl 1991;14:248.
42. Bebb RA, Bradley D, Anawalt R, Christensen RB, Paulsen CA, Bremner WJ, et al. Combined administration of levonorgestrel and testosterone induces more rapid and effective suppression spermatogenesis than testosterone alone: a promising male contraceptive approach. J Clin Endocrinol Metab 1996;81:757–62.
43. Wu FCW, Balasubramanian R, Mulders T, Coelinh-Bennink H. Oral progestogen combined with testosterone as a potential male contraceptive: additive effects between desogestrel and testosterone enanthate in suppression of spermatogenesis, pituitary testicular axis and lipid metabolism. J Clin Endocrinol Metab 1999; 84(1):112–22.
44. Merrigiola CM, Bremner WJ, Paulsen CA, Valdiserri A, Incorvaia L, Motta R, et al. A combined regimen of cuproterone acetate and testosterone enanthate as a potential highly effective male contraceptive. J Clin Endocrinol Metab 1996;81: 3018–23.
45. Merrigiola CM, Bremner WJ, Costantino A, Pavani A, Capelli M, Flamigni C. An oral regimen of cyproterone acetate and testosterone undecanoate for spermatogenic suppression in men. Fertil Steril 1997;68:844–50.
46. Nieschlag E, Behre HM, Weinbauer GF. Hormonal contraception: a real chance? In: Spermatogenesis–fertilization–contraception; molecular cellular and endocrine events in male reproduction. Nieschlag E, Habenicht U-F, eds. Schering Foundation Workshop (Vol. 4). Berlin: Springer-Verlag, 1992:477–501.
47. Pavlou S, et al. Mode of suppression of pituitary and gonadal function after acute or prolonged administration of a luteinizing hormone-releasing hormone antagonist in normal men. J Clin Endocrinol Metab 1989;68:446.
48. Pavlou SN, et al. Combined administration of a gonadotropin-releasing hormone antagonist and testosterone in men induces reversible azoospermia without loss of libido. J Clin Endocrinol Metab 1991;73:1360.
49. Tom L, Bhasin S, Salameh E, et al. Induction of azoospermia in normal men with combined Nal-Glu gonadotropin-releasing hormone antagonist and testosterone enanthate. J Clin Endocrinol Metab 1992;75:476.
50. Bagatell CJ, Matsumoto AM, Christensen RB, et al. Comparison of a gonadotropin releasing-hormone antagonist plus testosterone (T) versus T alone as a potential male contraceptive regimen. J Clin Endocrinol Metab 1993; 77:427.

51. Karten MJ, Rivier JE. Gonadotropin-releasing hormone analog design. Structure-function studies toward the development of agonists and antagonists: rationale and perspective. Endocrinol Rev 1986;7:44.
52. Anderson RA, Wallace AM, Wu FCW. Comparison between testosterone enanthate induced azoospermia and oligospermia in a male contraceptive study. 3. Higher 5 alpha reductase activity in oligospermic men administered supraphysiological doses of testosterone. J Clin Endocrinol Metab 1996;81:902–8.
53. World Health Organization Task Force on Methods for the Regulation of Male Fertility. Rates of testosterone-induced suppression to severe oligozoospermia or azoospermia in two multicentre clinical studies. Int J Androl 1995;18:157–65.
54. Santner SJ, Albertson B, Zhang GY, Zhang GH, Santulli M, Wang C, et al. Comparative rates of androgen production and metabolism in Caucasian and Chinese subjects. J Clin Endocrinol Metab 1998;83:2104–9.
55. Wang C, Berman N, Veldhuis JD, Der T, McDonald V, Steiner B, et al. Graded testosterone infusions ditsinguish gonadotrophin negative feedback responsiveness in Asian and white men—a clinical research center study. J Clin Endocrinol Metab 1998;83:870–76.
56. Johnson L, Barnard J, Rodriguez L, Smith E, Swerdloff R, Wang X, et al. Ethnic differences in testicular structure and spermatogenic potential may predispose testes of Asian men to a high sensitivity to steroidal contraceptives. J Androl 1998;19:348–57.

Part III

Genetics and Cell Biology of Spermatogenesis

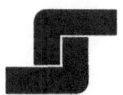

10

Developmental Genetics of Spermatogenesis in the Nematode *Caenorhabditis elegans*

STEVEN W. L'HERNAULT AND ANDREW W. SINGSON

Comparison of Spermatogenesis in Mammals and *C. elegans*

In both mammals and *C. elegans*, spermatogenesis is the process where a spermatogonial cell undergoes a series of divisions to produce a highly differentiated cell, *the spermatozoon*. Spermatogonial cellular divisions are incomplete in mammals so that all subsequent stages occur in a syncitium. The situation is similar in *C. elegans*, where spermatogonial nuclei initially share a common cytoplasm. Spermatogonial divisions in both mammals and *C. elegans* are regulated by signaling from gonadal accessory cells. In mammals, this process requires a series of accessory cell types, including Sertoli, peritubular myoid, and Leydig cells (1,2). In contrast, one somatic distal tip cell (Fig. 10.1) regulates exit of spermatogonia from mitosis in *C. elegans*, and it no longer participates in spermatogenesis after meiosis is initiated (3). Spermatogenesis occurs within a tubular structure in both mammals and *C. elegans*. Differentiation occurs along the length and across the radius of this tube (the seminiferous tubule) in mammals. The Sertoli accessory cell plays a crucial role in both the linear and radial aspects of mammalian spermatogenesis. At any given time, a single Sertoli cell can be in contact with up to 50 individual, developing germ cells that can be at four different stages of development (4). In each mammalian testis, spermatogenesis occurs within a "ball of yarn" composed of seminiferous tubules that, if unraveled, would be many meters long. The *C. elegans* gonadal tube is ~400 mm long (Fig. 10.1). and only linear differentiation is observed (5). After initiating meiosis, individual *C. elegans* spermatogonial cells bud from the syncitial testes and lineally complete development without the aid of accessory cells (6).

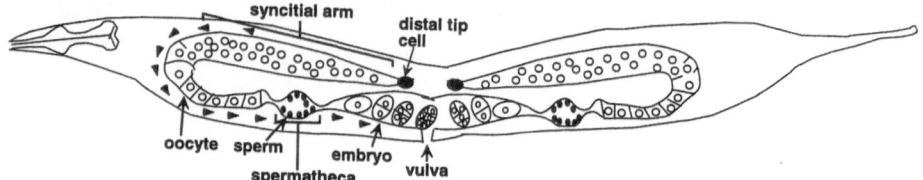

FIGURE 10.1. Schematic diagram of the *C. elegans* adult hermaphrodite reproductive tract. Anterior is left and dorsal is on top. Arrowheads indicate the direction of gamete movement and maturation in the germline. The hermaphrodite gonad is a double-armed structure and only the anterior arm is labeled in this figure.

The slow pace of mammalian spermatogenesis (weeks to months) and the complex histological milieu in which it occurs makes the study of this process challenging. Complex developmental processes can benefit from genetic analyses where mutant phenotypes yield insight into underlying mechanisms. Mammalian spermatogenesis is no exception; however, like other dioecious organisms, mammals have an inherent limit in their utility for large-scale genetic analyses of spermatogenesis because it is difficult to design simple screens for specific spermatogenesis mutants. In dioecious organisms suitable for genetic analyses (i.e., the mouse), the first step in such a screen is identification of mutant males that do not sire progeny. Many such mutant males fail to sire progeny for reasons (i.e., behavioral defects) other than spermatogenesis defects, and those that have detectable spermatogenesis defects also frequently show somatic defects (7). An experimental system is needed that somehow biases mutant hunts to favor recovery of those with specific defects in only spermatogenesis. The unusual reproductive biology of the nematode *C. elegans* contains such a bias and is especially suitable for the large-scale recovery of spermatogenesis-defective (*spe*) mutants (6).

C. elegans Reproductive Biology

Sexual reproduction requires production of two different gametes: *sperm* and *eggs*. In dioecious organisms, sperm are produced by males and eggs are produced by females. In contrast, wild-type *C. elegans* does not have a conventional female, but exists principally as a protandrous ("male first") hermaphrodite with an occasional male. Progeny can consequently result from self-fertilization in the hermaphrodite or cross-fertilization between a male and a hermaphrodite (Fig. 10.1) (8).

The hermaphrodite larva hatches with two germ cells that mitotically proliferate during larval stages I–III. Beginning during the third larval stage, germ cells exit mitosis and enter meiosis. The first approximately 50–75 germ cells become spermatocytes that form 200–300 spermatids during a brief time period where the hermaphrodite germline is a testis (5). The germline switches to oocyte production after the fourth stage larval hermaphrodite molts and becomes an adult. The first ovulation pushes spermatids out of what is now an ovary and into the spermathecae, where they rapidly become spermatozoa. The spermatheca is an organ in the reproductive tract where spermatozoa are stored (Fig. 10.1). Oocytes are ovulated into the spermatheca where they are fertilized by the stored spermatozoa (9). Ovulation, therfore, is both spatially and temporally coupled to fertilization. It is not surprising that virtually all ovulated oocytes produced by a young hermaphrodite are fertilized and the resulting shelled eggs are laid on the agar growth plate (9). This background, where nearly 100% self-fertilization occurs, makes it easy to identify any mutant hermaphrodite that lays unfertilized oocytes. Such self-sterile hermaphrodites usually arise because of defects in spermatogenesis. Cross-fertility after mating these mutant hermaphrodites to wild-type males confirms that their self-sterilization is due to defective sperm. The enormous advantage of this screening procedure is that an *spe* mutation is identified and recovered from one individual hermaphrodite. This simple screen has identified more than 40 genes that affect spermatogenesis (6).

Wild-type *C. elegans* spermatogenesis has been studied in detail, and this work is summarized in Figure 10.2 (6). This process is highly similar in males and hermaphrodites, except it occurs continually in males and only during a narrow time interval in hermaphrodites, as described earlier. The 4N primary spermatocyte buds off the rachis, which is a central syncitial cytoplasmic core, after entering pachytene and undergoes the first meiotic division. The primary spermatocyte can complete development in vitro without any exogenously supplied hormones or accessory cells (6). Secondary spermatocytes either completely separate or stay linked by a cytoplasmic bridge as they undergo the second meiotic division to yield a total of four haploid spermatids. Asymmetric cytoplasmic partitioning places spermatocyte ribosomes, actin, tubulin, and myosin into the residual body during spermatid formation. Resulting sessile apolar spermatids are activated to form motile bipolar spermatozoa in a 5–10 minute-differentiation process. Sperm activation does not require new macromolecular synthesis or contact with any other cell . Resulting *C. elegans* spermatozoa do not have a flagellum, rather, they crawl by directed membrane flow of a single pseudopod that is supported by a cytoskeleton of 10 nm filaments composed of major sperm protein (MSP) (10).

Asymmetric Partitioning of Cellular Components During *C. elegans* Spermatogenesis

Spermatogenesis in all species is characterized by a massive reorganization of the cytoplasm that is partly mediated by asymmetric partitioning during maturation. The process of asymmetric partitioning during *C. elegans* sper-

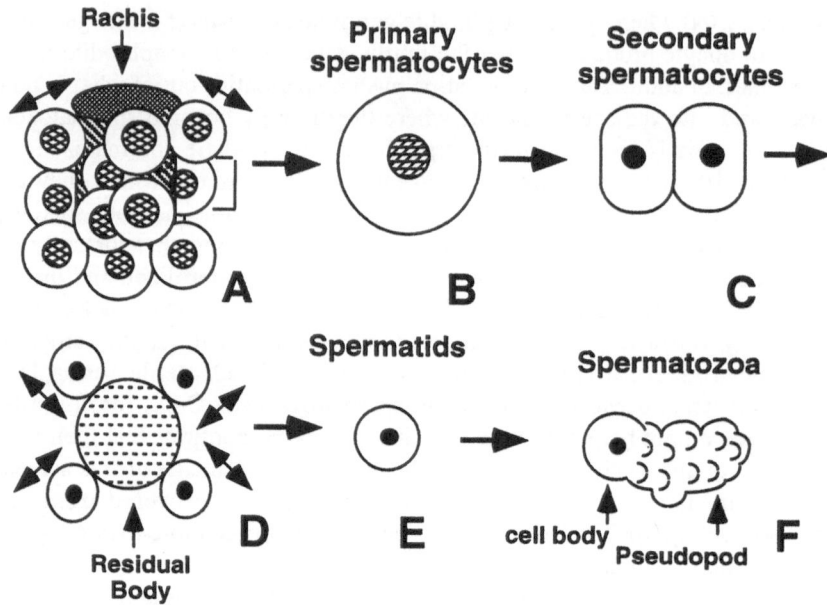

FIGURE 10.2. Schematic of *C. elegans* spermatogenesis. Asymmetric partitioning occurs at two points during *C. elegans* spermatocyte morphogenesis, as indicated by double-headed arrows in A and D.

matogenesis is structurally obvious during two stages (double arrowheads in Fig. 10.2). Asymmetric partitioning is especially dramatic when spermatids separate from an anucleate residual body (Fig. 10.2D). Most macromolecular components required by spermatids reside within large ER/Golgi-derived organelles called *the fibrous body–membranous organelles* (FB–MOs) that segregate exclusively into spermatids during their formation (11,12). In contrast, most voltage-gated ion channels, most tubulin, actin, and ribosomes segregate to the residual body during spermatid formation (11,13). As a result, asymmetric partitioning operates during this stage both within the cell and in its plasma membrane. FB–MO morphogenesis can be disrupted by mutations, and we have studied the genetic control of how these structures form.

An ER/Golgi-Derived Organelle That Mediates Asymmetric Partitioning

FB–MO development and its coordination with cellular stages during *C. elegans* spermatogenesis is summarized in Figures 10.2 and 10.3 (6). In syncitial pachytene spermatocytes (Fig. 10.2A), the MOs form from the Golgi apparatus; the FBs form a short time later in close association with the MOs (fb in Fig. 10.3A). The 4N primary spermatocyte (Fig. 10.2B) buds off the

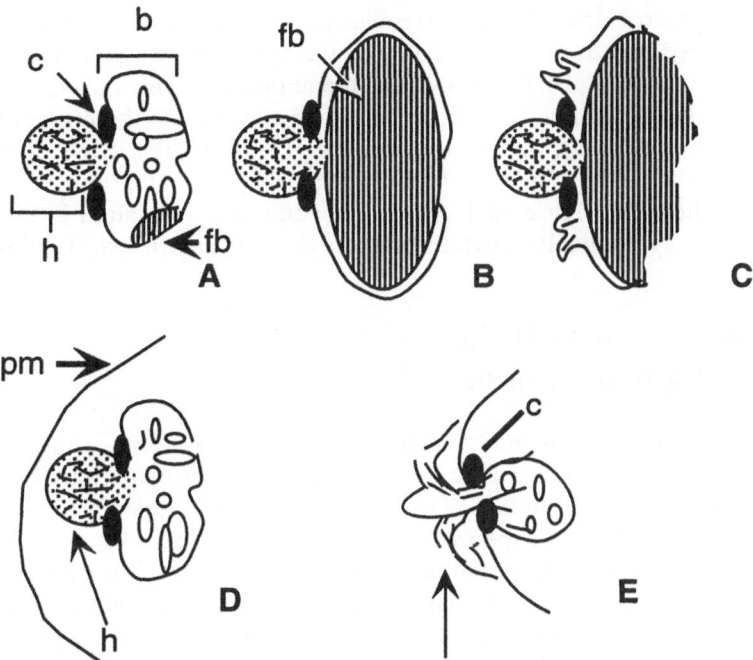

FIGURE 10.3. FB–MO morphogenesis. (A) The fibrous body (fb) forms within and is surrounded by the membranous organelle (MO) in a primary spermatocyte. A collar region (c) separates the MO into a head (h; speckled region at left) and body (b; right of the collar); (B) mature spermatocytes contain FB–MOs that have reached their maximum size. The fb is composed of major sperm protein filaments and is surrounded by a double layered MO-derived membrane; (C) membranes that surround the fb fold up as they retract and the filaments of the fb depolymerize and disperse after the residual body separates from spermatids; (D) each MO head (h) localizes near the spermatid plasma membrane (pm) after disappearance of the fbs; (E) exocytosis results in fusion of the MO head with the plasma membrane. MO contents (wavy lines at arrow) are placed onto the cell body surface. Each MO places a permanent fusion pore in the plasma membrane (each cell has many MOs).

rachis (a central, syncitial cytoplasmic core) and undergoes the first meiotic division. Growth of the FBs in primary spermatocytes occurs within an MO-derived membrane envelope during this stage (Fig. 10.3B). The FB–MO morphology remains as in Figure 10.3B in secondary spermatocytes (Fig. 10.2C). FB–MOs segregate exclusively to spermatids during budding from the residual body (Fig. 10.2D). Once the spermatid has completely separated from the residual body (Fig. 10.2E), the MO disassociates from the FB, the double membrane that surrounds the FB is retracted (Fig. 10.3C), and the filamentous contents (striped material in Fig. 10.3C), principally MSP, are depolymerized and dispersed throughout the cytoplasm. After the fibrous bodies have disappeared, the MOs localize near the plasma membrane (pm in Fig. 10.3D) in spermatids (Fig. 10.2E). When the spermatid is converted into the spermatozoon (Fig. 10.2F), MO head membranes (h, in Fig. 10.3D) fuse with the plasma membrane and deposit their contents on the plasma membrane of the cell body, but not the pseudopod (Fig. 10.3E). Each spermatocyte has many FB–MOs and all synchronously follow the developmental program shown in Figure 10.3. As the preceding data indicate, FB–MOs are convenient, cytologically obvious markers for asymmetric partitioning.

Two Mutants with Defects in FB–MO Morphogenesis

There are a number of mutants that affect FB–MO morphogenesis (Fig. 10.4), but only two that illustrate some important principles will be discussed (6). The *spe-4* mutant perturbs the normally intimate association of the FB with MO during spermatogenesis. The MOs and FBs are observed as discrete, unconnected structures in *spe-4* mutants, and it is presently unknown if there is ever an association between them in this mutant. The *spe-4* spermatocytes complete meiosis in the absence of cytokinesis and the resulting terminal spermatocyte contains distended, vacuolated MOs and separate FBs throughout its cytoplasm. The deduced protein sequence of *spe-4* reveals that it encodes an integral, multipass membrane protein located in the FB–MO during wild-type spermatogenesis (14,15). The SPE-4

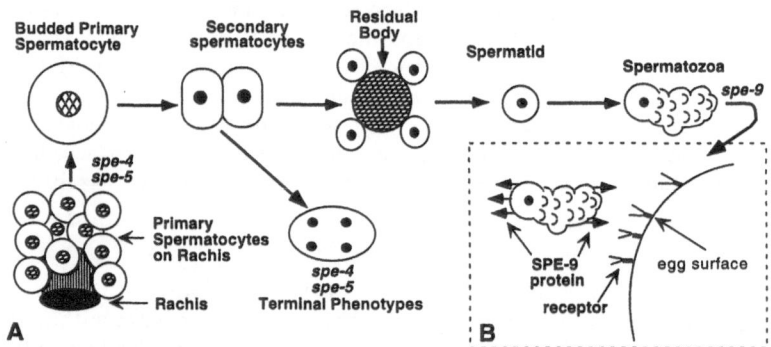

FIGURE 10.4. (A) Wild-type *C. elegans* spermatogenesis (top line) and representative mutants. Three of the more than 40 known genes are placed on the pathway at the earliest stage where ultrastructural or light microscopic defects are first evident. The last step (*spe-9*) of the pathway represents mutant spermatozoa that are cytologically normal but cannot enter oocytes. The *spe-4* and *spe-5* genes are placed on the pathway where they first show defects, and the terminal arrest stage is shown beneath the pathway. (B) Proposed mechanism of how the SPE-9 protein facilitates interaction between the sperm and egg.

protein is homologous to the presenilins for which nonnull mutations have been implicated in early onset Alzheimer's disease (16). Although mutant forms of these proteins cause a central nervous system disease in humans, they are normally expressed in plants and in many animal tissues, including testes (15). Furthermore, knockout loss of function mutant mice show neonatal lethality and die, presumably, because of defects in the rib cage that prevent proper breathing (17,18). The presenilins clearly perform an essential cellular function that is specific to multicellular organisms because homologues are not detectable in the complete *Saccharomyces cerevisiae* genomic DNA sequence.

Like *spe-4* mutants, *spe-5* mutants usually arrest spermatogenesis as terminal spermatocytes containing four haploid nuclei and defective FB–MOs. The cytological appearance of these *spe-5* terminal spermatocytes is similar to that observed for *spe-4* (see earlier). The FB–MO membranes are swollen and distended in *spe-5* primary spermatocytes, but, unlike *spe-4*, each FB retains an association with an MO. Although this association differs from wild-type, *spe-5* FB–MOs can occasionally function because spermatocytes can rarely form spermatids. A few *spe-5* spermatids can form spermatozoa that contain some MOs that fuse with the plasma membrane. These spermatozoa can fertilize eggs because putative *spe-5* null mutant hermaphrodites occasionally produce a few young (19,20).

An Integrated Hypothesis for FB–MO Function During Spermatogenesis

Meiosis, cell division, and asymmetric partitioning of organelles and macromolecules are usually coordinated during spermatogenesis so that spermatids always contain all required components in the right cellular location. The previously described analyses of mutants affecting sperm differentiation has begun to reveal how these processes are interrelated. Meiosis and cellular division are not interdependent because *spe-4* mutants always form, and *spe-5* mutants usually (but not always) form, four haploid nuclei within a single, terminal spermatocyte. The *spe-5* mutants can occasionally divide its spermatocytes to form spermatids that each contain a haploid nucleus. Because *spe-4* and *spe-5* mutants both exhibit severe disruption of FB–MO morphogenesis, this suggests that meiosis *per se* is not affected when FB–MOs do not form properly.

Even though the cellular location of the *spe-5*-encoded protein is not yet established, SPE-4 localizes exclusively to the FB–MOs (15). This indicates that all phenotypic defects in *spe-4* mutants result from defective FB–MO morphogenesis, and our working hypothesis is that SPE-5 will also localize exclusively to this organelle. Why can *spe-5* mutants form spermatids even though *spe-4* mutants cannot execute this step of spermatogenesis? One difference appears to be in how the FB–MOs are affected in these two different mutants. In *spe-5* mutants, unlike *spe-4* mutants, FB–MOs occasionally retain competency to associate with the spindle poles during meiosis II. This suggests that when FB–MOs are localized to the meiotic spindle poles during the second meiotic division, a spermatocyte can properly polarize to divide into spermatids. Positioning of the meiotic spindle apparently requires FB–MOs that are competent to associate with this structure, presumably via the astral microtubules. Only certain mutants with defective FB–MOs always affect asymmetric partitioning (e.g., *spe-4*), whereas other mutants show defects within FB–MOs that do not always affect partitioning (e.g., *spe-5*). The previously discussed data show that FB–MOs are key players in asymmetric partitioning. Our future studies will reveal how FB–MOs mediate asymmetric partitioning and how the meiotic spindle participates in FB–MO asymmetric partitioning.

C. elegans and the Genetics of Fertilization

The ultimate goal of spermatogenesis is to generate a male-derived gamete that can locate, interact with, and enter the egg during fertilization. A mutation that affects any of the numerous steps that occur during spermatogenesis can result in a spermatozoon that is unable to participate in fertilization. This fact makes it exceedingly difficult to identify the proteins designed to allow the sperm to interact with the egg. One example is the mouse protein calmegin, which is an ER resident chaperonin that presumably plays a role in protein folding. Although the calmegin knockout mouse mutant produces normal-appearing sperm that are incapable of participating in fertilization, this result did not reveal a spermatozoan plasma membrane candidate protein (21). Among genetically amenable animal species, *C. elegans* is well suited for analyses of mutants that specifically affect sperm during fertilization.

Fertilization Appears to Be the Only Defect in *spe-9* Mutant Spermatozoa

Spermatozoa from *spe-9* mutants are indistinguishable from wild-type spermatozoa when viewed by light and electron microscopy (19,22). Sessile, male-derived *spe-9* spermatids become bipolar, motile spermatozoa (spermiogenesis) after treatment with the in vitro activators pronase or triethanolamine, just like wild-type spermatids (22–24). The *spe-9* mutant hermaphrodites also produce spermatozoa that exhibit no morphological defects when compared with wild-type spermatozoa. The *spe-9* mutant hermaphrodites properly deposit their sperm in the spermatheca and they are still observed within this organ after many unfertilized oocytes are laid. This indicates that *spe-9* hermaphrodite-derived spermatozoa are motile and can maintain their position in the reproductive tract because ovulation tends to displace spermatozoa from the spermatheca. Passing oocytes have been observed in direct contact with *spe-9* mutant sperm without fertilizing them; this does not occur in the wild type, where every oocyte is fertilized.

When male and hermaphrodite worms are mated, the male-derived sperm take precedence over the hermaphrodite-derived sperm and outcross progeny are produced (9). This suggests that male-derived sperm have a competitive advantage over hermaphrodite-derived sperm. This bias in fertilization helps to ensure outcrossing in a predominantly self-fertilizing species. Male-derived sperm have this advantage because they are larger and can move faster or more vigorously than hermaphrodite sperm (25). This presumably allows them to displace hermaphrodite-derived sperm in the spermatheca and thus get used preferentially for fertilization. Sperm competition assays reveal that male derived *spe-9* spermatozoa outcompete hermaphrodite-derived wild-type spermatozoa. This results in wild-type hermaphrodites that are partially or fully sterilized after they have mated with *spe-9* males (26).

The *spe-9* gene encodes a putative transmembrane protein where the bulk of the extracellular domain consists of 10 cysteine-rich repeat motifs related to the epidermal growth factor (EGF) (22). EGF-like regions in proteins are involved in extracellular functions (e.g., adhesive and ligand–receptor interactions (27). Two missense mutations each affect residues critical for EGF motif folding or conformation, confirming the importance of this SPE-9 protein region. The overall structure of SPE-9 is similar to the Notch/LIN-12/GLP-1 receptor ligands Delta and Serrate from *Drosophila*, APX-1, and LAG-2 from *C. elegans* and the Jagged proteins from mammals (28). These ligand proteins all have similar placement of their signal sequence and transmembrane domain, all have a short cytoplasmic domain, and some have amino acid insertions in the EGF-like repeats that are never seen in the receptors. The SPE-9 structure and its conserved motifs are consistent with it playing a ligandlike role in cell adhesion and/or signaling during fertilization (Fig. 10.4B).

Conclusions

C. elegans has proven to be an outstanding system for genetic analyses, including spermatogenesis. The unusual *C. elegans* reproductive biology facilitates both the recovery of mutants and their subsequent analysis by a combination of in vivo and in vitro techniques. This collection of *spe* mutants includes those that affect sperm development and those that affect the role of sperm during fertilization. A number of *spe* genes encode conserved proteins that are implicated in critical roles during *C. elegans* spermatogenesis. A future challenge will be to determine if such proteins participate in similar processes during flagellated sperm development.

Acknowledgments. The authors thank Dr. Erwin Goldberg and the Organizing Committee for inclusion of our work in this symposium. We thank Dr. Grant MacGregor for comments on the manuscript. This work was supported by N.I.H. grant GM40697 and N.S.F. grant IBN-9808847 to S.W.L. and N.S.F. minority postdoctoral grant to A.W.S.

References

1. Skinner MK, Norton JN, Mullaney BP, Rosselli M, Whaley PD, Anthony CT. Cell-cell interactions and the regulation of testis function. Ann N Y Acad Sci 1991;637:354–63.

2. deRooij DG, Grootegoed JA. Spermatogonial stem cells. Curr Opin Cell Biol 1998;10:694–701.

3. Kimble J, White J. On the control of germ cell development in *Caenorhabditis elegans*. Dev Biol 1981;81:208–19.

4. Weber JE, Russell LD, Wong V, Peterson RN. Three-dimensional reconstruction of a rat Stage V Sertoli cell: II. Morphometry of Sertoli-Sertoli and Sertoli-germ-cell relationships. Am J Anat 1983;167:163–79.

5. Hirsh D, Oppenheim D, Klass M. Development of the reproductive system of Caenorhabditis elegans. Dev Biol 1976;49:200–19.

6. L'Hernault SW. Spermatogenesis. In: Riddle DL, Blumenthal T, Meyer BJ, Priess JR, eds. *C. Elegans* II. Cold Spring Harbor: Cold Spring Harbor Laboratory, 1997:271–94.

7. Okabe M, Ikawa M, Ashkenas J. Gametogenesis '98: male infertility and the genetics of spermatogenesis. Am J Hum Gen 1998;62:1274–81.

8. Brenner S. The genetics of *Caenorhabditis elegans*. Genetics 1974;77:71–94.

9. Ward S, Carrel JS. Fertilization and sperm competition in the nematode *Caenorhabditis elegans*. Dev Biol 1979;73:304–21.

10. Roberts TM, Stewart M. Nematode sperm locomotion. Curr Opin Cell Biol 1995;7:13–17.

11. Ward S. The asymmetric localization of gene products during the development of *Caenorhabditis elegans* spermatozoa. In: Gall J, ed. Gametogenesis and the early embryo. New York: Alan R. Liss, 1986:55–75.

12. Roberts TM, Pavalko FM, Ward S. Membrane and cytoplasmic proteins are transported in the same organelle complex during nematode spermatogenesis. J Cell Biol 1986;102:1787–96.

13. Machaca K, DeFelice LJ, L'Hernault SW. A novel chloride channel localizes to *Caenorhabditis elegans* spermatids and chloride channel blockers induce spermatid differentiation. Dev Biol 1996;176:1–16.

14. L'Hernault SW, Arduengo PM. Mutation of a putative sperm membrane protein in *Caenorhabditis elegans* prevents sperm differentiation but not its associated meiotic divisions. J Cell Biol 1992;119:55–68.

15. Arduengo PM, Appleberry OK, Chuang P, L'Hernault SW. The presenilin protein family member SPE-4 localizes to an ER/Golgi derived organelle and is required for proper cytoplasmic partitioning during *Caenorhabditis elegans* spermatogenesis. J Cell Sci 1998;111:3645–54.

16. Hardy J. Amyloid, the presenilins and Alzheimer's disease. Trends Neurosci 1997;20:154–59.

17. Shen J, Bronson RT, Chen DF, Xia W, Selkoe DJ, Tonegawa S. Skeletal and CNS defects in *presenilin-1*-deficient mice. Cell 1997;89:629–39.
18. Wong PC, Zheng H, Chen H, et al. Presenilin 1 is required for *Notch1* and *Dll1* expression in the paraxial mesoderm. Nature 1997;387:288–92.
19. L'Hernault SW, Shakes DC, Ward S. Developmental genetics of chromosome *I* spermatogenesis-defective mutants in the nematode *Caenorhabditis elegans*. Genetics 1988;120:435–52.
20. Machaca K, L'Hernault SW. The *Caenorhabditis elegans spe-5* gene is required for morphogenesis of a sperm-specific organelle and is associated with an inherent cold-sensitive phenotype. Genetics 1997;146:567–81.
21. Ikawa M, Wada I, Kominami K, et al. The putative chaperone calmegin is required for sperm fertility. Nature 1997;387:607–11.
22. Singson A, Mercer KB, L'Hernault SW. The *C. elegans spe-9* gene encodes a sperm transmembrane protein that contains EGF-like repeats and is required for fertilization. Cell 1998;93:71–79.
23. Nelson GA, Ward S. Vesicle fusion, pseudopod extension and amoeboid motility are induced in nematode spermatids by the ionophore monensin. Cell 1980;19:457–64.
24. Ward S, Hogan E, Nelson GA. The initiation of spermiogenesis in the nematode *Caenorhabditis elegans*. Dev Biol 1983;98:70–79.
25. LaMunyon CW, Ward S. Larger sperm outcompete smaller sperm in the nematode *Caenorhabditis elegans*. Proc R Soc Lond B Biol Sci 1998;265:1997–2002.
26. Singson A, Hill KL, L'Hernault SW. Sperm competition in the absence of fertilization in *Caenorhabditis elegans*. Genetics 1999;152:201–8.
27. Campbell ID, Bork P. Epidermal growth factor-like modules. Curr Opin Struct Biol 1993;3:385–92.
28. Weinmaster G. The ins and outs of notch signaling. Mol Cell Neurosci 1997;9:91–102.

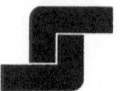

11

Regulation of Meiosis and Spermatid Differentiation in *Drosophila* Primary Spermatocytes

Ting-Yi Lin, M. Jodeane Pringle, and Margaret T. Fuller

Spermatogenesis in *Drosophila* is an excellent model system for exploring the mechanisms that mediate and regulate the differentiation of male gametes. The cellular events of *Drosophila* spermatogenesis are well characterized at the ultrastructural level (1–3) Most stages are easily visualized by light microscopy, either in unfixed squashed preparations (Fig. 11.1) or by immunofluorescence with specific markers (e.g., see Ref. 4). Many male sterile mutants that affect different specific aspects of spermatogenesis have already been identified. The events affected by existing male sterile mutations include germline stem-cell proliferation, the spermatogonial divisions, the spermatocyte growth phase, entry into the meiotic divisions, completion of meiosis, cytokinesis and formation of intercellular bridges, nuclear elongation, and individualization (reviewed in Ref. 5). These male sterile mutations bring the power of genetic analysis in *Drosophila* to investigations of the molecular mechanisms that underlie the dramatic morphological changes of male gametogenesis.

The process of spermatogenesis in flies bears many striking similarities to spermatogenesis in mammals. As in mammals, *Drosophila* male germ cells undergo three different types of cell cycles: stem-cell–type asymmetric divisions, mitotic amplification divisions during the spermatogonial stages, and the specialized cell cycle of meiosis. In both mammals and *Drosophila,* the meiotic cell cycle features an extended G2 period (i.e., the meiotic prophase) during which male germ cells grow substantially in volume. This extended period of spermatocyte growth is characterized by an extensive and novel transcription program (5,6) because spermatocytes accumulate many mRNAs for use during subsequent spermatid differentiation. At the completion of the primary spermatocyte period transcription decreases dramatically (6,7). In flies, as in mammals, spermiogenesis involves a series of

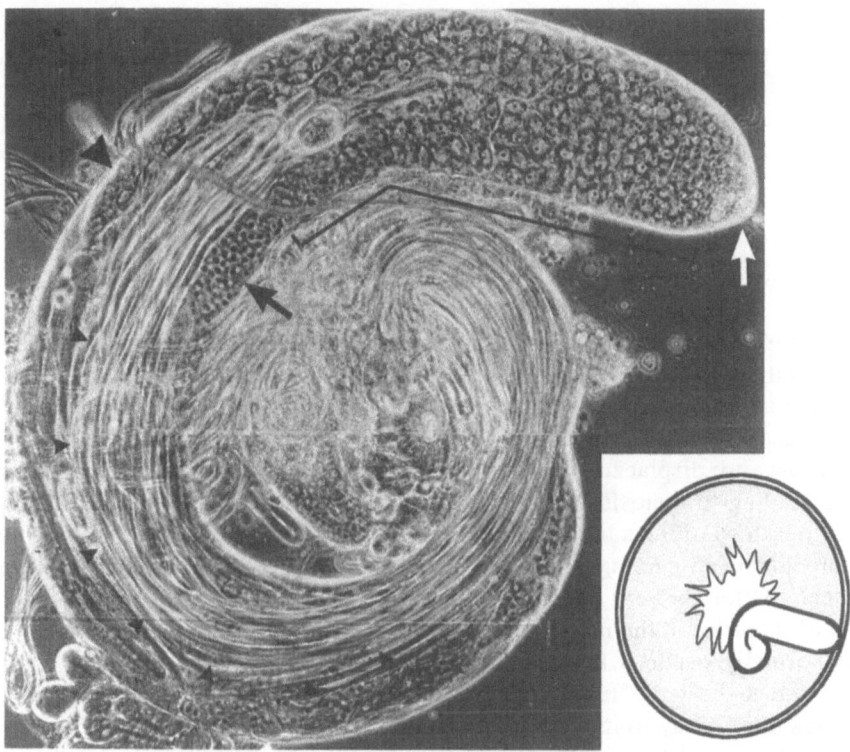

FIGURE 11.1. Differentiating male germ cells in *Drosophila*. Whole adult wild-type *Drosophila* testis viewed by phase contrast light microscopy. Germ cells in the first half of spermatogenesis are visible in rough developmental order along the testis wall, proceeding from stem cells and spermatogonia at the apical tip, through growing primary spermatocytes, to cells in meiosis and early round spermatids. White arrow: germ cells undergoing mitotic divisions. Bracket: primary spermatocytes. Black arrow: haploid spermatid cells. Large arrowhead: germ cells undergoing meiotic division. Small arrowheads: elongated bundles of spermatids, which extend up the lumen of the testis as they differentiate. Inset: diagram showing comparison of *Drosophila* testis to a mammalian seminiferous tubule (not to scale): Mammalian germline stem cells are located at the periphery of the seminiferous tubule and the developing germ cells progress toward the lumen of the seminiferous tubule as they differentiate. From (17).

dramatic morphogenetic events, producing highly elongate, flagellated cells in which almost every subcellular component has been extensively remodeled. In both cases, much of spermatid differentiation occurs after most transcription has been shut down. Finally, in *Drosophila* as in mammals, the process of male gametogenesis takes place in a collaborative unit consisting of the differentiating germ cells and intimately associated somatic cells, which may contribute crucial signals that regulate germ-cell differentiation.

The fundamental similarities in the cellular events of spermatogenesis between mammals and *Drosophila* raise the possibility that morphogenetic mechanisms, regulatory pathways, and even the function of specific genes may be conserved. Thus, results gleaned from genetic and molecular analysis in *Drosophila* may illuminate the mechanistic basis of similar events during mammalian spermatogenesis.

Spermatogenesis in *Drosophila*

The *Drosophila* spermatogenesis program is initiated late in embryogenesis and continues throughout larval and adult life. The adult *Drosophila* testis is shaped as a long coiled tube (Fig. 11.1). The male germline stem cells are located at the apical tip of the testis. As the germ cells initiate differentiation, they are displaced away from the testis tip. The stages of spermatogenesis leading to meiosis are displayed roughly in developmental order along the first third of the adult testis, with the early stages at the apical tip and the more advanced moving down along the testis wall (Fig. 11.1). The resulting linear spatial gradient of maturity is reminiscent of the radial spatial gradient of maturity in the mammalian seminiferous tubule (Fig. 11.1) (8). Meiosis normally occurs when *Drosophila* germ cells are about one third of the way down the testis tube. During spermiogenesis, the differentiating spermatids move away from the testis wall and lie with their nuclei toward the base of the testis and their elongating tails extending up through the testis lumen back toward the apical tip. At the base of the testis, the interconnected mature spermatids are individualized and coiled into packets, ready to enter the seminal vesicle, where mature motile sperm are stored. The entire developmental program from the primary spermatogonial cell to mature sperm lasts approximately 250 hours (3) in *Drosophila melanogaster* so that mature sperm are available at or soon after eclosion of the adult fly from the pupal case.

Male germline stem cells in *Drosophila* reside in a structure called the *germinal proliferation center* at the testis apical tip. At the third larval instar stage, there are 16–18 germline stem cells in each testis. By the third day after eclosion, however, only stem cells are maintained per adult testis (9). The stem cells are in close contact with a group of densely packed apical cells that form the central hub (reviewed in Ref. 5). Surrounding the male germline stem cells at the apical tip of the testis are somatically derived cyst progenitor cells that act as stem cells (9,10), giving rise to support cells that accompany the germ cells through the process of differentiation.

Spermatogenesis is initiated when a male germline stem cell divides asymmetrically to produce a new stem cell and a primary spermatogonial cell (Fig. 11.2). The daughter cell that remains in contact with the hub normally retains stem-cell character, wheres the daughter cell displaced away from the hub becomes a primary spermatogonial cell (9). The cyst progenitor cells also divide asymmetrically, giving rise to new cyst progenitor cells and daugh-

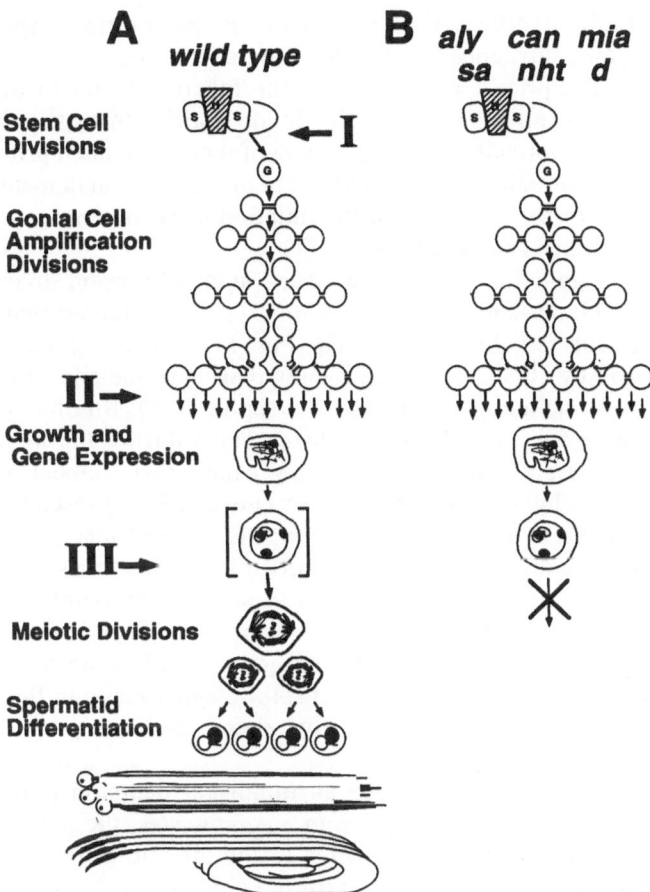

FIGURE 11.2. Phenotype of *Drosophila* meiotic arrest mutants. (A) Major events of wild-type *Drosophila* spermatogenesis. The three major switch points in the development of the male germline are: (I) A stem cell produces the single primary spermatogonial cell by asymmetrical division. The gonial cells then undergo mitotic divisions, producing a cyst of 16 interconnected cells. (II) Onset of the meiotic cell cycle. Premeiotic S occurs early in the 16-cell stage, marking the initiation of meiosis and the primary spermatocyte program of gene expression and cell growth. Note: Only one of the 16 synchronously developing primary spermatocytes is shown. (III) The 16 mature primary spermatocytes exit meiotic prophase and enter the meiotic divisions. Bracket: cell undergoing the G2/M transition of meiosis I. The resulting 64 haploid spermatids then undergo spermatid differentiation. (B) Stages of spermatogenesis in flies mutant for any one of the meiotic arrest genes. Germ cells arrest at the G2/M transition of meiosis I, with partially condensed chromosomes (33). No cells in the meiotic divisions and no stages of spermatid differentiation are visible in the mutant testes. Adapted from (17).

ter cells that initiate differentiation as cyst cells. Each primary spermatogonial cell becomes surrounded by a pair of somatically derived cyst cells (9). Together they comprise a cyst, which is the functional unit of differentiation. The two cyst cells do not normally divide again; rather, they enclose all the mitotic and meiotically derived progeny of their associated primary spermatogonial cell through the entire program of differentiation to mature sperm. The cyst cells express a series of differentiation markers temporally coordinated with the germ cells they enclose (11).

The primary gonial cell undergoes four rounds of mitotic divisions with incomplete cytokinesis to produce a cyst of 16 cells interconnected by stable intercellular bridges called *ring canals* (Fig. 11.2). The ring canals appear to be produced by stabilization of proteins that mark the site of contractile ring formation, including anillin and the septins (12). Similar incomplete cytokinesis and ring canal assembly takes place during the meiotic divisions. At the ultrastructural level, the ring canals that connect mitotically and meiotically related male germ cells in *Drosophila* (1) resemble the ring canals that connect male germ cells in mammals. Intercellular bridges formed during the meiotic divisions may be important in mammalian spermatid cells to ensure that all spermatids have access to products of Y-linked genes and of both alleles of autosomal genes expressed during the haploid stages (13,14). Intercellular bridges between developing germ cells in both mammals and *Drosophila* may also play an important role in synchronizing the events of differentiation in cohorts of mitotically related spermatogonia or meiotically related spermatids.

The 16-cell stage appears to be an important decision point in male germ cell differentiation. In *Drosophila melanogaster*, the germ cells normally cease mitotic division and switch to the meiotic differentiation program at the 16-cell stage. The switch from spermatogonial mitotic amplification to primary spermatocyte growth and gene expression requires wild-type function in the germ cells of at least two *Drosophila* genes; *bag of marbles (bam)* and *benign gonial cell neoplasm (bgcn)*. In males mutant for either *bam* or *bgcn*, spermatogonia continue to undergo the mitotic amplification program, producing cysts of 32, 64, and more interconnected, synchronously dividing cells (15). The 16-cell stage may be a decision point in mammalian spermatogenesis as well. Interconnected Type A spermatogonial cells appear to pause mitotic proliferation at the 16-cell stage before resuming mitotic amplification divisions to produce the large number of mitotically related spermatogonia characteristic of mammals (see Chap. 5 this volume).

The decision to stop mitotic division and initiate the terminal differentiation program of meiosis in *Drosophila* also involves signals from the somatic cyst cells. Wild-type function of *schnurri* and *punt*, which are both known components of the TGF-β signaling pathway, is necessary within the cyst cells for the germ cells they enclose to enter meiosis (16). The pathway connecting *schnurri* and *punt* function in the somatic cyst cells and *bam* and *bgcn* function in the germ cells to regulate the switch from spermatogonia to primary spermatocyte in *Drosophila* has not yet been elucidated (see Ref. 17 for a more detailed discussion). If *Drosophila* cyst cells are the functional equivalent of Sertoli cells in mammals, it may be that Sertoli cells play an analogous role in regulating crucial transitions in germ-cell differentiation in mammals.

The 16 germ cells within a late spermatogonial *Drosophila* cyst initiate meiosis synchronously with premeiotic DNA replication, then enter an extended (90-hour) G2 phase comprising meiotic prophase (Fig. 11.2). Meiotic prophase in *Drosophila* is unusual in that there is no recombination, synaptonemal complex formation, or the classic chromosomal events that normally allow meiotic prophase to be staged. Male germ cells in *Drosophila* undergo dramatic growth during the extended G2 period of meiotic prophase, as in mammals (18,19). Primary spermatocytes mature to their maximum volume during this time. As in mice, the primary spermatocyte period lasts for approximately one third of the total time required for the entire process of spermatogenesis: In *Drosophila,* the primary spermatocyte phase lasts 3.5 of the total of 10 days, whereas the primary spermatocyte period lasts 11 out of the total of 36 days required for completion of the entire program in mice.

During the extended G2 period of meiotic prophase, the growing primary spermatocytes within the cyst undergo a period of robust gene expression. At the completion of meiotic prophase, mature primary spermatocytes in *Drosophila* shut down most transcription (7,20). It is crucial, therefore, that the G2/M transition of meiosis I is delayed long enough to allow the accumulation of all of the transcripts required for the progression of meiosis and postmeiotic differentiation. Although transcription of many spermatid differentiation genes occurs during the primary spermatocyte growth period, translation of the resulting messages often does not take place until after meiosis (21), which suggests that translational control is an important mechanism for timing expression of gene products during differentiation in *Drosophila* spermatogenesis. Translational control also plays an important role in regulating the timing of gene expression during spermatogenesis in mammals (22). For example, the expression of a protamine of mice is delayed until elongating spermatid stages by a translational control mechanism that acts through sequences in the 3'UTR of the mRNA (23). If expression of the protamine protein is forced to occur in round spermatids, the germ-cell nuclei condense prematurely and spermatogenesis is disrupted (24).

The 16 mature primary spermatocytes proceed through the two meiotic divisions in synchrony, producing a cyst of 64 interconnected haploid round spermatids (Fig. 11.2). Elongated spermatids are formed by a series of dramatic morphological changes, including fusion and remodeling of the mitochondria (25,26), flagellar elongation, and microtubule-based nuclear shaping (reviewed in Refs. 3,5). Each of the 64 interconnected spermatids is ultimately tightly invested in its own plasma membrane, and much of the cytoplasm is displaced into a waste bag by a head-to-tailward progression of a novel actin-based structure—the investment cone (27,28), which produces individualized mature sperm.

The Primary Spermatocyte
Program of Gene Expression

In *Drosophila*, most of the genes required for the meiotic divisions and postmeiotic spermatid morphogenesis are transcribed in primary spermatocytes during the extended G2 period corresponding to meiotic prophase. Many genes transcribed at this time are expressed only during the spermatocyte stage and not expressed in any other cell type of the developing organism (reviewed in Ref. 5). Many other genes that are more widely expressed employ testis-specific promoters for expression in primary spermatocytes. Similar extensive transcription of genes required for meiosis and postmeiotic morphogenesis takes place during the primary spermatocyte period in mice (reviewed in Refs. 6,19). In mice, as in *Drosophila*, many genes are expressed in primary spermatocytes from novel, spermatocyte specific promotors (29–31). In both flies and mice, several testis-specific transcripts have been shown to have *cis*-acting sequences that confer testis expression on the gene (and/or reporter constructs) that are situated very close to the promoter region, and in some cases within 100 base pairs of the transcription start site. The mouse *lactate dehydrogenase-c* promoter (31) and the fly *beta-2 tubulin* promoter (32) are two examples of genes with promoter-proximal testis-specific *cis*-regulatory sequences. The similar unusual characteristics of the primary spermatocyte gene expression program in mice and flies raises the question of whether primary spermatocytes utilize novel mechanisms to regulate transcription that might be conserved from insects to mammals.

Genes That Coordinately Regulate Meiotic Cell
Cycle Progression and Spermatid Differentiation

We are utilizing the *Drosophila* system to investigate the mechanisms that regulate expression of spermatid differentiation genes in primary spermatocytes. One striking result of our findings to date is that progression of the meiotic cell cycle through the G2/M transition of meiosis I is coordinately regulated with expression of spermatid differentiation genes.

Progression of the meiotic cell cycle and onset of spermatid differentiation during *Drosophila* male gametogenesis are coordinately controlled by the action of several meiotic arrest genes. Loss of function of *always early (aly)*, *cannonball (can)*, *meiosis I arrest (mia)*, or *spermatocyte arrest (sa)*

(33), or any of at least four additional genes, including *no hitter (nht)* and *d* (Hiller, MacQueen, Moreno, White-Cooper, and Wood, personal communication), results in cell cycle arrest at the G2/M transition of meiosis I and failure of spermatid differentiation (Fig. 11.2B). In testis from males mutant for any one of these genes, cells at the early stages of spermatogenesis are present and appear normal. Mature primary spermatocytes with partially condensed chromatin, however, accumulate to fill the testis, and no cells in meiotic division and no cells in the spermatid differentiation stages are visible (33). The meiotic arrest mutants characterized to date appear to have no effect on viability or female fertility, suggesting that the genetic pathway they define is required only in males.

Analysis of gene expression in mutant spermatocytes revealed that *aly, can, mia,* and *sa* are needed for normal transcription in primary spermatocytes of several spermatid differentiation genes (34). Most of these target genes, including but not limited to *fuzzy onion, Mst87F, Mst84D, Mst98C, janB,* and *don juan,* are involved in postmeiotic spermatid differentiation (34). One of the target genes, *fuzzy onion,* encodes a novel GTPase that mediates mitochondrial fusion in early postmeiotic spermatids (26). The *Mst87F, Mst84D,* and *Mst98C* genes encode sperm tail components (35,36). *don juan* is a component of the sperm tail, but it may also associate with chromatin in sperm heads (37). Although the exact function of *janB* is currently unknown, the *janB* message is transcribed in primary spermatocytes, but it is not translated until days after completion of the meiotic divisions (38).

Analysis of effects of the meiotic arrest mutants on expression of a number of genes normally transcribed in primary spermatocytes led to a model for the wild-type function of the genes during spermatogenesis (34, Fig. 11.3). *can, mia, sa, nht* and *d,* appear to act together or in a pathway to turn on normal levels of transcription in primary spermatocytes of a set of spermatid differentiation genes. *Aly* appears to act at a different point in the pathway, because the wild-type function of *aly* is also needed for transcription in primary spermatocytes of several genes required for meiotic cell cycle progression. Although they play an important role in regulated transcription of spermatid differentiation genes, *aly, can, mia,* and *sa* are not needed for general transcription in spermatocytes: Transcripts from many nonspermatocyte specific genes are expressed normally in spermatocytes from the mutant testes.

The *aly* gene appears to act upstream or in parallel with *can, mia,* and *sa* because all transcripts identified to date that require *can, mia,* and *sa* for normal levels of transcription also require *aly.* Wild-type function of *aly* may directly or indirectly regulate the expression or activity of *can, mia, sa, nht,* or *d.* On the other hand, *aly* may directly act as or be indirectly responsible for a cofactor that acts with *can, mia, sa, nht,* or *d* to regulate transcription of target genes.

Wild-type function of *can, mia, sa, nht,* and *d* are also required for progression of the meiotic cell cycle through the G2/M transition of meiosis I (33). Analysis of expression of the cell cycle phosphatase *twine,* the cdc25 homologue that triggers the G2/M transition of meiosis I, suggested a mecha-

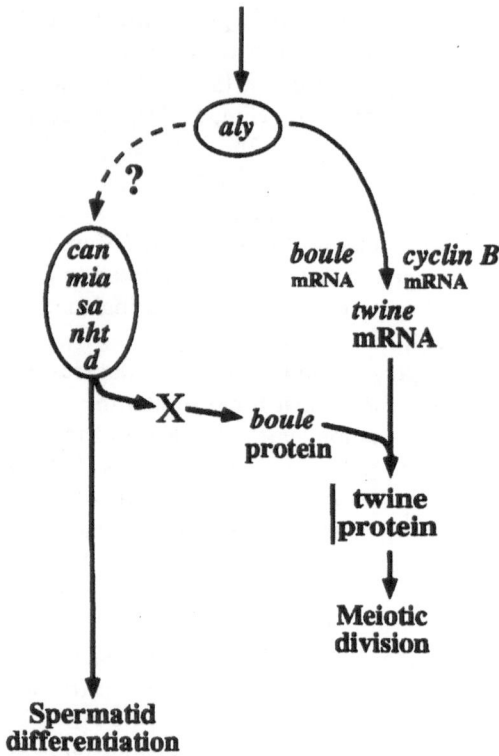

FIGURE 11.3. Model for the role of the meiotic arrest genes in coordinating meiotic divisions with spermatid differentiation. The products of the *can*, *mia*, *sa*, *nht*, and *d* genes act together or in a pathway to activate transcription of a set of target genes required for spermatid differentiation. At least one of these target genes (denoted by X) is required for the translation or stabilization of the *boule* protein (Cheng and Wasserman, personal communication), which is a *Drosophila* homolog of the human *Deleted in Azoospermia (DAZ)* protein (39). The *boule* protein is required for expression of normal levels of the *twine* protein (40), which is a cell-cycle phosphatase that activates the *cdc2/cyclin* kinase to allow the G2/M transition of meiosis I. This cross-regulatory arm of the pathway thus acts to ensure that spermatocytes do not progress through the G2/M transition of meiosis I until the *can-*, *mia-*, *sa-*, *nht-* and *d*-dependent transcription of genes required for spermatid differentiation has been turned on. *aly* appears to act upstream, possibly through *can*, *mia*, *sa*, *nht*, and *d*, to regulate the spermatid differentiation pathway. Wild-type function of *aly* is also required for transcription of the cell cycle control genes *twine*, *cyclin B*, and *boule* in primary spermatocytes. Adapted with permission from (34).

nism by which wild-type function of the *can*, *mia*, *sa*, *nht*, and *d* genes might control cell cycle progression. Although the *twine* mRNA was expressed normally in *can*, *mia*, and *sa* mutant testes, a *twine-lacZ* reporter fusion protein was not expressed, which indicates a requirement for the *can*, *mia*, and *sa* functions for the accumulation of *twine* protein (34). We have postulate that one or more of the target genes regulated by *can*, *mia*, and *sa* is required for the translation of *twine* and perhaps other critical gene products needed for the G2/M transition of meiosis I (indicated by the cross bar in Fig. 11.3). This cross-regulatory mechanism would thus ensure that spermatocytes cannot enter G2/M transition of meiosis I until they have received information that transcription of spermatid differentiation genes has initiated successfully.

One likely component of this cross-regulatory mechanism is the *Drosophila boule* gene, which encodes a homolog of the human DAZ gene implicated in azoospermia in man. The *boule* and *DAZ* genes encode homologous proteins with conserved domains suggestive of RNA binding activity (39). Wild-type function of *boule* is required for accumulation of normal levels of the *twine-lacZ* fusion protein, but not for accumulation of *twine* mRNA (40). Furthermore, exogenous expression of *twine* protein in primary spermatocytes from a chimeric message in which the 5' and 3' UTRs of the *twine* transcript were replaced with those of the *Beta2-tubulin* gene partially rescued the meiotic arrest phenotype of *boule* mutants (40). These data suggest that *boule* may act to allow the G2/M transition of meiosis I by alleviating translational repression of the *twine* message. Expression of *boule* protein is itself under control of the meiotic arrest genes. The *boule* mRNA does not accumulate in spermatocytes from males mutant for *aly*. *boule* mRNA accumulates normally in spermatocytes from males mutant for *can*, *mia*, or *sa* (34). Accumulation of the *boule* protein, however, requires wild-type function of at least *sa* and *mia* (Cheng and Wasserman, personal communication).

Our work on the meiotic arrest genes of *Drosophila* has revealed outlines of the genetic circuitry that regulates and coordinates primary spermatocyte gene expression, meiotic cell cycle progression and spermatid differentiation in *Drosophila*. To elucidate the molecular mechanisms that underlie this coordinate regulation we are cloning the *aly*, *can*, and *nht* genes.

One goal of future work will be to determine if the genetic circuitry that regulates spermatogenesis in *Drosophila* is conserved and important in regulating male germ-cell differentiation in mammals. Two observations suggest that this may indeed be so: the finding that expression of *boule*, the *Drosophila* homolog of DAZ, is regulated by the meiotic arrest genes (discussed earlier) and the comparison of the *Drosophila* meiotic arrest mutant phenotype with the clinical description of meiosis I maturation arrest in man.

The phenotype of meiotic arrest mutants in flies bears striking resemblance to the clinical description of a human male infertility syndrome, meiosis I maturation arrest. Approximately 15% of couples attempting to conceive are infertile, and one third to one half of these cases can be attributable to the male partner (41,42). Approximately 3–4% of male infertility cases are due to defects in sperm production (43,44), ranging from oligozoospermia, which is a reduction in sperm count, to azoospermia, which is a total absence of sperm in semen. Testicular biopsies revealed that nearly half of the cases of infertile men with azoospermia were associated with a pathology described as meiosis I maturation arrest (45–47). Testicular biopsies of patients with meiosis I maturation arrest showed a cytological pathology similar to the phenotype of *Drosophila* meiotic arrest mutants. The early stages of spermatogenesis were typically abundant and appeared normal, but postmeiotic stages of spermatogenesis were absent (48). Instead, mature primary spermatocytes with abnormal, partially condensed chromatin accumulate in the testis. The similarities between the clinical features of meiosis I maturation arrest in humans and the phenotype of mutants in meiotic arrest genes in flies suggest a possible genetic basis for the human syndrome. Our results, that recessive mutations in at least eight and probably several more autosomal genes in *Drosophila* can lead to the meiotic arrest phenotype are consistent with a relatively high frequency of occurrence of the phenotype among infertile human males.

Acknowledgments. We are grateful to members of the Fuller Lab, past and present, for stimulating discussions. This work was supported by NICHD research grant 1R01-HD32936 to M.T.F. T.-Y. L. was supported by NIGMS Medical Scientist Training Program 5 T32 GM07365-24. M. J. P. is supported by a Human Genome Fellowship Training Grant NIH/NRSA 5 T32 GM07790.

References

1. Tates AD. Cytodifferentiation during spermatogenesis in *Drosophila melanogaster*: an electron microscope study. Rijksuniversiteit: Leiden, 1971.
2. Stanley HP, Bowman JT, Romrell LJ, Reed SC, Wilkinson RF. Fine structure of normal spermatid differentiation in *Drosophila melanogaster*. J Ultrastruct Res 1972;41:433–66.
3. Lindsley D, Tokuyasu KT. Spermatogenesis. In: Ashburner M, Wright TRF, eds. Genetics and biology of *Drosophila*; second ed. New York: Academic Press, 1980:225–94.
4. Cenci G, Bonaccorsi S, Pisano C, Verni F, Gatti M. Chromatin and microtubule organization during premeiotic, meiotic and early postmeiotic stages of *Drosophila melanogaster* spermatogenesis. J Cell Sci 1994;107:3521–34.
5. Fuller MT. Spermatogenesis. In: Bate M, Martinez-Arias A, ed. The development of drosophila, Vol. 1. Cold Spring Harbor: Cold Spring Harbor Laboratory Press, 1993:712–147.
6. Hecht NB. Gene expression during male germ cell development. In: Desjardins C, Ewing LL, eds. Cell and molecular biology of the testis. New York: Oxford University Press; 1993:400–32.
7. Gould-Somero M, Holland L. The timing of RNA synthesis for spermiogenesis in organ cultures of *Drosophila melanogaster* testes. Wilhelm Roux' Arch 1974;174: 133–48.
8. Niederberger CS, Lamb DJ. Spermatogenesis in the adult. In: Lipshultz LI, Howards SS, eds. Infertility in the male. St. Louis: Mosby-Year Book, 1997:106–22.
9. Hardy RW, Tokuyasu KT, Lindsley DL, Garavito M. The germinal proliferation center in the testis of *Drosophila melanogaster*. J Ultrastruct Res 1979;69: 180–90.

10. Gönczy P, DiNardo S. The germline regulates somatic cyst cell proliferation and fate during *Drosophila* spermatogenesis. Development 1996;122:2437–47.

11. Gönczy P, Viswanathan S, DiNardo S. Probing spermatogenesis in *Drosophila* with P-element enhancer detectors. *Development* 1992;114:89–98.

12. Hime GR, Brill JA, Fuller MT. Assembly of ring canals in the male germline from structural components of the contractile ring. J Cell Sci 1996;109:2779–88.

13. Braun RE, Behringer RR, Peschon JJ, Brinster RL, Palmiter RD. Genetically haploid spermatids are phenotypically diploid. Nature 1989;337:373–76.

14. Caldwell KA, Handel MA. Protamine transcript sharing among postmeiotic spermatids. Proc Natl Acad Sci USA 1991;88:2407–11.

15. Gönczy P, Matunis E, DiNardo S. *bag-of-marbles* and *benign gonia cell neoplasm* act in the germline to restrict proliferation during *Drosophila* spermatogenesis. Development 1997;124:4361–71.

16. Matunis E, Tran J, Gonczy P, Caldwell K, DiNardo S. *punt* and *schnurri* regulate a somatically derived signal that restricts proliferation of committed progenitors in the germline. Development 1997;124:4383–91.

17. Fuller MT. Genetic control of cell proliferation and differentiation in *Drosophila* spermatogenesis. In: Bellve AR ed. The male germ cell: migration to fertilization. Cell Dev Biol 1998;9:433–44.

18. de Kretzer DM, Kerr JB. The cytology of the testis. In: Knobil E, Neill JD, eds. The physiology of reproduction. New York: Raven Press, 1998:837–932.

19. Handel MA. Genetic control of spermatogenesis in mice. In: Hennig W, ed. Spermatogenesis: genetic aspects, Vol. 15. Berlin:Springer-Verlag, 1987:1–62.

20. Olivieri G, Olivieri A. Autoradiographic study of nucleic acid synthesis during spermatogenesis in *Drosophila melanogaster*. Mutat Res 1965;2:366–80.

21. Schafer M, Nayernia K, Engel W, Schafer U. Translational control in spermatogenesis. Dev Biol 1995;172:344–52.

22. Braun RE. Post-transcriptional control of gene expression during spermatogenesis. In: Bellve A ed. The male germ cell: migration to fertilization, Vol. 9. London: Academic Press, 1998:483–89.

23. Braun RE, Peschon JJ, Behringer RR, Brinster RL, Palmiter RD. Protamine 3′ untranslated sequences regulate temporal translational control and subcellular localization of growth hormone in spermatids of transgenic mice. Genes Dev 1989;3:793–802.

24. Lee K, Haugen HS, Clegg CH, Braun RE. Premature translation of protamine 1 mRNA causes precocious nuclear condensation and arrests spermatid differentiation in mice. Proc Nat Acad Sci USA 1995;92:12451–55.

25. Tokuyasu KT. Dynamics of spermiogenesis in *Drosophila melanogaster*. VI. Significance of "onion" nebenkern formation. J Ultrastruct Res 1975;53:93–112.

26. Hales KG, Fuller MT. Developmentally regulated mitochondrial fusion mediated by a conserved novel predicted GTPase. Cell 1997;90:121–29.

27. Tokuyasu KT, Peacock WJ, Hardy RW. Dynamics of spermiogenesis in *Drosophila melanogaster*. I. Individualization process. Z Zellforsch Mikrosk Anat 1972;124:479–506.

28. Fabrizio JJ, Hime G, Lemmon SK, Bazinet C. Genetic dissection of sperm individualization in *Drosophila melanogaster*. Development 1998;125:1833–43.

29. Willison K, Ashworth A. Mammalian spermatogenic gene expression. Trend Gen 1987;3:351–55.

30. Goldberg E. Transcriptional regulatory strategies in male germ cells. J Androl 1996;17:628–32.

31. Zhou W, Goldberg E. A dual-function palindromic sequence regulates testis-specific transcription of the mouse *lactate dehydrogenase c* gene *in vitro*. Biol Reprod 1996;54:84–90.
32. Michiels F, Gasch A, Kaltschmidt B, Renkawitz-Pohl R. A 14 bp promoter element directs the testis specificity of the *Drosophila* β2-tubulin gene. EMBO J 1989; 8:1559–65.
33. Lin T, Visvanathan S, Wood C, Wilson PG, Wolf N, Fuller MT. Coordinate developmental control of the meiotic cell cycle and spermatid differentiation in *Drosophila* males. Development 1996;122:1331–41.
34. White-Cooper H, Schafer MA, Alphey LS, Fuller MT. Transcriptional and post-transcriptional control mechanisms coordinate the onset of spermatid differentiation with meiosis I in *Drosophila*. Development 1998;125:125–34.
35. Kuhn R, Schafer U, Schafer M. Cis-acting regions sufficient for spermatocyte-specific transcriptional and spermatid-specific translational control of the *Drosophila melanogaster* gene *mst(3)gl-9*. EMBO J 1988; 7:447–54.
36. Schafer M, Borsch D, Hulster A, Schafer U. Expression of a gene duplication encoding conserved sperm tail proteins is translationally regulated in *Drosophila melanogaster*. Mol Cell Biol 1993;13:1708–18.
37. Santel A, Winhauer T, Blümer N, Renkawitz-Pohl R. The *Drosophila don juan* (*dj*) gene encodes a novel sperm specific protein component characterised by an unusual domain for repetitive amino acid motif. Mech Dev 1997;64:19–30.
38. Yanicostas C, Lepesant JA. Transcriptional and translational cis-regulatory sequences of the spermatocyte-specific *Drosophila janusB* gene are located in the 3′ exonic region of the overlapping *janusA* gene. Mol Gen Genet 1990;224:450–58.
39. Eberhart CG, Maines JZ, Wasserman SA. Meiotic cell cycle requirement for a fly homologue of human *Deleted in Azoospermia*. Nature 1996;381:783–85.
40. Maines JZ, Wasserman SA. Post-transcriptional regulation of the meiotic Cdc25 protein twine by the DAZ orthologue Boule. Nat Cell Biol 1999;1:171–74.
41. de Kretser DM. Male infertility. Lancet 1997;349:787–90.
42. World Health Organization. Towards more objectivity in diagnosis and management of male infertility. Int J Androl 1997;7(Suppl.):1–53.
43. van Zyl JA, Menkveld R, van Kotze TJ, Retief AE, van Niekerk WA. Oligospermia: a seven-year survey of the incidence, chromosomal aberrations, treatment and pregnancy rate. Int J Fertil 1975;20:129–32.
44. Hull MG, Glazener CM, Kelly NJ, Conway DI, Foster PA, Hinton RA, et al. Population study of causes, treatment, and outcome of infertility. Br Med J 1985; 291:1693–97.
45. Wong TW, Straus FH, Warner NE. Testicular biopsy in the study of male infertility. Arch Pathol 1973;95:151–59.
46. Colgan TJ, Bedard YC, Strawbridge TG, Buckspan MB, Klotz PG. Reappraisal of the value of testicular biopsy in the investigation of infertility. Fertil Steril 1980;33:56–60.
47. Meyer JM, Maetz JL, Rumpler Y. Cellular relationship impairment in maturation arrest of human spermatogenesis: an ultrastructural study. Histopathology 1992; 21:25–33.
48. Soderstrom K-O, Suominen M. Histopathology and ultrastructure of meiotic arrest in human spermatogenesis. Arch Pathol Lab Med 1980;104:476–82.

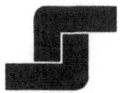

12

HSP70 Chaperones in Spermatogenesis

EDWARD M. EDDY, WILLIAM D. WILLIS,
KIYOSHI MIKI, AND CHISATO MORI

HSP70 Proteins of Spermatogenic Cells

The HSP70 heat-shock proteins serve as molecular chaperones that assist other proteins as they undergo folding, transport, and assembly into multiprotein complexes within cells (1–3). There are at least seven HSP70 proteins present in spermatogenic cells, including GRP78, which is present within the endoplasmic reticulum (4), and GRP75, which is found within mitochondria (5). Most HSP70 proteins, however, are located within the cytoplasm. They include constitutively expressed HSC70 (6,7), stress-induced HSP70-1 and HSP70-3 (8–10), and two members of this family, HSP70-2 and HSC70T, found only within spermatogenic cells.

Expression of the Hsp70-2 *Gene*

Northern blot studies indicate that the *Hsp70-2* gene is expressed at significant levels only in spermatogenic cells (11,12). The *Hsp70-2* transcript is abundant in pachytene spermatocytes and round spermatids, and is first detected by northern analysis in the testes of juvenile mice on day 10 (12). This coincides with the earliest appearance of leptotene spermatocytes that occurs during the nearly synchronous first wave of spermatogenesis in prepubertal mice (13). In situ hybridization studies indicated that *Hsp70-2* transcript levels rise above background in leptotene spermatocytes (14). Biosynthetic labeling (15) and immunohistochemical studies (12,14), however, suggested that HSP70-2 protein synthesis begins in preleptotene spermatocytes. Although the mRNA and protein are present in spermatids (8,9,12), there appears to be little HSP70-2 protein synthesis during the postmeiotic phase (15). In situ studies indicate that *Hsp70-2* transcripts are abundant in pachytene spermatocytes and step 1–7 spermatids, but not detected in step 8–16 spermatids (Mori et al., unpublished observations).

The promoter region responsible for regulating expression of the *Hsp70-2* gene was defined using transgenic mice. It was found that a 640–base pair promoter fragment, but not a 318–base pair promoter fragment, was sufficient to direct expression of a bacterial β-galactosidase reporter gene in preleptotene spermatocytes (14). This strongly suggested that the *cis* regulatory elements necessary for cell type–specific and stage-specific expression of the *Hsp70-2* gene are within 640 base pairs of the translation start site (14). Further analysis by band shift assays indicated that expression of this gene is probably regulated by transcription factors that bind to two promoter regions approximately 360 and 80 base pairs from the translation start codon (Gotoh and Eddy, unpublished observations).

Expression of the Hsc70t *Gene*

Northern blot analysis indicated that *Hsc70t* transcripts are present at significant levels only in spermatogenic cells and are not found until the postmeiotic phase of spermatogenesis (16,17). This was confirmed by in situ hybridization, with *Hsc70t* mRNA being seen first in round spermatids of adult mice (18). Transcripts were also detected first by northern analysis in testes of 22-day-old juvenile mice (Willis, Miki, and Eddy, unpublished observations) soon after round spermatid development begins (13). HSC70T protein, however, was not found until the appearance of elongated spermatids (18; Willis, Miki, and Eddy, unpublished observations). This indicates that HSC70T, like several others proteins synthesized in postmeiotic germ cells (19) is under translational control, which results in a delay between transcription and synthesis of the protein (18).

Roles of HSP70-2 Protein

Targeted Gene Disruption

The specificity of the cell type and the stage of germ cell development when the protein is produced led to the hypothesis that HSP70-2 is a chaperone essential for the process of meiosis. When this was tested using the gene knockout approach, it was found that male mice homozygous for a mutation that disrupted the gene (*Hsp70-2*[-/-]) were infertile (20). Female *Hsp70-2*[-/-] mice were fertile, however, indicating that the protein is not required during oogenesis. No other effects of the mutation were seen, which is consistent with prior findings that the *Hsp70-2* gene is expressed at significant levels only in spermatogenic cells (12,14). Further analysis determined that infertility occurred in *Hsp70-2*[-/-] males because spermatocytes failed to complete meiosis and underwent apoptosis. Testis weight was less than one half that in wild-type males, postmeiotic germ cells were rare, and spermatozoa were not present in the epididymis (20; Mori et al., unpublished observations).

Disruption of Desynapsis

The synaptonemal complex (SC) forms during the zygotene phase of meiotic prophase between each pair of homologous chromosomes as they synapse in spermatocytes and oocytes (21). The SCs are composed of two lateral elements connected by transverse filaments and a ladderlike central element. They persist throughout pachytene spermatocyte development, which is a period of approximately 1 week in the mouse, and then separate and disassemble at the end of the diplotene stage as the homologous chromosomes desynapse and condense in preparation for the first meiotic division. HSP70-2 is present in the lateral elements of the SC and in the attachment plaques that anchor the ends of the chromosomes to the nuclear envelope in spermatocytes (7,20). The SCs form in zygotene spermatocytes of *Hsp70-2$^{-/-}$* mice, but fragment in diplotene spermatocytes rather than undergo disassembly (7,20). These findings indicate that HSP70-2 is required either directly or indirectly for desynapsis. One hypothesis suggested by these results is that HSP70-2 is a structural component of the SC, with its absence destabilizing the SC and leaving it prone to fragmentation before desynapsis can occur.

An alternate hypothesis is that HSP70-2 is a chaperone required for the orderly disassembly of the SC, with this process failing in the absence of HSP70-2. Synaptonemal complex 1 (SCP1) protein is present in the transverse filaments of the SC, and this protein has a domain in the carboxy-terminal portion that is a potential target site for phosphorylation by the Cdc2 kinase (22,23). Phosphorylation can lead to disassembly of protein complexes (24), and lack of Cdc2 kinase activity (see later) could alter disassembly of the SC. An additional hypothesis is that HSP70-2 chaperone activity is required to form complexes of proteins associated with the SC that are involved in DNA recombination and repair. Such proteins include recombinase A homologue 51 (RAD51), MutL homologue 1 (MLH1), putative mutS-related protein 2 (PMS2), DNA topoisomerase II, breast cancer-associated protein 1 (BRCA1), mutated in ataxiatelangiectasia (ATM), ATM-related (ATR), polymerase β, and ubiquitin-conjugating enzyme 9 (UBC9) (25, and references therein). Failure of such proteins to form functional complexes could alter their interactions with the SC, the SC and DNA loops that attach to the SC, or with the SC and other proteins of the nuclear matrix involved in SC integrity, thereby destabilizing the SC (26).

Disruption of Meiosis

The process of meiosis begins after completion of the last DNA synthesis associated with chromosome duplication (S phase of the cell cycle) in preleptotene spermatocytes. During meiotic prophase (G2 phase of the cell cycle), the homologous chromosomes synapse in zygotene spermatocytes, recombine in pachytene spermatocytes, and desynapse in diplotene spermatocytes. This is followed by two meiotic divisions (M phase of the cell cycle) that occur in rapid succession to produce haploid spermatids. Spermatogenesis fails in $Hsp70-2^{-/-}$ mice at the G2 to M-phase transition (20). This transition in other cells is known to require the activity of a protein kinase, consisting of a dimer of a catalytic subunit (Cdc2) and a regulatory subunit (cyclin B) (27). Cdc2 acquires kinase activity by undergoing changes in phosphorylation prior to and during dimerization with cyclin B. The highest concentration of cyclin B1 in the mouse testis is in pachytene spermatocytes and Cdc2 kinase activity is present mainly in pachytene spermatocytes (28). This suggests that Cdc2 kinase activity enables pachytene spermatocytes to progress from the G2 to the M-phase of meiosis.

Because of the failure of the G2 to M-phase transition in spermatocytes, it was hypothesized that HSP70-2 is a chaperone involved in Cdc2-cyclin B1 assembly required for Cdc2 activation (29). It was found that both Cdc2 and cyclin B1 are present in homogenates of testis from $Hsp70-2^{-/-}$ mice, and that HSP70-2 associates with Cdc2, but not with cyclin B1 or the Cdc2-cyclin B1 complex. This suggested that HSP70-2 is a chaperone for Cdc2, but not for cyclin B1. It was also determined that the Cdc2 in the testis of $Hsp70-2^{-/-}$ mice lacks kinase activity and does not undergo the changes in phosphorylation seen in wild-type mice (29). Addition of recombinant HSP70-2 protein to a homogenate of testis from $Hsp70-2^{-/-}$ mice resulted in assembly of the Cdc2-cyclin B1 heterodimer and in Cdc2 becoming an active kinase. These results supported the hypothesis that HSP70-2 is a chaperone for Cdc2 and further suggested that their interaction allows Cdc2 to acquire the appropriate conformation to heterodimerize with cyclin B1, leading to the development of Cdc2 kinase activity. The absence of this activity in $Hsp70-2^{-/-}$ mice appears to be a major cause of failure to complete the G2 to M-phase transition at the end of meiotic prophase.

Apoptosis

Another effect of the $Hsp70-2$ gene knockout was that it caused most spermatogenic cells to undergo apoptosis at the end of meiotic prophase (20). The nuclei of late spermatocytes were often found to have highly condensed chromatin suggestive of apoptosis. Further evidence of apoptosis was seen using the TUNEL method (terminal deoxynucleotidyl transferase-mediated dUTP biotin nick end labeling) on histology sections. These studies indicated that fragmented DNA was present in the nuclei of many late pachytene spermatocytes in the testis of $Hsp70-2^{-/-}$ mice (20,30,31). In addition, analysis of genomic DNA from the testes of these mice demonstrated the presence of DNA ladders caused by internucleosomal chromatin degradation (20,31), and provided strong evidence that apoptosis was occurring.

Apoptosis is a natural event during spermatogenesis and occurs most frequently in spermatogonia (32,33) where it has been estimated to result in the loss of the majority of the progeny of type A1 spermatogonia (34). To examine the possible role of HSP70-2 in this process, the frequency of apoptosis in spermatogenic cells was compared for *Hsp70-2*-/- and wild-type mice. Apoptosis for both was higher between postnatal days 8 and 22 than at other periods, with most of the cell death occurring in spermatogonia (31). There were no apparent differences between *Hsp70-2*-/- and wild-type mice in the frequency of apoptosis during the first 2 weeks of life; however, the number of apoptotic cells was slightly higher in *Hsp70-2*-/- than in wild-type mice on postnatal day 15, and substantially higher on day 17 (30,31). These results suggest that HSP70-2 may have a minor chaperone role during the middle part of meiotic prophase, but that it is essential for completion of meiotic prophase.

It is unknown if disruption of desynapsis, failure of meiosis, and triggering of apoptosis in spermatocytes are linked or occur independently in the absence of HSP70-2 protein. Heat-shock proteins have been suggested to have integral roles in cell-cycle events and in apoptosis. For example, HSP70 proteins may regulate the cell cycle by interacting with other cellular proteins in a cell-cycle–dependent manner (35), and HSP70 overexpression shortens drug-induced cell-cycle arrest in the G2 phase (36). In addition, even though heat shock and other stresses can trigger apoptosis, increasing HSP70 levels can reduce apoptosis (37,38) and reducing HSP70 expression can enhance apoptosis (39). A hypothesis suggested by these results is that the lack of Cdc2 kinase activity and failure to phosphorylate SCP1 leads to disruption of desynapsis, and failure to phosphorylate other proteins required for the G2 to M-phase transition leads to disruption of meiosis, with these events in turn triggering apoptosis. HSP70-2, however, associates with other proteins in addition to Cdc2 in spermatogenic cells (7). Another hypothesis suggested by these data is that apoptosis is triggered by the failure of at least one other protein to undergo appropriate folding or assembly into complexes in the absence of HSP70-2. Additional studies will be required to determine if one of the hypotheses is correct.

Acrosome Formation

Most late spermatocytes in *Hsp70-2*-/- mice undergo apoptosis, but it was found that a few undergo the first and sometimes the second meiotic division and begin acrosome formation (Mori et al., unpublished observations). It was initially observed that cells with an acrosomelike structure were occasionally present in sections of testes of juvenile and adult *Hsp70-2*-/- mice. To determine if these structures were acrosomes, sections were stained with the periodic acid-Schiff (PAS) reagent. This histochemical reagent is commonly used to stain acrosomes to define the steps of spermatid development (40,41) and the structures were found to be PAS positive. They were also found to immunostain with monoclonal antibody MN7, which has been shown to be specific for acrosomes (42,43). These structures were confirmed to be acrosomes by electron microscopy and some of the cells containing them had condensing nuclei typical of step 8–9 spermatids. The nucleus and cell body of acrosome-containing cells in *Hsp70-2^{-/-}* mice were often larger and usually had twice as much DNA as did spermatids in wild-type mice. In addition, meiotic metaphase I and II chromosome spreads were observed at low frequency in spermatogenic cells from *Hsp70-2^{-/-}* mice. These results indicated that a few spermatocytes in *Hsp70-2^{-/-}* mice undergo one or sometimes two meiotic divisions and begin acrosome formation and nuclear condensation. They also indicate that completion of meiosis is not essential for initiation of acrosome formation (Mori et al., unpublished observations).

Spermatid development without the completion of meiosis also occurs in *Drosophila* with mutations in *cdc2* (44,45) or *twine*, a Cdc25 homologue (46,47). Cdc25 is a protein phosphatase that participates in activation of the Cdc2 kinase at the G2 to M-phase transition of the cell cycle (48). The spermatogenic cells in mutant flies undergo flagellar elongation and changes in nuclear shape and condensation typical of spermatid differentiation. This is of particular interest because of the finding that Cdc2 kinase activity is lacking in spermatocytes of *Hsp70-2^{-/-}* mice; however, there is a significant difference between initiation of spermatid development in mutant flies and in *Hsp70-2^{-/-}* mice. Both meiotic divisions are bypassed in mutant flies, whereas one or two meiotic divisions may occur in *Hsp70-2^{-/-}* mice. Nevertheless, mouse cells without Cdc2 activity can be coaxed from G2 into mitosis in vitro by treatment with exogenous phosphatase inhibitors, which suggests that other kinases may function during the G2 to M-phase of the cell cycle (49). In that case other kinases of *Hsp70-2^{-/-}* mice might compensate for the absence of Cdc2 kinase activity in an occasional spermatocyte and allow that cell to progress through one or two meiotic divisions.

Role of the HSC70T Protein

A monoclonal antibody developed against a spermatogenic cell protein extracted from two-dimensional polyacrylamide gels recognized a protein highly similar by electrophoretic mobility, isoelectric point, western blotting, and ATP-binding characteristics to HSC70 (6). The protein was detected only in postmeiotic germ cells and was labeled biosynthetically in spermatids cultured in the presence of [³⁵S]methionine. The antibody was used to isolate cDNA clones that were found to be identical in sequence to *Hsc70t* (Willis, Miki, and Eddy, unpublished observations), a member of the HSP70 family in the mouse whose mRNA is present only in spermatids (16). An antibody to a deduced peptide sequence in HSP70T was specific for testis by western blotting and detected HSC70T by immunohistochemistry only in condensing spermatids (Willis, Miki, and Eddy, unpublished observations); however, the mRNA was detected in testes from 22-day old mice, when the developmentally most advanced germ cells are round spermatids (13). This indicates that *Hsc70t* is subject to translational regulation (Willis, Miki, and Eddy, unpublished observations) and confirms another report (18).

The specificity of cell type and the stage of germ-cell development when HSP70T is synthesized led to the hypothesis that it is a chaperone for proteins with unique roles during the postmeiotic phase of spermatogenesis. As was done for HSP70-2, this hypothesis was tested using the gene targeting approach to disrupt the *Hsc70t* gene. A genomic clone for *Hsc70t* was isolated and used to engineer a targeting construct, the gene was disrupted in ES cells, and chimeras were produced that transmitted the mutated gene to their offspring. Immunohistochemistry indicated that spermatids of males homozygous for the mutation (*Hsc70t*$^{-/-}$) lacked HSC70T. Postmeiotic germ cell development was not disrupted, however, and mating studies determined that male *Hsc70t*$^{-/-}$ mice were fertile and sired litters of normal size (Willis, Miki, and Eddy, unpublished observations). The process of spermiogenesis appeared to be unaffected in the absence of HSC70T protein by these criteria.

The lack of an apparent effect of this mutation suggests either that another HSP70 protein compensates for the absence of HSC70T protein, or that HSC70T does not have a significant role in the usual events of spermiogenesis. The two other cytoplasmic members of the HSP70 protein family that might compensate for the absence of HSC70T are HSC70, which is constitutively expressed, and HSP70-2, which is synthesized mainly in spermatocytes, but is present in spermatids. The level of HSC70 protein, however, is relatively low in spermatids, and there did not appear to be a compensatory increase in this protein in *Hsc70t*$^{-/-}$ mice. In addition, male *Hsc70t*$^{-/-}$ mice that had only one intact *Hsp70-2* allele and would be predicted to have a reduced level of HSP70-2 protein also had normal fertility (Willis, Miki, and Eddy, unpublished observations). Although disruption of the *Hsc70t* gene does not appear to have overt effects on postmeiotic germ cell development or function, it is hypothesized that postmeiotic germ cells from male *Hsc70t*$^{-/-}$ mice may be more susceptible to damage by stress than those from wild-type mice. Further studies will be necessary to test this hypothesis.

Conclusions

Many genes are expressed in spermatogenic cells that encode unique proteins, are developmentally regulated, and are either transcribed only in male germ cells or produce mRNAs specific to these cells (50,51). It is hypothesized that such genes encode proteins with key structural or functional roles in the successive mitotic, meiotic, and postmeiotic phases of spermatogenesis. Some of these proteins are spermatogenic cell-specific members of protein families, some are products of alternative transcripts produced by cell-specific promoter or exon-utilization processes, and yet others are products of unique genes that are not homologous to genes expressed in other cell types. *Hsp70-2* and *Hsc70t* are members of the HSP70 family and were hypothesized to serve chaperone roles unique to spermatogenic cells. Strong evidence in support of this has been gained for HSP70-2 using gene targeting to disrupt protein production. As was hypothesized, HSP70-2 is a chaperone essential for the process of meiosis. The gene targeting approach, however, has not yet provided insight into the role of HSC70T in postmeiotic germ cells. It remains to be determined if spermatids lacking this protein are more susceptible to damage by heat-shock or other stresses than are spermatids from wild-type mice.

References

1. Georgopoulos C, Welch WJ. Role of the major heat shock proteins as molecular chaperones. Ann Rev Cell Biol 1993;9:601–34.
2. Hendrick JP, Hartl F-U. Molecular chaperone functions of heat-shock proteins. Ann Rev Biochem 1993;62:349–84.
3. Hendrick JP, Hartl F-U. The role of molecular chaperones in protein folding. FASEB J 1995;9:1559–69.
4. Munro S, Pelham HRB. An Hsp70-like protein in the ER: identity with the 78 kd glucose–regulated protein and immunoglobulin heavy chain binding protein. Cell 1986;46:291–300.
5. Mizzen LA, Change C, Garrels J, Welch WJ. Identification, characterization and purification of two mammalian stress proteins present within mitochondria: one related to hsp70 and the other to the bacterial GroEL protein. J Biol Chem 1989;264:20664–75.
6. Maekawa M, O'Brien DA, Allen RL, Eddy EM. Heat-shock cognate protein (hsc71) and related proteins in mouse spermatogenic cells. Biol Reprod 1989;40:843–52.
7. Allen JW, Dix DJ, Collins BW, Merrick BA, He C, Selkirk JK, et al. HSP70-2 is part of the synaptonemal complex in mouse and hamster spermatocytes. Chromosoma 1996;104:414–21.
8. Allen RL, O'Brien DA, Eddy EM. A novel hsp70-like protein (P70) is present in mouse spermatogenic cells. Mol Cell Biol 1988;8:828–32.
9. Allen RL, O'Brien DA, Jones CC, Rockett DL, Eddy EM. Expression of heat shock proteins by isolated mouse spermatogenic cells. Mol Cell Biol 1988;8:3260–66.
10. Sarge KD. Male germ cell-specific alteration in temperature set point of the cellular stress response. J Biol Chem 1995;270:18745–48.
11. Zakeri ZF, Wolgemuth DJ, Hunt CR. Identification and sequence analysis of a new member of the mouse HSP70 gene family and characterization of its unique cellular and developmental pattern of expression in the male germ line. Mol Cell Biol 1988;8:2925–32.
12. Rosario MO, Perkins SL, O'Brien DA, Allen RL, Eddy EM. Identification of the gene for the developmentally expressed 70 kDa heat-shock protein (P70) of mouse spermatogenic cells. Dev Biol 1992;150:1–11.
13. Bellve AR, Cavicchia JC, Millette CF, O'Brien DA, Bhatnagar YM, Dym M. Spermatogenic cells of the prepubertal mouse: isolation and morphological characterization. J Cell Biol 1977;74:68–85.
14. Dix DJ, Rosario-Herrle M, Gotoh H, Mori C, Goulding EH, Barrett CV, et al. Developmentally regulated expression of *Hsp70-2* and a *Hsp70-2/lacZ* transgene during spermatogenesis. Dev Biol 1996;174:310–21.

15. O'Brien DA. Stage-specific protein synthesis by isolated spermatogenic cells throughout meiosis and early spermiogenesis in the mouse. Biol Reprod 1987;37;147–57.
16. Matsumoto M, Fujimoto H. Cloning of a *hsp70*-related gene expressed in mouse spermatids. Biochem Biophys Res Commun 1990;166:43–49.
17. Matsumoto M, Kurata S, Fujimoto H, Hoshi M. Haploid specific activations of protamine 1 and hsc70t genes in mouse spermatogenesis. Biochem Biophys Acta 1993;1174:274–78.
18. Tsunekawa N, Matsumoto M, Tone S, Nishida T, Fujimoto H. The *Hsp70* homolog gene, *Hsc70t*, is expressed under translational control during mouse spermiogenesis. Mol Reprod Dev 1999;52:383–91.
19. Kleene KC. Patterns of translational regulation in the mammalian testis. Mol Reprod Dev 1996;43:268–81.
20. Dix DJ, Allen JW, Collins BW, Mori C, Nakamura N, Poorman-Allen P, et al. Targeted gene disruption of Hsp70-2 results in failed meiosis, germ cell apoptosis, and male infertility. Proc Natl Acad Sci USA 1996;93:3264–68.
21. Moens PB, Pearlman RE, Heng HHQ, Traut W. Chromosome cores and chromatin at meiotic prophase. In: Handel MA, ed. Meiosis and gametogenesis. Current topics in developmental biology, vol. 37. San Diego: Academic Press, 1998:241–62.
22. Meuwissen RLJ, Offenberg HH, Dietrich AJJ, Riesewijk A, Van Iersel M, Heyting C. A coiled-coil related protein specific for synapsed regions of meiotic prophase chromosomes. EMBO J 1992;11:5091–100.
23. Dobson MJ, Pearlman RE, Karaiskakis A, Spyropoulos B, Moens PB. Synaptonemal complex proteins: occurrence, epitope mapping and chromosome disjunction. J Cell Sci 1994;107:2749–60.
24. Draetta G, Beach D. Activation of cdc2 protein kinase during meiosis in human cells: cell cycle-dependent phosphorylation and subunit rearrangement. Cell 1988;54:17–26.
25. Ashley T, Plug A. Caught in the act: deducing meiotic function from protein immunolocalization. In: Handel MA, ed. Meiosis and gametogenesis. Current topics in developmental biology, vol. 37. San Diego: Academic Press, 1998:201–39.
26. Eddy EM. Role of heat shock protein HSP70-2 in spermatogenesis. Rev Reprod 1999;4:23–30.
27 Dunphy WG, Brizuela L, Beach D, Newport J. The Xenopus homolog of cdc2 is a component of MPF, a cytoplasmic regulator of mitosis. Cell 1988;54:423–31.
28. Chapman DL, Wolgemuth DJ. Regulation of M-phase promoting factor activity during development of mouse germ cells. Dev Biol 1994;165:500–6.
29. Zhu D, Dix DJ, Eddy EM. HSP70-2 is required for CDC2 kinase activity in meiosis I of mouse spermatocytes. Development 1997;124:3007–14.
30. Dix DJ, Allen JW, Collins BW, Poorman-Allen P, Mori C, Blizard DR, et al. HSP70-2 is required for desynapsis of synaptonemal complexes during meiotic prophase in juvenile and adult mouse spermatocytes. Development 1997;124:4595–603.
31. Mori C, Nakamura N, Dix DJ, Fujioka M, Nakagawa S, Shiota K, et al. Morphological analysis of germ cell apoptosis during postnatal testis development in normal and *Hsp70-2* knockout mice. Dev Dynamics 1997;208:125–36.
32. Allen DJ, Harmon BV, Roberts SA. Spermatogonial apoptosis has three morphologically recognizable phases and showns no circadian rhythm during normal spermatogenesis in the rat. Cell Prolif 1992;25:241–50.
33. Bartke A. Apoptosis of male germ cells, a generalized or a cell type-specific phenomenon? Endocrinology 1995;128:3–4.

34. Huckins C. The morphology and kinetics of spermatogonial degeneration in normal adult rats: an analysis using a simplified classification of the germinal epithelium. Anat Rec 1978;190:905–26.
35. Milarski KL, Welch WJ, Morimoto RI. Mutational analysis of the human HSP70 protein: distinct domains for nucleolar localization and adenosine triphosphate binding. J Cell Biol 1989;109:1947–62.
36. Karlseder J, Wissing D, Holzer G, Orel L, Sliutz G, Auer H, et al. HSP70 overexpression mediates the escape of a doxorubicin-induced G2 cell cycle arrest. Biochem Biophys Res Commun 1996;220:153–59.
37. Wei Y, Kariya Y, Fukata H, Teshigawara K, Uchida A. Induction of apoptosis by quercetin: involvement of heat shock protein. Cancer Res 1994;54:4952–57.
38. He L, Fox MH. Variation of heat shock protein 70 through the cell cycle in HL-60 cells and its relationship to apoptosis. Exp Cell Res 1997;232:64–71.
39. Wei Y, Zhao X, Kariya Y, Teshigawara K, Uchida A. Inhibition of proliferation and induction of apoptosis by abrogation of heat-shock protein (HSP) 70 expression in tumor cells. Cancer Immunol Immunother 1995;40:73–78.
40. Leblond CP, Clermont Y. Definition of the stages of the cycle of the seminiferous epithelium in the rat. Ann NY Acad Sci 1952;55:548–73.
41. Russell LD, Ettlin RA, Sinha Hikim AP, Clegg ED. Histological and histopathological evaluation of the testis. Clearwater: Cache River Press, 1990.
42. Tanii I, Araki S, Toshimori K. Intra-acrosomal organization of a 90-kilodalton antigen during spermiogenesis in the rat. Cell Tissue Res 1994;277:61–67.
43. Tanii I, Araki S, Toshimori K. Further characterization of intra-acrosomal MN7 and MC41 antigens, with special reference to immunoelectron microscopic comparison of releasing process during the acrosome reaction in the mouse. Acta Histochem Chytochem 1995;28:447–52.
44. Sigrist S, Ried G, Lener CF. Dmcdc2 kinase is required for both meiotic division during *Drosophila* spermatogenesis and is activated by the Twine/cdc25 phosphatase. Mech Dev 1995;53:247–60.
45. Stern B, Ried G, Clegg NJ, Grigliatti TA, Lehner CF. Genetic analysis of the *Drosophila* cdc2 homolog. Development 1993;117:219–32.
46. Lin T-Y, Viswanathan S, Wood C, Wilson PG, Wolf N, Fuller MT. Coordinate developmental control of the meiotic cell cycle and spermatid differentiation in *Drosophila* males. Development 1996;122:1331–41.
47. White-Cooper H, Alphey L, Glover DM. The *cdc25* homologue *twine* is required for only some aspects of the entry into meiosis in *Drosophila*. J Cell Sci 1993; 106:1035–44.
48. Jackman JR, Pines JN. Cyclins and the G_2/M transition. In: Kastan MB, ed. Cancer Surveys, vol. 29. Oxford: Oxford University Press, 1997: 47–73.
49. Gowdy PM, Anderson HJ, Roberg M. Entry into mitosis without Cdc2 kinase activation. J Cell Sci 1998;111:3401–10.
50. Eddy EM. Chauvinist genes of male germ cells: gene expression during mouse spermatogenesis. Reprod Fertil Develop 1995;7:695–704.
51. Eddy EM, O'Brien DA. Gene expression during mammalian meiosis. In: Handel MA, ed. Meiosis and gametogenesis. Current topics in developmental biology, vol. 37. San Diego: Academic Press, 1998:141–200.

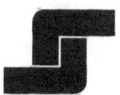

13

Characterization of the Testicular Histone-Binding Protein, NASP

MICHAEL G. O'RAND, IGLIKA N. BATOVA, AND RICHARD T. RICHARDSON

The nuclear autoantigenic sperm protein (NASP) was first recognized because of its autoantigenicity in males and immunological cross-reactivity with the sperm-specific autoantigen RSA (1). NASP was initially described as a highly immunogenic testis and sperm-specific protein, which was present in the postacrosomal region of mature spermatozoa and in the nucleus of developing spermatogenic cells (1,2). From DNA sequence comparisons, NASP appears to have evolved from the N1/N2 gene expressed in oocytes of *Xenopus laevis* (3,4). Indeed, the 3' untranslated sequence identity between the rabbit and *Xenopus* mRNAs reaches approximately 60%, implying that mammalian NASP is a true homologue of N1/N2.

Elucidation of the DNA and protein sequences of rabbit NASP revealed a number of its seminal characteristics. These have since proven to be present in testicular NASP (tNASP) proteins from three different species as well as in discovered somatic NASP (sNASP) from a variety of different adult and embryonic tissues (5). Figure 13.1 shows the characteristic histone binding sites and the nuclear localization signal of all known NASP proteins. The consensus sequence from rabbit, human and mouse NASP for histone-binding site I (HBS-I) is EEEEGEKTE-. Located close to the N-terminal of NASP, HBS-I is completely conserved, except for the last position, in all three species. The consensus HBS-II, located in the C-terminal portion of NASP, is KEGEETEGSEE-D-ENDK—EE-PN-SVLE-KSL-ENE and is not as highly conserved as HBS-I. Both HBS-I and HBS-II are present in the *Xenopus* oocyte protein N1/N2 (6,7). A third histone binding site (HBS-III) was first recognized in human NASP (8) and is located between HBS-I and HBS-II (Fig. 13.1). It is not present in *Xenopus* N1/N2 and appears to be the least conserved of the three sites. Moreover, it is not present in sNASP (5).

NASP's nuclear localization signal (NLS), VRKKRK, is identical to that in *Xenopus* N1/N2 and in several other nuclear proteins (9,10). A leucine

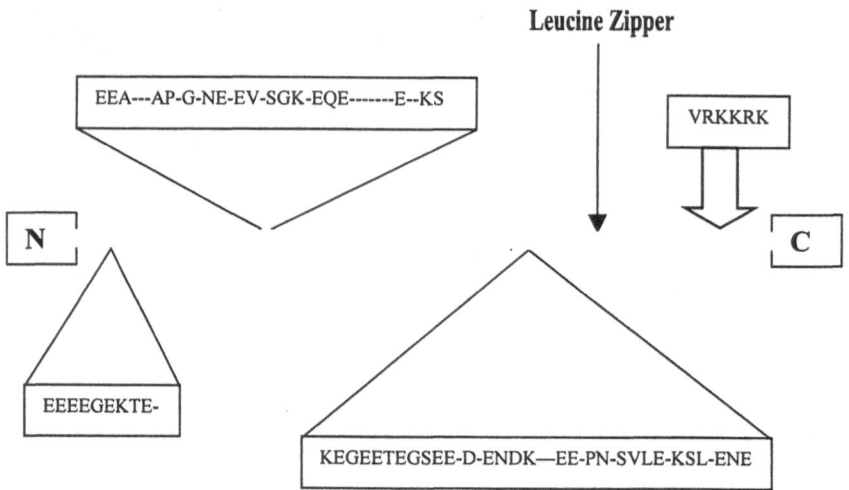

FIGURE 13.1. Diagrammatic representation of the nuclear autoantigenic sperm protein (NASP). The consensus sequence from rabbit, human and mouse testicular NASP sequences is shown for each histone binding site (HBS). HBS-I is EEEEGEKTE-. HBS-II is KEGEETEGSEE-D-ENDK—EE-PN-SVLE-KSL-ENE. HBS-III is EEA—AP-G-NE-EV-SGK-EQE————E—KS. The dashes represent amino acid residues that were not identical in all three species. The nuclear localization signal is VRKKRK. The arrow indicates the position of the leucine zipper. N = amino terminal. C = carboxy terminal.

zipper sequence is also conserved in all NASP proteins (Fig. 13.1; L-LQEQYLEAHDRLLAETHYQL) that may facilitate dimerization and play a role in NASP's interaction with DNA. Leucine zippers are characteristic of several gene regulatory proteins (11). An ATP/GTP-binding site is present in each NASP protein, although the location within each sequence differs and mouse testicular NASP has three separate sites. It is interesting that *Xenopus* N1/N2 does not have a consensus ATP/GTP-binding site; however, this could be due to the utilization of a different sequence motif by *Xenopus*. The presence of these conserved features in mammalian NASP strongly suggests the evolution of a protein with an important function in the binding and transport of histones during meiosis and mitosis.

Characterization of NASP from rabbit testes indicated that it is a highly acidic protein (73.5 kDa, pI = 4.06) with a predominance of α-helical secondary structures containing heptad repeat patterns that are often associated with the presence of intermolecular coiled-coil structures. Consistent with its highly acidic nature, 25% of the amino acids are either glutamic or aspartic acid. It is consequently not surprising that the observed molecular weight after SDS-PAGE is 130 kDa, which is in considerable excess of the predicted 73.5 kDa (1). Other nuclear proteins often display this anomalous migration characteristic after SDS-PAGE (4,12).

Human NASP (13) is also an acidic protein (pI = 4.02), encoded by a 3.2 kb mRNA that is somewhat larger than the 2.5 kb mRNA of rabbit NASP. The human protein is larger than the rabbit NASP (85.19 kDa vs. 73.5 kDa), primarily because of an additional 100 amino acids at the N-terminal. The additional N-terminal sequence present in human NASP allowed a proper alignment analysis of the two mammalian NASP proteins—rabbit and human—with the *Xenopus* N1/N2 protein (13). This analysis clearly showed a 53% identity between human NASP and *Xenopus* N1/N2 and an 85% identity between human and rabbit NASP. As shown in Figure 13.1 and described earlier, HBS-I and HBS-II are conserved in human NASP. Sequencing of mouse NASP (5) has indicated that it, too, is an acidic protein (pI = 4.16) similar in size to human NASP (83.9 kDa, 773 amino acids vs. 85.19 kDa, 787 amino acids in human), and containing the conserved histone binding sites (Fig. 13.1).

Studies on the localization of NASP mRNA during spermatogenesis in mice, rats, and rabbits (2), and NASP protein in rabbits (2), humans (13), and most recently in mice, have revealed a consistent pattern of synthesis. Rat testicular NASP mRNA is not present in sexually immature animals and begins its appearance on day 16 after birth, doubling by day 21, and reaching 48% of the adult level by day 26. By day 36 the adult level of NASP mRNA is reached and remains relatively constant throughout sexual maturity (2). In mice, NASP mRNA was first detected on day 14 after birth (2) when primary spermatocytes are present. In situ hybridization studies of rabbit testis detected NASP mRNA only in the cytoplasm of primary spermatocytes (2). Consistent with the appearance of NASP mRNA in primary spermatocytes of mice, rats, and rabbits, NASP protein is first detected in leptotene and zygotene spermatocyte nuclei and becomes progressively more concentrated in the nucleus throughout the pachytene stage. It is of interest that NASP appears to accumulate in patches that are often associated with the inner aspect of the nuclear membrane. As development proceeds, the patches increase in size and the nucleus fills with NASP. The first meiotic division eventually occurs and NASP can be clearly seen dispersed in the cytoplasm. Observations in mice indicate that some NASP might be associated with the spindle microtubules during the division of primary to secondary spermatocytes, but NASP has never been observed associated with the condensed chromosomes.

The behavior of NASP during cell division is similar to that of the nuclear lamins (14–18) and some other nuclear matrix proteins. If the presence of a leucine zipper in NASP indeed indicates that it is associated with DNA, then NASP's association with DNA would have to be terminated during chromosome condensation in preparation for division. At the completion of each division, NASP reappears in the nucleus in its characteristic peripheral nuclear patches. At this point it would presumably reestablish itself with DNA. With the formation of the haploid round spermatid, NASP again appears as patches within the nucleus. As nuclear condensation begins, however, NASP seems to begin a posterior shift in location, away from the developing acrosome. This observation may indicate that NASP is functional in primary and secondary spermatocytes, and in round spermatids through step 8, prior to the beginning of significant chromatin changes in spermatids (steps 9–12; 19–21).

Immunogold labeling of testis sections for electron microscopy confirmed the localization of NASP throughout spermatogenesis (22). At the ultrastructural level NASP is first seen in the rough endoplasmic reticulum and Golgi regions of primary spermatocytes, and, subsequently, in the nucleus. During spermiogenesis NASP can be observed in the nucleus, throughout the acrosome, and in the subacrosomal space. In late spermatids with condensing nuclei, NASP is located primarily in the nucleus, but the acrosome still retains some NASP. Although it was speculated that NASP might be associated with nuclear pores (2), no specific association between NASP and nuclear pores could be observed in the electron microscope (22). Further studies will be required to determine if NASP is associated with other nuclear proteins.

NASP was also initially associated with the postacrosomal region of mature spermatozoa (2). It was clearly present from ultrastructural studies in the condensed nuclei of spermatozoa (22). Western blots of rabbit spermatozoa, however, did not reveal a 130 kDa NASP; rather, they showed two sets of triplet bands of lower molecular weight proteins (1). Whether or not these are breakdown products of full-length testicular NASP and are truly in the nucleus remains to be determined. In human spermatozoa NASP appears to be present both before and after the acrosome reaction (13). Immunofluorescence studies of spermatozoa, however, may not detect NASP that is sequestered within the condensed sperm nucleus and may therefore reflect only residual NASP present in the sperm acrosome, subacrosomal space, or postacrosomal cytoplasm. Nevertheless, because of NASP's presence in spermatozoa, it was of interest to ask whether or not the fertilizing spermatozoon would carry NASP into the unfertilized egg (13). To begin these studies immunolabeling of histological sections of mouse ovaries for the presence of NASP were undertaken. In the course of these studies, contrary to expectations, NASP was present in the germinal vesicle of mouse oocytes in primary and secondary follicles. Moreover, granulosa cells surrounding the zona pellucida and lining the antrum were also positive for NASP. Subsequent sequencing of an ovarian cDNA library revealed the somatic form of NASP (sNASP; 5). As described by Richardson et al. (5), sNASP is a shorter version of tNASP and retains the conserved features of NASP (Fig. 13.1) except for HBS-III. Studies are currently under way to elucidate NASP's role in somatic cells.

The defining characteristic of NASP is its ability to bind and transport histones. Although the NLS (Fig. 13.1) is completely conserved from the *Xenopus* N1/N2 protein, it is necessary to confirm that it is functional in the mammalian protein. Further investigation of NASP's NLS (23) has revealed that amino acids 701–722 can function as a discrete nuclear import sequence and translocate full-length NASP as well as a heterologous protein into the nucleus. Using *Xenopus laevis* oocytes as a test system, a chimeric protein of β-galactosidase fused to NASP's NLS efficiently moved the construct into the nucleus after translation in the cytoplasm. In addition, using a myc-epitope–tagged full-length NASP, this construct accumulated in the nuclei of *Xenopus* oocytes. In contrast, truncated mutants lacking the NLS remained in the cytoplasm. The NLS domain of NASP is therefore both necessary and sufficient to direct nuclear import of NASP.

The histone-binding properties of NASP were initially inferred from the sequence similarity to the histone-binding sites first reported for the *Xenopus* N1/N2 protein (3,4). Subsequent experimental investigations of recombinant human NASP (8) using full-length and various deletion constructs spanning the entire sequence demonstrated that the two HBS conserved from N1/N2 were functional. Moreover, Western blotting and ELISA-binding assays demonstrated the presence of a third HBS (8). This study also found that there are stretches of negatively charged amino acids in the NASP sequence that do not bind histones, leading to the conclusion that the negatively charged HBS must exhibit some sequence-specific binding. Similar regions of negatively charged amino acids are found in a number of other nuclear proteins (24). Studies (23) have demonstrated a direct physical interaction of recombinant mouse NASP with linker as well as core histones, purified from mouse testis or translated in vitro.

The demonstration of a functional NLS and a functional interaction between NASP and mouse testicular histones (23) is important because it indicates that NASP could translocate histones into the nucleus. After DNA synthesis for meiosis has finished (19,25,26), the synthesis of both testis-specific histones (26–30) and NASP continues during the primary spermatocyte stage. In most cells DNA synthesis is coupled to histone synthesis; however, this is not the case in the testis. Studies of the stored non–DNA-bound histone pools in *Xenopus laevis* oocytes have shown that the non–chromatin-bound histones H3/H4 are tightly associated with the core histone-binding protein N1/N2, whereas H2A/H2B are selectively complexed with nucleoplasmin (31). The binding of histones to N1/N2 and nucleoplasmin in *Xenopus* eggs creates a soluble storage complex and provides a mechanism for assembling nucleosomes during cell replication in the early embryo. Thus, NASP could serve as a storage site for histones in the nucleus such that as somatic histones are removed, possibly by ubiquitination (21), testis histones would be immediately available to replace them. NASP could alternatively transport testis histones to the nucleus and transfer them immediately to DNA.

Regardless of whether NASP stores histones or transfers them to DNA immediately, there is a striking correlation between the appearance of histone H1t and NASP in mouse primary spermatocytes (27,32). The simplest conclusion from this timing correlation is that NASP binds and transports

H1t into the nuclei of primary spermatocytes. It has been suggested that H1t might be involved in the condensation of metaphase I chromosomes (32) and that consequently, both H1t and NASP may be critical for chromatin reorganization prior to meiosis.

In addition to NASP, other distinct histone-binding proteins have been identified that differentially transport histones into the nucleus. The nucleosome assembly protein, NAP-1, in *Drosophila* binds H2A and H2B and is cytoplasmic in G2 and nuclear in S phase (33). In yeast NAP-1 also binds linker histones and high mobility group (HMG) proteins (34). It has been suggested that NAP-1 and a chromatin assembly factor (CAF-1) act together in the presence of histones to arrange nucleosomes in a regular pattern on DNA (33,35). Neither NAP-1 nor CAF-1 has been identified in spermatogenic cells and it remains to be seen if they might play a role in nucleosome reorganization during spermatogenesis.

The association of NASP in vitro and in vivo with core and linker histones as well as its functional NLS suggests that NASP operates as a transport molecule facilitating their delivery and deposition and/or exchange in chromatin remodeling during spermatogenesis. The implication of these observations in all three species is that NASP's role must be one of interaction with chromatin during G1 and G2 of the cell cycle. It will be interesting to examine NASP in more detail for any DNA-binding sites from which it could play a more direct role in chromatin remodeling.

Acknowledgments. This research was supported by NICHD/NIH through cooperative agreement U54HD35041 as part of the Specialized Cooperative Centers Program in Reproductive Research.

References

1. Welch JE, Zimmerman LJ, Joseph DR, O'Rand MG. Characterization of a sperm-specific nuclear autoantigenic protein. I. Complete sequence and homology with the *Xenopus* protein N1/N2. Biol Reprod 1990;43:559–68.
2. Welch JE, O'Rand MG. Characterization of a sperm-specific nuclear autoantigenic protein. II. Expression and localization in the testis. Biol Reprod 1990;43:569–78.
3. Krohne G. Immunological identification of the karyophilic, histone-binding proteins N1 and N2 in somatic cells and oocytes of diverse amphibia. Exp Cell Res 1985;158:205–22.
4. Kleinschmidt JA, Dingwall C, Maier G, Franke WW. Molecular characterization of a karyophilic histone binding protein: cDNA cloning, amino acid sequence and expression of nuclear protein N1/N2 of *Xenopus laevis*. EMBO J 1986;5:3547–52.
5. Richardson RT, Batova I, O'Rand MG. Characterization of testicular and somatic NASP, mouse histone binding proteins. Mol Bio Cell 1998;9(Suppl.):178a.
6. Kleinschmidt JA, Fortkamp E, Krohne G, Zentgraf H, Franke WW. Co-existence of two different types of soluble histone complexes in nuclei of *Xenopus laevis* oocytes. J Biol Chem 1985;260:1166–76.

7. Kleinschmidt JA, Seiter A. Identification of domains involved in nuclear uptake and histone binding of protein N1 of *Xenopus laevis*. EMBO J 1988;7:1605–14.

8. Batova I, O'Rand MG. Histone binding domains in a human nuclear autoantigenic sperm protein. Biol Reprod 1996;54:1238–44.

9. Smith AE, Kalderon D, Roberts BL, Colledge WH, Edge M, Gillett P, et al. The nuclear localization signal. Proc R Soc Lond 1985;226:43–58.

10. Robbins J, Dilworth SM, Laskey RA, Dingwall C. Two interdependent basic domains in nucleoplasmin nuclear targeting sequence: identification of a class of bipartite nuclear targeting sequence. Cell 1991;64: 615–23.

11. Pabo CO, Sauer RT. Transcription factors: structural families and principles of DNA recognition. Ann Rev Biochem 1992;61:1053–95.

12. Lapeyre B, Bourbon H, Amalric F. Nucleolin, the major nucleolar protein of growing eukaryotic cells: an unusual protein structure revealed by the nucleotide sequence. Proc Natl Acad Sci USA 1987;84:1472–76.

13. O'Rand MG, Richardson RT, Zimmerman LJ Widgren EE. Sequence and localization of human NASP: conservation of a *Xenopus* histone binding protein. Dev Biol 1992;154:37–44.

14. Gerace L, Blobel G. The nuclear envelope is reversibly depolymerized during mitosis. Cell 1980;19:277–87.

15. Maul GG, French BT, Bechtol KB. Identification of lamins during nuclear differentiation in mouse spermatogenesis. Dev Biol 1986;115:68–77.

16. Moss SB, Donovan MJ, Bellve AR. The occurrence and distribution of lamin proteins during mammalian spermatogenesis and early development. Ann NY Acad Sci 1987;513:74–89.

17. Furukawa K, Hotta Y. cDNA cloning of a germ cell specific lamin B3 from mouse spermatocytes and analysis of its function by ectopic expression in somatic cells. EMBO J 1993;12:97–106.

18. Furukawa K, Inagaki H, Hotta Y. Identification and cloning of an mRNA coding for a germ cell-specific A-type lamin in mice. Exp Cell Res 1994;212:426–30.

19. Meistrich ML. Histone and basic nuclear protein transitions in mammalian spermatogenesis. In: Hnilica LS, Stein GS, Stein JL, eds. Histones and other basic nuclear proteins. Boca Raton, FL: CRC Press, 1989:165–82.

20. Oko RJ, Jano V, Wagner CL, Kistler WS, Hermo LS. Chromatin reorganization in rat spermatids during the disappearance of testis-specific histone, H1t, and the appearance of transition proteins TP1 and TP2. Biol Reprod 1996;54:1141–57.

21. Chen HY, Sun JM, Zhang Y, Davie JR, Meistrich ML. Ubiquitination of histone H3 in elongating spermatids of rat. J Biol Chem 1998;273:13165–69.

22. Lee YH, O'Rand MG. Ultrastructural localization of a nuclear autoantigenic sperm protein in spermatogenic cells and spermatozoa. Anat Rec 1993;236:442–48.

23. Batova I, Ingledue TC, Richardson RT, Marzluff WF, O'Rand MG. Nuclear translocation and histone binding of mouse testis NASP. Mol Bio Cell 1998;9 (Suppl.):178a.

24. Earnshaw WC. Anionic regions in nuclear proteins. J Cell Biol 1987;105:1479–82.

25. Meistrich ML, Bucci LR, Trostle-Weige PK, Brock WA. Histone variants in rat spermatogonia and primary spermatocytes. Dev Biol 1985;112:230–40.

26. Kim YJ, Hwang I, Tres LL, Kierszenbaum AL, Chae CB. Molecular cloning and differential expression of somatic and testis-specific H2B histone genes during rat spermatogenesis. Dev Biol 1987;124:23–34.

27. Kremer EJ Kistler WS. Localization of mRNA for testis-specific histone H1t by in situ hybridization. Exp Cell Res 1991;197:330–32.
28. Moss SB, Orth JM. Localization of a spermatid-specific histone 2B protein in mouse spermiogenic cells. Biol Reprod 1993;48:1047–56.
29. Unni E, Zang Y, Kangasniemi M, Saperstein W, Moss SB, Meistrich M. Stage-specific distribution of the spermatid-specific histone 2B in the rat testis. Biol Reprod 1995;53:820–26.
30. Trostle-Weige PK, Meistrich ML, Brock WA, Nishioka K. Isolation and character-ization of TH3, a germ cell-specific variant of histones in rat testis. J Biol Chem 1984;259:8769–76.
31. Dilworth SM, Black SJ, Laskey RA. Two complexes that contain histones are re-quired for nucleosome assembly in vitro: role of nucleoplasmin and N1 in *Xenopus* egg extracts. Cell 1987;51:1009–18.
32. Cobb J, Cargile B, Handel MA. Acquisition of competence to condense metaphase I chromosomes during spermatogenesis. Dev Biol 1999;205:49–64.
33. Ito T, Bulger M, Kobayashi R, Kadonaga JT. *Drosophila* NAP-1 is a core histone chaperone that functions in ATP-facilitated assembly of regularly spaced nucleo-somal arrays. Mol Cell Biol 1996;16:3112–24.
34. McQuibban GA, Commisso-Cappelli CN, Lewis PN. Assembly, remodeling, and histone binding capabilities of yeast nucleosome assembly protein 1. J Biol Chem 1998;273:6582–90.
35. Kaufman PD, Kobayashi R, Kessler N, Stillman B. The p150 and p60 subunits of chromatin assembly factor I: a molecular link between newly synthesized histones and DNA replication. Cell 1995;81:1105–14.

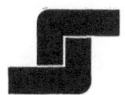

14

The Actin-Bundling Protein Espin and Its Role in the Ectoplasmic Specialization

JAMES R. BARTLES, LILI ZHENG,
MIN WANG, AND BIN CHEN

Introduction

The ectoplasmic specialization is thought to anchor and position spermatids within the seminiferous epithelium throughout much of spermiogenesis. It may also contribute to the "blood–testis" barrier between Sertoli cells (1,2). These activities are believed to depend critically on the ectoplasmic specialization junctional plaque, which is characterized by a layer of parallel actin bundles sandwiched between the Sertoli-cell plasma membrane and a cistern of endoplasmic reticulum (1,2). The parallel actin bundles are believed to act both as a scaffold that supports and stabilizes an adhesive domain within the overlying Sertoli-cell plasma membrane and indirectly, via the cistern of endoplasmic reticulum, as a link to an underlying network of microtubules to allow for changes in the position of the ectoplasmic specialization–spermatid complex (1,2).

To gain a better understanding of the structure and function of the ectoplasmic specialization, we have undertaken a molecular-level analysis of the junction. By preparing antibodies to a subcellular fraction enriched in ectoplasmic specializations, we have identified a novel ~110-kD protein of the ectoplasmic specialization that we have named "espin" (ectoplasmic specialization + -in) (3). The localization and properties of espin suggest that it is a major actin-bundling protein of the ectoplasmic specialization and could, therefore, be responsible for the formation of the parallel actin bundles that characterize the ectoplasmic specialization junctional plaque. Through the discovery of espin-related proteins in association with actin filament-rich structures in other cell types [e.g., brush border microvilli (4)], we have ascertained that espin is the founding member of a new family of actin-binding/bundling proteins.

Results and Discussion

Identification, Cloning, and Sequencing of Espin and Small Espin, Two Splice-Isoforms That Are Members of a New Family of Actin-Binding/Bundling Proteins

The first espin isoform to be identified was the ~110-kD isoform ("espin") of Sertoli cell ectoplasmic specializations, which we discovered using a monoclonal antibody raised to isolated rat spermatids (3). This monoclonal antibody was used to isolate an espin cDNA from a rat testis cDNA library. The espin cDNA was used to prepare a bacterial fusion protein that included only the C-terminal part of espin. This espin fusion protein was used to prepare and affinity purify polyclonal antibodies in rabbits (our "pan-espin" antibody). An ~30-kD isoform of espin ("small espin") was discovered because its mRNA was found to hybridize with a ^{32}P-labeled espin cDNA probe in preparations of RNA isolated rat small intestine and kidney (3). On western blots, the pan-espin antibody was found to react with a single band of ~110-kD in homogenates of rat testis and a closely spaced doublet of ~30-kD in homogenates of rat small intestinal mucosa or kidney (4). Upon cDNA sequence analysis, espin was found to be a novel protein that contained a unique assortment of motifs for protein–protein interaction (e.g., ankyrinlike repeats and proline-rich peptides) and a potential P-loop for binding and/or hydrolyzing ATP or GTP that can be found as peptide elements in other proteins (3; GenBank Accession number U46007) (Fig. 14.1).

The cDNA sequence analysis of small espin indicated that it shared a C-terminal 167-amino acid peptide with espin, but that its N-terminus was lacking the ankyrinlike repeats and proline-rich peptides of espin; in their

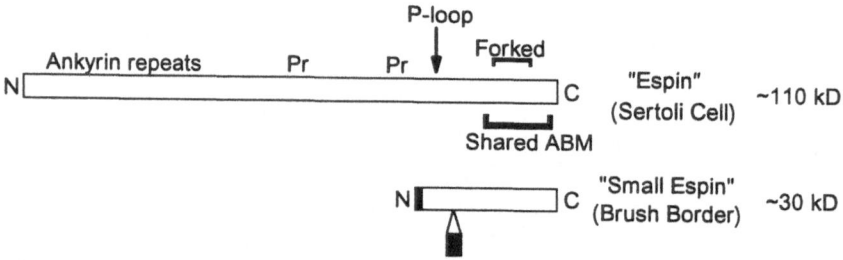

FIGURE 14.1. Stick-figure diagram depicting the sequence relationships between espin and small espin. Peptide segments of small espin that are shared with espin are shown as open, whereas those unique to small espin are filled. (Pr, proline-rich peptide; Forked, 66-amino acid forked homology peptide; Shared ABM, C-terminal actin-bundling module shared between espin and small espin.)

place, the N-terminus of the small isoform contained two unique small peptides that were interrupted with another short peptide that was shared with
espin (4; GenBank Accession number AF076856) (Fig. 14.1). We have now
confirmed that the different espin isoforms arise through differential splicing through southern blot tests for gene multiplicity and partial gene sequence analyses in the rat and mouse. The C-terminal peptide shared by the
two isoforms contained a 66-amino acid peptide that was 39% identical to a
peptide in the putative actin-bundling proteins encoded by the forked gene
in Drosophila, and the larger isoforms of the forked proteins are known to
contain ankyrinlike repeats at their N-terminus (5). Outside of this limited,
yet nonetheless intriguing sequence similarity to the forked proteins, however, the espins showed no signficant sequence similarity to other proteins
known or suspected to bind actin.

Localization at the Light Microscopic Level: Espin and Small Espin Are Localized to Structures That Contain Parallel Actin Bundles, and the Proteins Accumulate in a Developmentally Regulated Fashion

By immunofluorescence, the affinity-purified rabbit polyclonal pan-espin
was found to react with the junctional plaques of ectoplasmic specializations, which can be visualized as a phase-dense cap or "hat" on the heads of
spermatids released from the seminiferous epithelium by mechanical dissociation (3). The pattern of labeling observed with the espin antibody was
coincident with that of the actin filaments in the ectoplasmic specialization
junctional plaque, as revealed through double labeling with fluorescent phalloidin. When localized on paraffin sections of adult rat testis, the immunoperoxidase reaction product was found to accumulate at the site of the ectoplasmic specialization in a developmental fashion (3). Espin was first detected at the Sertoli cell–spermatid head interface during midspermiogenesis,
coinciding with the time when ectoplasmic specializations are known to form,
and it remained there until near the end of spermiogenesis when the ectoplasmic specialization is known to disassemble, apparently through the formation of a related structure, the tubulobulbar complex (1,2). Another type
of structure labeled with the espin antibody was present in the basal compartment of the seminiferous epithelium and took the form of intermittent
stripes or a "scalloped" pattern that appeared to pass around or between
adjacent cells (3). This pattern was similar to those observed for F-actin and
vinculin at the sites of those ectoplasmic specializations that are part of the
junctional complexes between adjacent Sertoli cells (1,2).

When paraffin sections of rat small intestine and kidney were labeled with pan-espin antibody, the immunoperoxidase reaction product showed the highest levels of accumulation over the brush borders of the enterocytes and the proximal tubular epithelial cells (4). Like the plaque of the Sertoli cell ectoplasmic specialization, the brush border also contains parallel actin bundles (6). It is interesting that the labeling of enterocyte precursors in the crypts of Lieberkuhn was considerably less than that observed for the mature enterocytes on the intestinal villi, which suggests that the accumulation of small espin in the brush border was developmentally regulated. In fact, intense labeling of small espin was not observed until enterocytes approached the crypt–villus junction, which suggests that it accumulated after villin and fimbrin/plastin, the other two actin-bundling proteins known to be involved in forming the parallel actin bundles at the core of brush border microvilli (6). This observation of a relatively late time of accumulation in the brush border has caused us to hypothesize that small espin might be involved in one of the later stages of brush border assembly (e.g., the terminal elongation of microvilli), and/or that it might confer a special property on a largely already-constructed core actin bundle. On the basis of the in vitro properties of recombinant small espin (see later), one possibility is that it supplies a high-affinity cross-link that is not sensitive to changes in the concentration of calcium ion.

Localization at the Electron Microscopic Level: Espin and Small Espin Are Localized to Parallel Actin Bundles

When localized on isolated rat spermatid–ectoplasmic specialization complexes by pre-embedment immunogold electron microscopy, espin was found to be localized to the parallel actin bundles of the ectoplasmic specialization junctional plaque (3). Postembedment immunogold electron microscopy was used to localize small espin on isolated rat small intestinal brush borders. The small espin was found to be localized over the parallel actin bundles of the microvillus core, including the microvillar rootlets (4). It was not, however, detected at significant levels in the terminal web or in the antiparallel actin bundle of the zonula adherens belt. Pre-embedment immunogold labeling indicated that a significant pool of small espin along the microvilli proper (but apparently not that associated with the rootlets) was accessible to the pan-espin antibody and to secondary antibody–colloidal gold conjugate in isolated brush borders that had been fixed with paraformaldehyde and permeabilized with Triton X-100 before labeling (4). The localization of espin and small espin to parallel actin bundles is consistent with the fact that they both appear to be associated with the cytoskeleton by the operational criterion of resisting extraction with Triton X-100 and that these proteins can to bind to and bundle F-actin in vitro and in transfected cells (see later). Quantitative western blot analysis indicated that espin is a major component of the Triton X-100-resistant cytoskeletal fraction of the ectoplasmic specialization, where it is present at approximately 5 million copies per ectoplasmic specialization, which translates into around 1 espin for every 25 actin monomers.

Binding to Actin Filaments In Vitro: Recombinant Espin and Small Espin Bind to F-actin with High Affinity

Because espin and small espin proved to be difficult to extract from their natural sources without the use of denaturants, we chose to examine the properties of recombinant forms of the proteins produced in *E. coli* (4). For this purpose, we used the ProEX HT vectors (Life Technologies, Gaithersburg, MD), which introduce a 22-amino acid extension at the N-terminus that includes a 6 × His tag, a short spacer peptide, and a protease cleavage site for the highly specific Tobacco Etch Virus protease. The recombinant espin isoforms were completely soluble and could be isolated to homogeneity under nondenaturing conditions using one-step batchwise affinity chromatography on Ni-NTA agarose (Qiagen, Santa Clarita, CA). We have even examined the recombinant small espin by circular dichroism spectroscopy and found it to be a highly folded polypeptide with a high percentage of α-helical secondary structure (4). Both small espin and espin were found to bind to preformed filaments of actin and to elicit the formation of parallel actin bundles under physiological conditions of ionic strength, pH, and temperature (4). Identical results were obtained with or without prior removal of the N-terminal extension peptide by treatment with 6 × His-tagged recombinant Tobacco Etch Virus protease followed by removal of 6 × His-tagged protease, uncleaved protein, and released extension peptide by a second brief challenge with Ni-NTA agarose. The dissociation constant (K_d) for the binding of small espin to filaments of rabbit skeletal muscle actin (the reference standard actin) or human platelet nonmuscle actin was determined to be approximately 150 nM and approximately 50 nM, respectively (4). The K_d for the binding of espin constructs to filaments of rabbit skeletal muscle actin was approximately 10–25 nM (3), corresponding to a 6- to 15-fold higher binding affinity than that exhibited by the small isoform (see later). These data imply that the espins bind to actin filaments with affinities that are one to two orders of magnitude greater than that exhibited by the other known actin-bundling proteins (7–9). The binding of small espin saturated at approximately 1 small espin for every three to four actin monomers. This value is typical of actin-bundling proteins and reflects the upper limit on cross-linking for hexagonally packed filaments allowed by the helical pitch of the actin filament (10).

Bundling of Actin Filaments In Vitro: Recombinant Espin and Small Espin Elicit the Formation of Parallel Actin Bundles

The incubation of recombinant espin or small espin with preformed actin filaments under physiological conditions like those described earlier in the binding assays caused the solutions to become noticeably turbid. Furthermore, when centrifuged under low-speed conditions that were not sufficient to pellet actin filaments, large percentages of the actin filaments and recombinant espin present in the mixtures were recovered in the pellet (4). When these mixtures were examined by negative staining electron microscopy, it became evident that the recombinant espins were incredibly efficient at eliciting the formation of parallel actin bundles in these mixtures (4). A close examination of these bundles revealed that they were partially ordered [i.e., they displayed the cross-striations at intervals of approximately 12 nm (and integral multiples) characteristic of maximally cross-linked, hexagonally packed parallel actin bundles] (10), but these ordered segments were not in perfect alignment across the width of the bundles. Consistent with the fact that espin was observed to bind to actin filaments with a higher affinity than small espin, espin also appeared to be more efficient at causing bundles to form. Unlike other actin-bundling proteins (e.g., villin and fimbrin) the bundling activity of the espin isoforms was not inhibited by calcium ion (4).

Interactions with the Actin Cytoskeleton In Vivo: Green-Fluorescent-Protein-Tagged Espins Decorate Actin Fibers in Transfected Cells and Appear to Bring About Their Accumulation and/or Bundling

When expressed ectopically in cells of the baby hamster kidney fibroblastic line by transient transfection using the pEGFP-C vectors (Clontech, Palo Alto, CA), both green-fluorescent-protein-small espin and green-fluorescent-protein-espin were observed to decorate stress fiberlike structures (4). This result was obtained whether examining living cells or fixed cells. It was readily evident that the fibers labeled with green-fluorescent-protein-tagged espin derivatives contained filamentous actin upon double labeling of the fixed cells with fluorescent phalloidin (4). It is interesting that the cells expressing a green-fluorescent-protein-tagged espin derivative consistently showed much higher levels of labeling with fluorescent phalloidin than did the corresponding untransfected control cells, which suggests that the espins might also bring about an accumulation and/or bundling of actin filaments in vivo. Consistent with our observation that espin binds to actin filaments with a higher affinity than does small espin (and is a more efficient bundler) in vitro (see earlier), green-fluorescent-protein-espin appeared to elicit the formation of a higher percentage of coarse stress fiberlike structures than did green-fluorescent-protein-small espin in the transfected cells. All of the results in these transfection experiments were independent of the green-fluorescent-protein moiety because identical results were obtained when the espin isoforms were expressed without green-fluorescent-protein using the pcDNA3 vector (Invitrogen, Carlsbad, CA) and localized by immunofluorescence.

The Mechanism of Espin-Induced Actin Bundling: Small Espin Is a Monomer with an Actin-Bundling Module That "Defines" the Espin Family Present in a Shared C-Terminal 116-Amino Acid Peptide

Certain cations and cationic small peptides can bundle actin filaments at relatively low ionic strength by a mechanism called *counterion condensation* (11). The observations that the recombinant small espin and espin could bundle actin filaments at physiological ionic strength (0.1–0.15 M KCl) and that the bundling was not inhibited by relatively high concentrations of anions (e.g., 10 mM ATP) suggested that espin-mediated bundling is not the result of counterion condensation, but instead involves specific binding sites. Upon sedimentation equilibrium analysis, small espin proved to be a monomer (4). This suggested that it contained at least two such specific actin-binding sites to mediate the cross-linking of filaments into a bundle. The supposition that the actin-binding sites in question might be present in the C-terminal peptide shared by the two isoforms was, in fact, borne out by experiment: Deletion mutagenesis demonstrated that the C-terminal 116-amino acid peptide of the espins was sufficient for maximum bundling activity (4). Further deletions from either end of this peptide resulted in a loss of bundling activity. The simplest interpretation is that this C-terminal 116-amino acid peptide contains two actin-binding sites and that these binding sites are disposed roughly at opposite ends of the peptide. It is interesting that the loss of bundling activity upon further deletion from the N-terminal end of the 116-amino acid peptide coincided with the loss of approximately the N-terminal half of the espins' 66-amino acid forked homology peptide.

Although many actin-binding proteins have been identified, a large number of them appear to have arisen through the mutation and duplication of a relatively small number of actin-binding motifs or modules (e.g., calponin, gelsolin, or ADF homology domains; 12). Because the C-terminal 116-amino acid actin-bundling module has been identified in every espin isoform we have sequenced to date, our data suggest that this shared C-terminal actin-bundling module, with its constituent actin-binding sites, are the defining characteristic for membership in this new family of actin-binding/bundling proteins. The observation, however, that the C-terminal 116-amino acid peptide is all that is needed for efficient bundling of actin filaments begs the question of why different parallel actin bundle-containing structures contain different espin splice-isoforms, in which this shared C-terminal actin-bundling module is linked to a different N-terminal peptide.

Differences Between the Espin and Small Espin in Their Interactions with Actin: The Unique N-Terminus of Espin Contains a Second Actin-Bundling Module

One possible explanation for the presence of different N-termini on espin and small espin is that they influence the ways that the proteins interact with actin. As mentioned earlier, espin was found to bind to filaments of rabbit skeletal muscle actin with a 6- to 15-fold higher affinity than small espin. It also appeared to be more efficient at forming bundles in vitro and showed a higher percentage of coarse espin– and F-actin–containing fibers in transfected BHK cells. We have now determined the reason for these differences. Through deletion mutagenesis, we have determined that there is a second actin-bundling module positioned roughly between the two proline-rich peptides in the unique N-terminus of espin (Fig. 14.1). Thus far, we have been able to map the second actin-bundling module to a 28-amino acid peptide that presumably contains two (or possibly more) actin-binding sites. This peptide does not show significant sequence similarity to the actin-binding sites of other proteins, including those in the shared C-terminal actin-bundling module of the espins. The reason for having a second actin-bundling module is not clear, but it must certainly explain why the large isoform of espin appears to be such a "super binder and bundler." One possibility is that the presence of more than one actin-bundling module allows for a single espin molecule to bind at two or more sites along a single filament. From a theoretical standpoint, this would be expected to have a stabilizing effect on both filaments and bundles. Furthermore, if the two actin-binding sites for a single filament were spaced a nonintegral number of actin monomers apart, it could also lead to bending of the actin bundle.

The Search for Espin-Binding Proteins Other Than Actin: The Yeast Two-Hybrid Method Yields a Number of Promising Candidates for Binding to Espin

A second possible explanation for why espin and small espin have different N-termini is that they are needed to interact with different complements of espin-associated proteins. This would especially appear to be likely for espin, which has multiple motifs for protein–protein interaction (ankyrinlike repeats and proline-rich peptides) in its N-terminus. Possible candidates for espin-associated proteins might include structural proteins that link espin-containing actin bundles to membranes or other cytoskeletal systems and, therefore, are additional components of the supramolecular complexes that contain the espins. They might alternatively include regulatory proteins that modify the activity or location of the espin in response to input within a specific signal transduction pathway. To identify espin-binding proteins other than actin, we have been carrying out yeast two-hybrid screens using the GAL4-based Matchmaker Two-Hybrid System 2 (Clontech), employing espin missing its two actin-bundling modules as "bait," and screening a mouse testis Matchmaker 2 cDNA library in the pACT-2 vector. Thus far, we have identifed 13 very promising cDNA clones that have withstood the huge battery of control experiments needed to ensure that they are true positives (our unpublished observations). Two of the three cDNA clones we have sequenced to date encode known signal transduction proteins: a tyrosine kinase substrate (four independent clones) and a multifunctional SH3 domain-containing protein (two independent clones). The third is unlike any protein in the database. When co-expressed with espin in baby hamster kidney fibroblastic cells by transient transfection (4), green-fluorescent-protein-tagged versions of each of these proteins become targeted, along with the espin (4), to actin stress fiberlike structures. Whereas, when introduced by transfection in the absence of espin, these green-fluorescent-protein-labeled proteins are either distributed homogenously throughout the cytoplasm or become concentrated in discrete foci within the nucleus (our unpublished observations). These data suggest that these proteins do indeed interact with espin in the cytoplasmic compartment of cultured mammalian cells. We are currently preparing the corresponding bacterial fusion proteins to examine candidate protein–espin interactions in vitro and to make antibodies in rabbits for use in comparing the localizations of the candidate proteins with that of espin in Sertoli cells in situ.

The Role of Espin in Ectoplasmic Specializations

Taken together our results support the hypothesis that espin is a major actin-bundling protein involved in the formation of the layer of parallel actin bundles within the ectoplasmic specialization junctional plaque. As such, espin might be expected to play a critical role in spermatogenesis. As one means to test this hypothesis directly, we are currently preparing mice in which key functional parts of the espin gene has been deleted by gene targeting. In addition, we are continuing to use espin as a molecular "handle" with which to gain further insight into the organization and function of this important intercellular junction.

Acknowledgments. We gratefully acknowledge support by NIH R01 HD35280 and Independent Scientist Award K02 HD01210 awarded to James R. Bartles. We also wish to thank Dennis Wang, Allison Wierda, and Anli Li for their contributions to aspects of this work.

References

1. Vogl AW, Pfeiffer DC, Redenbach DM. Ectoplasmic ("junctional") specializations in mammalian Sertoli cells: influence on spermatogenic cells. Ann NY Acad Sci 1991;637:175–202.
2. Russell LD, Peterson RN. Sertoli cell junctions: morphological and functional correlates. Int Rev Cytol 1985;94:177–211.
3. Bartles JR, Wierda A, Zheng L. Identification and characterization of espin, an actin-binding protein localized to the F-actin-rich junctional plaques of Sertoli cell ectoplasmic specializations. J Cell Sci 1989;109:1229–39.
4. Bartles JR, Zheng L, Li A, Wierda A, Chen B. Small espin: a third actin-bundling protein and potential forked protein ortholog in brush border microvilli. J Cell Biol 1998;143:107–19.
5. Hoover KK, Chien AJ, Corces VG. Effect of transposable elements on the expression of the forked gene of *Drosophila melanogaster*. Genetics 1993;135:507–26.
6. Heintzelman MB, Mooseker M. Assembly of the intestinal brush border cytoskeleton. Curr Top Dev Biol 1992;26:93–122.
7. Glenney JR Jr, Kaulfus P, Matsudaira P, Weber K. F-actin binding and bundling properties of fimbrin, a major cytoskeletal protein of microvillus core filaments. J Biol Chem 1981;256:9283–88.
8. Burgess DR, Broschat KO, Hayden JM. Tropomyosin distinguishes between the two actin-binding sites of villin and affects actin-binding properties of other brush border proteins. J Cell Biol 1987;104:29–40.
9. Pollard TD. Actin and actin-binding proteins. In: Kreis T, Vale R, eds. Guidebook to the cytoskeletal and motor proteins. Oxford: Oxford University Press, 1993:3–11.
10. Tilney LG, Tilney MS, Guild GM. F-Actin bundles in *Drosophila* bristles. I. Two filament cross-links are involved in bundling. J Cell Biol 1995;130:629–38.
11. Tang JX, Janmey PA. The polyelectrolyte nature of F-actin and the mechanism of actin bundle formation. J Biol Chem 1996;271:8556–63.
12. Puius Y, Mahoney NM, Almo SC. The modular structure of actin-regulatory proteins. Curr Opin Cell Biol 1998;10:23–34.

Part IV

Epididymal Maturation and Fertilization

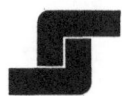

15

Regulation of Epididymal Function by Testicular Factors: The Lumicrine Hypothesis

BARRY T. HINTON, ZI JIAN LAN, R. JOHN LYE, AND JACQUELYN C. LABUS

The Lumicrine Hypothesis

It is very clear that the mammalian epididymis needs androgens to be fully functional. During the 1980s and 1990s, however, it became evident that factors passing into the epididymal duct that originate from the testis appear to play an equal role in maintaining a functional epididymis. There have been very few studies, however, that examined the identification of such factors and the mechanisms by which they act. The mechanism of action of testicular factors cannot be classified as either endocrine or autocrine, although it may be considered paracrine in nature. The term *lumicrine* has been coined to define the regulation of cells by factors secreted and/or produced by an upstream set of cells through a luminal or ductal system (Fig. 15.1). Lumicrine is not new, and has been used to define a novel neuroendocrine intracellular signaling pathway (1). In this case, the pathway involves the lumen of the intracellular secretory pathway (e.g., the endoplasmic reticulum and the Golgi apparatus). Lumicrine regulation, however, can occur both intracellularly and extracellularly.

Among the first examples of lumicrine regulation observed in the male reproductive tract were the studies published by Skinner and Rowson (2,3). These investigators showed that following unilateral vasectomy, the ampulla of the vas deferens on the ipsilateral side weighed less, was smaller in diameter, and contained less fructose compared with the intact contralateral ampulla. The investigators suggested that the vasectomy prevented the flow of testosterone from the testis to the ampulla. To test this hypothesis, testosterone was perfused into the vas deferens of a surgically castrated ram, and the investigators noted that the ampulla on the perfused side was found to be twice as large and heavy when compared with the untreated side. The amounts

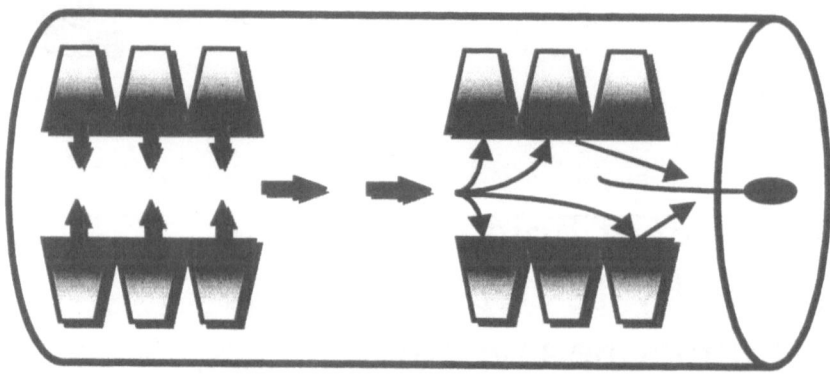

FIGURE 15.1. The Lumicrine Hypothesis. The term *lumicrine* has been coined to define the regulation of cells by factors secreted and/or produced by an upstream set of cells through a luminal or ductal system. Putative lumicrine testicular factors include androgens, androgen-binding protein, and growth factors such as bFGF.

of fructose and citric acid were also greater in the ampulla of the perfused side compared with the untreated side.

Testicular Factors Are Needed for Normal Epididymal Morphology and Metabolic Activity

Maintenance of an intact and normal epithelial-cell morphology of the proximal regions of the epididymis, especially the initial segment, is dependent upon the presence of testicular factors (4–10). In particular, the epithelial cells within zones 1A, B, and C of the rat initial segment (11) are altered following efferent duct ligation (8–10). Longer-term efferent duct ligation (> 20 days) caused a decrease in cell height, loss of endoplasmic cytoplasm in the apical region of the cells, and loss of Golgi function, but maintenance of pinocytosis within the initial segment of the rat epididymis (6,8). Apoptosis of the initial segment epithelium, however, was observed following shorter-term efferent duct ligation (1–5 days) (9). Apoptosis was seen primarily within zone 1A of the initial segment with cytoplasmic regression, necrotic cells, and focal degeneration in the epithelium. Nicander et al. (9) suggested that because the initial segment epithelial cells have a higher mitotic rate than do the distal epididymal cells, they may then be more dependent upon the presence of a mitogenic factor taken up from the luminal fluid. It was suggested that the factor responsible is nonandrogenic and is a growth factor of Sertoli-cell origin.

The study by Nicander et al. (9) has been confirmed and extended by Fan and Robaire (12) and by Turner et al. (13). Using the TUNEL technique and DNA fragmentation analysis, both of these studies also demonstrated apoptosis in the initial segment, especially zone 1A, following short-term efferent duct ligation. Fan and Robaire (12) showed that apoptosis resulted in the cells of all epididymal regions following orchiectomy. Androgen replacement, however, prevented apoptosis in the distal epididymal regions, but not in the initial segment, again, providing evidence that a testicular factor is necessary to prevent apoptosis in the initial segment. The investigators suggest that high intraluminal androgens may be responsible for preventing apoptosis. Evidence against higher androgen levels preventing apoptosis comes from the earlier studies of Fawcett and Hoffer (8). They showed that high doses of testosterone administration to rats that had undergone efferent duct ligation failed to prevent cell degeneration within the initial segment (8). The circulating levels of androgens within this group of animals were about 8–10 times higher than were the controls. A more convincing argument, however, would have been made had the intraluminal androgen levels been measured and shown to be equivalent to that of controls.

Ligating the efferent ducts of rats caused changes in the metabolic activity of the proximal epididymis, but not in the distal epididymal regions (14). Six-week EDL resulted in lowering of tissue weight, respiration rate, glycolytic rate, and phosphofructokinase activities in the initial segment compared with control. A lower tissue weight, carnitine content, acetylcarnitine glycolytic rate, and pyruvate carboxylase activities were also lowered in the caput epididymidis as compared with control (14). Brooks (14) suggested that the critical component in testicular fluid is not related to ABP. Preventing ABP from entering the epididymis caused negligible changes in tissue weight or in the activities of either pyruvate carboxylase or phosphofructokinase.

Testicular Factors Are Needed to Maintain Protein Secretion and Expression of Epididymal Genes

The synthesis and secretion of specific proteins by the epididymis has been shown to be dependent upon the presence of testicular factors (15–23). One of the most well-characterized proteins that has been shown to be regulated by testicular factors might be 5α-reductase (15,16,23,24). Following orchiectomy, 5α-reductase activity and mRNA levels decline and do not return to normal levels following administration of testosterone, which results in higher-than-normal circulating levels of androgen.

Several other epididymal genes that are also regulated by testicular factors include: proenkephalin (25), retinoic acid binding protein (26), cystatin related epididymal specific (CRES) gene (27), gamma glutamyl-transpeptidase (GGT) mRNA IV (28), A-raf (29), glutathione peroxidase (GPX5; 21,30), polyomavirus enhancer activator 3 (PEA3; 31), and a disintegrin and metalloprotease (ADAM) 7 (32). Expression of many of these genes, including GGT mRNA IV, PEA3, 5α-reductase, and proenkephalin, is high in zone 1A (11) of the rat initial segment, and all are affected by loss of testicular factors. It is interesting that the promoter region of some of these genes have PEA3 binding motifs. Proenkephalin promoter sequence has been fused with a β-galactosidase reporter gene to generate transgenic mice. Although the transgene is highly expressed in the proximal epididymis, no experiments were performed to examine the regulation of the transgene by testicular factors (33).

Identification of Putative Testicular Factors

Composition of Rete Testis Fluid

Testicular fluid (rete testis fluid) entering the initial segment comprises spermatozoa and fluid, so either component can be considered to regulate epididymal function. The composition of rete testis fluid (RTF) is distinctly different from that of either seminiferous tubular fluid or blood plasma (see Refs. 34, 35 for reviews). For most mammalian species RTF contains 7–14 mM potassium, 118–143 mM sodium, 122–140 mM chloride, 0.8–1.2 mM calcium, 0.39–0.5 mM magnesium, 7–21 mM bicarbonate, 2.5–5.7 mM inositol, 1mg/ml total protein, 0.85–22.4 ng/ml pregnenolone, 1.2–3.7 ng/ml progesterone, 0.5–21 ng/ml dehydroepiandrosterone, 1.1–17 ng/ml 5-androstene-3,17-dione, 3–88 ng/ml testosterone, 1–32.7 ng/ml dihydrotestosterone, and 0.02–0.248 ng/ml total estrogen. Proteins include immunoglobulins, clusterin, androgen-binding protein, transferrin, malate dehydrogenase, aspartate aminotransferase, albumin, acid phosphatase, uridine 5'-diphosphate galactose:N-acetylglucosamine galactosyltransferase, α-lactalbuminlike protein, Muellerian inhibiting substance, and various growth factors including bFGF, mitogenic growth factor, and Sertoli-cell-derived growth factor. RTF from rats contains approximately 3×10^7 spermatozoa/ml (see Ref. 34 for review). Hence, any of the preceding ions, organic solutes, and macromolecules can be considered to be potential testicular factors that regulate epididymal function.

One of the first and most convincing experiments to suggest that secretagogue activity is present in RTF might come from the study by Sujarit et al. (36). Protein synthesis and secretion was shown to be stimulated in Zone 1A of the rat initial segment following luminal microperfusion of ovine RTF. The study showed that the secretagogue was not extracted by charcoal, was sensitive to protease digestion, and was greater than 10,000 kDa. Studies outlined later present evidence that putative testicular factors that regulate epididymal function include spermatozoa, ABP, and growth factors.

Spermatozoa

Work by Garrett et al. (25) suggested that testicular spermatozoa may be important regulators of epididymal gene expression. Their study showed that loss of developing germ cells following bulsulphan treatment in rats also caused a reduction in the expression of proenkephalin mRNA in the initial segment compared with controls. The reduction in expression of proenkephalin mRNA, however, may have also been the result of either a direct effect of the drug on transcription, or an effect of the drug on the synthesis and secretion of a putative testicular factor(s). Further studies are obviously needed to test the hypothesis that spermatozoa can regulate epididymal gene expression.

Androgen-Binding Protein

Androgen-binding protein (ABP) has been considered to be one of the putative testicular factors that regulate epididymal function (8,9,22,23,37), even though Brooks (14) had suggested that ABP might not be important in the regulation of certain epididymal proteins. The exact role played by ABP is not known, although Robaire and Viger (23) suggested that it may play a critical role in the regulation of nuclear 5α-reductase within the cells of the initial segment. The enzyme would in turn provide high concentrations of dihydrotestosterone, the active androgen, to mediate androgen action in this epididymal region. Evidence that ABP may play a role in the caput epididymidis, which is a site more distal to the initial segment, comes from the studies of Turner et al. (22). Sex-hormone binding globulin (SHBG), an ABP analogue, stimulated protein synthesis and secretion by the cells of the caput epididymidis following introduction of SHBG into the caput lumen. The precise mechanism of this cellular response is not known, but it does provide evidence for a possible physiological role of ABP.

Growth Factors—Basic Fibroblast Growth Factor

The idea that growth factors may play an important role in the regulation of epididymal function, especially within the initital segment, may have originally been suggested by Nicander et al. (9), although other investigators had suggested that other unknown factors, not androgen nor ABP, may play a role (8,14). Studies in our laboratory have focused on the regulation of expression of GGT mRNA IV as a means to identify putative testicular factors (28,31,38,39). Futhermore, these studies have examined the mechanisms by which such putative testicular factors regulate epididymal gene expression (39,40). GGT (EC 2.3.2.2) is an important enzyme involved in the metabolism of glutathione (GSH; gamma-gly-cys-gly), an important antioxidant (see Ref. 41 for review). The rat epididymis expresses three (II, III, and IV) of the four GGT mRNAs that are transcribed in various rat tissues. The three mRNAs are expressed in a region-dependent manner, and only one—GGT mRNA IV—is highly expressed in the initial segment and is specifically regulated by testicular factors (28).

Following 1-day EDL, the steady-state level of GGT mRNA IV within the initial segment declined to about 50% of control levels (28). The decline in transcript was due to both a reduction in transcription rate and decreased stability (42). Hence, under normal physiological conditions testicular factors act to maintain transcription and to stabilize messages. To understand the mechanisms responsible for changes in transcription, the promoter region of GGT mRNA IV was analyzed using the Genetics Computer Group sequence analysis software package to identify potential *cis* and *trans* regulatory elements. Several conserved PEA3-binding motifs were identified. PEA3 is a member of the Ets (E26 transformation specific) transcription family that has DNA binding activity to the motif 5'-AGGAAG-3' (43). To summarize our studies, we have shown that: (1) PEA2 mRNA is highly expressed in the initital segment, (2) is regulated by testicular factors, (3) binds to GGT promoter IV, and (4) activates the promoter (31,39,44). Further studies have shown that bFGF is present in rete testis and epididymal fluid, and regulates GGT activity (44). Hence, it is proposed that bFGF is a candidate testicular factor that regulates epididymal function (Fig. 15.2). It is hypothesized specifically that bFGF interacts with its receptor (39,40) on the apical membrane of zone 1A initial segment cells, whereupon it initiates a signal transduction pathway, the ras, raf, MAPK, MAPKK pathway. PEA3 is phosphorylated by appropriate kinases, whereupon it binds to the promoter region of GGT mRNA IV for transactivation, leading to GGT protein synthesis and trafficking to the apical membrane. Basic FGF may also directly regulate GGT protein synthesis and enzyme activity. In view of the importance of this growth factor in the development and differentiation of the mamma-

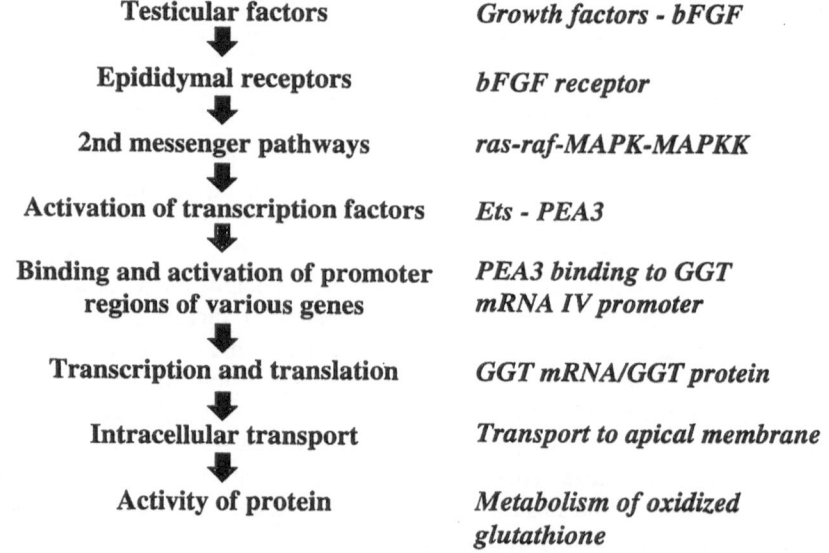

Testicular factors	Growth factors - bFGF
Epididymal receptors	bFGF receptor
2nd messenger pathways	ras-raf-MAPK-MAPKK
Activation of transcription factors	Ets - PEA3
Binding and activation of promoter regions of various genes	PEA3 binding to GGT mRNA IV promoter
Transcription and translation	GGT mRNA/GGT protein
Intracellular transport	Transport to apical membrane
Activity of protein	Metabolism of oxidized glutathione

FIGURE 15.2. Schematic representation of our working hypothesis showing how epididymal function can be maintained and regulated by a lumicrine mechanism. The left-hand side outlines a general pathway by which protein activity in the epididymis is maintained by testicular factors. The right-hand side shows putative candidates that may be involved in this pathway in Zone 1A (11) of the initial segment. Reproduced by kind permission of the *Journal of Reproduction and Fertility* from (40).

lian epididymis (45), it is anticipated that bFGF will regulate other initial segment genes.

The mechanisms by which testicular factors act to stabilize transcripts in the initial segment is not clear. When allowed to decay, GGT mRNA IV was shown to decay in a biphasic manner (42). There was an initial rapid decay rate with a half-life of less than 1 hour, followed by a slower decay rate with a half-life of approximately 8 hours. Secondary structure models of GGT mRNA IV suggest that there are two families (α and β) of folding patterns for the 5' untranslated region (UTR). Analyses revealed that one 5' UTR folding pattern (α family) was more thermodynamically stable than the other (β family). Hence, it was postulated that the GGT mRNA IV α family decayed during the first hour after loss of testicular factors (42). As a result, and presumably during the first hour as well, the GGT mRNA IV β family decayed, but at a much slower rate. The mechanisms to account for differences in stability of the two families may involve differential binding of stabilizing complexes to each configuration, or that each family was more or less susceptible to cellular nucleases.

Other Mechanisms of Regulation by Testicular Factors

Components within RTF also act to repress the expression of certain epididymal genes and/or the synthesis and secretion of proteins. Brooks (46) showed that two proteins not normally synthesized in the initial segment were synthesized and secreted following orchiectomy. If androgens were administered following orchiectomy, these two proteins were still synthesized and secreted. Brooks (46) concluded that a factor(s) originating from the testis was responsible for the downregulation of these proteins. Studies by Holland et al. (20) clearly showed the appearance of a 40 kDa protein within the mouse proximal epididymis following EDL.

Testicular factors appear to play a dual role in maintaining the phosphorylation state of epididymal proteins. Loss of testicular factors causes dephosphorylation of MAPK in the initial segment (Hinton and Labus, unpublished observations), but several other initial segment cytoplasmic and nuclear proteins have been shown to be phosphorylated following the removal of testicular factors (40). These findings would suggest that testicular factors play a key role in maintaining a balance of kinase and phosphatase activities within the initial segment.

The Importance of the Initial Segment Toward Sperm Maturation

It is very clear from the studies outlined herein that testicular factor appear to play a vital role in the functioning of a very defined region of the epididymis, the initial segment. It seems that the function of zone 1A is highly dependent upon the presence of testicular factors, for the rat initial segment. This would suggest that this epididymal region is vital for sperm maturation. Evidence supporting the importance of the initial segment comes from the studies of Sonnenberg-Riethmacher et al. (47). The investigators generated an orphan tyrosine kinase receptor, c-ros, knock-out male mouse that resulted in an undeveloped initial segment and an infertility phenotype. The infertility appears to be due to abnormal sperm motility (48) and is assumed to be the result of the undeveloped initial segment and an infertility phenotype. The infertility appears to be due to abnormal sperm motility (48) and is assumed to be the result of the undeveloped initial segment. The mechanisms by which the initial segment contributes to sperm motility is not clear, but warrants further studies on the role and regulation of this important epididymal region.

Acknowledgments. Studies presented in this paper were supported by NIH Grants HD32979 (BTH), and P-30 HD28934 Center for Cellular and Molecular Studies in Reproduction, from The Rockefeller Foundation and the Ernst Schering Research Foundation.

References

1. Schiller MR, Mains RE, Eipper BA. A novel neuroendocrine signaling pathway. Mol Endocrinol 1997;11:1846–57.
2. Skinner JD, Rowson LEA. Effect of unilateral cryptorchidism on sexual development in the pubescent male animal. J Reprod Fertil 1967;14:349–50.
3. Skinner JD, Rowson LEA. Some effects of unilateral cryptorchidism and vasectomy on sexual development of the pubescent ram and bull. J Reprod Fertil 1968;42:311–21.
4. Gustafsson B. Luminal contents of the bovine epididymis under conditions of reduced spermatogenesis, luminal blockage and certain sperm abnormalities. Acta Vet Scand 1966;17(Suppl.):1–80.
5. Prasad MRN, Rajalakshmi M, Gupta G, Karkun T. Control of epididymal function. J Reprod Fertil 1973;18(Suppl.):215–22.
6. Danzo BJ, Cooper TG, Orgebin-Crist M-C. Androgen binding protein (ABP) in fluids collected from the rete testis and cauda epididymidis of sexually mature and immature rabbits and observations on morphological changes in the epididymis following ligation of the ductuli efferentes. Biol Reprod 1977;17:64–77.
7. Moniem KA, Glover TD, Lubicz-Nawrocki CW. Effects of duct ligation and orchiectomy on histochemical reactions in the hamster epididymis. J Reprod Fertil 1978;54:173–76.
8. Fawcett DW, Hoffer AP. Failure of exogenous androgen to prevent regression of the initial segments of the rat epididymis after efferent duct ligation or ochiectomy. Biol Reprod 1979;20:162–81.
9. Nicander L, Osman DI, Ploen L, Bugge HP, Kvisgaard KN. Early effects of efferent ductule ligation on the proximal segment of the rat epididymis. Int J Androl 1983;6:91–102.

10. Abe K, Takano H, Ito T. Interruption of the luminal flow in the epididymal duct of the corpus epididymidis in the mouse, with special reference to differentiation of the epididymal epithelium. Arch Histolog Jap 1984;47:137–47.
11. Reid BL, Cleland KW. The structure and function of the epididymis: histology of the rat epididymis. Aust J Zool 1957;5:223–46.
12. Fan XP, Robaire B. Orchiectomy induces a wave of apoptotic cell death in the epididymis. Endocrinology 1998;139:2124–36.
13. Turner TT, Riley TA. p53 independent, region-specific epithelial apoptosis is induced in the rat epididymis by deprivation of luminal factors. Mol Reprod Dev 1999;53:188–97.
14. Brooks DE. Influence of testicular secretions on tissue weight and on metabolic and enzyme activities in the epididymis of the rat. J Endocrinol 1979;82:305–13.
15. Robaire B, Ewing LL, Zirkin BR, Irby DC. Steroid Δ^4-5α-reductase and 3α-hydroxysteroid dehydrogenase in the rat epididymis. Endocrinology 1977;101:1379–90.
16. Pujol A, Bayard F, Louvet J-P, Boulard C. Testosterone and dihydrotestosterone concentrations in plasma, epididymal tissues, and seminal fluid of adult rats. Endocrinology 1976;98:111–13.
17. Brooks DE, Higgins SJ. Characterization and androgen-dependence of proteins associated with luminal fluid and spermatozoa in the rat epididymis. J Reprod Fertil 1980;59:363–75.
18. Jones R, Brown CR, von Glos KI, Parker MG. Hormonal regulation of protein synthesis in the rat epididymis: characterization of androgen-dependent and testicular fluid dependent proteins. Biochem J 1980a;188:776–76.
19. Jones R, von Glos KI, Brown CR. The synthesis of a sperm-coating protein in the initial segment of the rat epididymis is stimulated by factors in testicular fluid. IRCS Med Sci 1980b;8:193–9.
20. Holland MK, Vreeburg JTM, Orgebin-Crist M-C. Testicular regulation of epididymal protein secretion. J Androl 1992;13:266–73.
21. Rigaudiere N, Ghyselinck NB, Faure J, Dufaure J-P. Regulation of the epididymal glutathione peroxidase-like protein in the mouse: dependence upon androgens and testicular factors. Mol Cell Endocrinol 1992;89:67–77.
22. Turner TT, Miller DW, Avery EA. Protein synthesis and secretion by the rat caput epididymidis in vivo: influence of the luminal microenvironment. Biol Reprod 1995;52:1012–19.
23. Robaire B, Viger RS. Regulation of epididymal epithelial cell functions. Biol Reprod 1995;52:226–36.
24. Robaire B. Effects of unilateral orchiectomy on rat epididymal Δ^4-5'-reductase and 3α-hydroxysteroid dehydrogenase. Can J Physiol Parmacol 1979;57:998–1003.
25. Garrett JE, Garrett SH, Douglass J. A spermatozoa-associated factor regulates proenkephalin gene expression in the rat epididymis. Mol Endocrinol 1990;4:108–18.
26. Zwain IH, Grima J, Cheng CY. Rat epididymal retinoic acid-binding protein: development of a radioimmunossay, its tissue distribution, and its changes in selected androgen-dependent organs after orchiectomy. Endocrinology 1992;131:1511–26.
27. Cornwall GA, Orgebin-Crist M-C, Hann SR. The CRES gene: a unique testis-regulated gene related to the cystatin family is highly retricted in its expression to the proximal region of the mouse epididymis. Mol Endocrinol 1992;6:1653–64.

28. Palladino MA, Hinton BT. Expression of multiple gamma-glutamyl transpeptidase messenger ribonucleic acid transcripts in the adult rat epididymis is differentially regulated by androgens and testicular factors in a region-specific manner. Endocrinology 1994;135:1146–56.

29. Winer MA, Wolgemuth DJ. The segment-specific pattern of A-raf expression in the mouse epididymis is regulated by testicular factors. Endocrinology 1995; 136:2561–72.

30. Vernet P, Faure J, Dufaure J-P, Drevet JR. Tissue and developmental distribution, dependence upon testicular factors and attachment to spermatozoa of GPX, a murine epididymis-specific glutathione peroxidase. Mol Reprod Deve 1997;47: 87–98.

31. Lan Z-J, Palladino MA, Rudolph DB, Labus JC, Hinton BT. Identification, expression and regulation of the transcription factor polyomavirus enhancer activator 3 and its putative role in regulating the expression of gamma-glutamyl transpeptidase mRNA-IV in the rat epididymis. Biol Reprod 1997;57:186–93.

32. Cornwall GA, Hsia N. ADAM 7, a member of the ADAM (A Disintegrin and Metalloprotease) gene family is specifically expressed in the mouse anterior pituitary and epididymis. Endocrinology 1997;138:4262–72.

33. Borsook D, Rosen H, Collard M, Dressler H, Herrup K, Comb MJ, Hyman SE. Expression and regulation of a proenkephalin β-galactosidase fusion gene in the reproductive system of transgenic mice. Mol Endocrinol 1997;6:1502–12.

34. Setchell BP, Maddocks S, Brooks DE. Anatomy, vasculature, innervation, and fluids of the male reproductive tract. In: Knobil E, Neill JD, eds. The physiology of reproduction, second ed. New York: Raven Press, 1994:1063–175.

35. Hinton BT, Setchell BP. Fluid secretion and movement. In: Russell LD, Griswold MD, eds. The Sertoli cell. Vienna, IL: Cache River Press, 1993:249–67.

36. Sujarit S, Jones RC, Setchell BP, Chaturapnich G, Lin M, Clulow J. Stimulation of protein secretion in the initial segment of the rat epididymis by fluid from the ram rete testis. J Reprod Fertil 1990;88:315–21.

37. Danzo BJ, Eller BC, Orgebin-Crist M-C. Studies on the site of origin of the androgen binding protein present in epididymal cytosol from mature intact rabbits. Steroids 1974;24:107–22.

38. Palladino MA, Laperche Y, Hinton BT. Multiple forms of gamma-glutamyl transpeptidase messenger ribonucleic acid are expressed in the adult rat testis and epididymis. Biol Reprod 1994;50:320–28.

39. Lan Z-J, Lye RJ, Holic N, Labus JC, Hinton BT. The involvement of polyomavirus enhancer activator 3 (PEA3), an *ets* transcription factor, in the regulation of gamma-glutamyl transpeptidase mRVA-IV in the rat epididymis. Biol Reprod 1999;60:664–73.

40. Hinton BT, Lan ZJ, Rudolph DB, Labus JC, Lye RJ. Testicular regulation of epididymal gene expression. J Reprod Fert Suppl 1999;53:47–57.

41. Hinton BT, Palladino MA, Rudolph DB, Lan ZJ, Labus JC. The role of the epididymis in the protection of spermatozoa. In: Pederson RA, Schatten GP, eds. Current Topics in Developmental Biology, vol. 33. New York: Academic Press, 1996: 61–102.

42. Rudolph DB, Hinton BT. Stability and transcriptional regulation of gamma-glutamyl transpeptidase mRNA expression in the initial segment of the rat epididymis. J Androl 1997;18:501–12.

43. Xin JH, Cowie A, Lachance P, Hassell JA. Molecular cloning and characterization of PEA3, a new member of the Ets oncogene family that is differentially expressed in mouse embryonic cells. Genes Dev 1992;6:481–96.
44. Lan Z-J, Labus JC, Hinton BT. Regulation of gamma-glutamyl transpeptidase catalytic activity and protein level in the initial segment of the rat epididymis by testicular factors: role of basic fibroblast growth factor. Biol Reprod 1998;58:197–206.
45. Alarid ET, Cunha GR, Young P, Nicoll CS. Evidence for an organ- and sex-specific role of basic fibroblast growth factor in the development of the fetal mammalian reproductive tract. Endocrinology 1991;129:2148–54.
46. Brooks DE. Effect of androgens on protein synthesis and secretion in various regions of the rat epididymis, as analysed by two-dimensional gel electrophoresis. Mol Cell Endocrinol 1983;29:255–70.
47. Sonnenberg-Riethmacher E, Walter B, Riethmacher D, Godecke S, Birchmeier C. The c-ros tyrosine receptor controls regionalization and differentiation of epithelial cells in the epididymis. Genes Dev 1996;10:1184–93.
48. Yeung CH, Sonnenberg-Riethmacher E, Cooper TG. Receptor tyrosine kinase c-ros knock-out mice as a model for the study of epididymal regulation of sperm function. J Reprod Fert Suppl 1999;53:137–47.

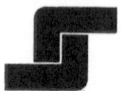

16

Aging Causes Structural
and Functional Alterations
in the Epididymis

BERNARD ROBAIRE AND VALERIE SERRE

The development of the epididymis between birth and adulthood has been the subject of many histological, histochemical, and biochemical studies. It has generally been assumed that once adult structure and functions are established in this tissue, they remain unaltered thereafter; however, we know little about changes in the appearance of this tissue or in the ability of the tissue to impart proper motility characteristics and fertilizing ability to spermatozoa during aging. Understanding changes that take place in this tissue beyond the attainment of adulthood is of particular interest for two major reasons. The first is the increasing age at which individuals are choosing to have a family, and thus the potential effects of aging on progeny outcome. The second is the ability to study aging in a system that is not essential for survival of the organism, thus providing a tool to understand the intrinsic mechanisms by which a tissue ages.

A difficulty with most studies designed to study aging of the male reproductive system is the inability to dissociate aging of the male reproductive tract from degenerative conditions in other tissues that may indirectly cause the reproductive tract to deteriorate. The brown Norway (BN) rat has the advantage of remaining in excellent health throughout its long lifespan. Age-related pathologies consist mostly of cardiac lesions (7%); these rats do not develop testicular, liver, or pituitary tumors (1,2). Thus, it is possible to distinguish changes related to aging per se, from changes induced by a specific disease. Several age-related changes occurr in the reproductive tract of the BN rats that are very similar to those found in men. With increasing age, BN rats exhibit an atrophy of the seminiferous tubules, thickening of the basement membrane, decreased steroidogenesis, changes in secretory patterns of leutenizing hormone (LH) and follicle-stimulating hormone (FSH), and decreased spermatogenesis (3–8).

Using the BN rat as a model, Zirkin and collaborators have shown that the age-related decreases in serum and testicular testosterone concentrations were due to Leydig cell failure (9–11). In addition to changes in Leydig cell structure and function, changes in gene expression in both seminiferous tubules and epididymis have been found to occur as animals age (3,4,12). As a result, the BN rat provides an excellent tool for the study of aging, and new exciting data on the mechanism of aging are emerging rapidly. We will focus on structural and functional changes taking place in the epididymis during aging, as well as on the ability of spermatozoa from aging rats to produce normal offspring.

Structural Changes in the Epididymis During Aging

One of the few studies that has described morphological changes in the epididymis during aging was done by Cran and Jones in 1979 (13) using the rabbit as the animal model. They found that, in aged animals, there was an absence of spermatozoa in the epididymal lumen, an accumulation of lipofuscin in principal and basal cells, occasional cytoplasmic vacuoles, and intranuclear inclusions. Several studies in other species (e.g., rat, monkey, and human) have also provided data suggesting decreases in epididymal sperm count, appearance of lipofuscin, lymphocyte infiltration, and emergence of sperm autoantibodies (14–20). We have undertaken a series of studies designed to assess systematically the effects of age on each segment of the epididymis of BN rats.

The Basement Membrane and Epithelial Cells

The epididymides of BN rats ranging in age from 3 to 24 months were assessed by light and electron microscopy. Evaluation of the effect of age on the luminal diameter, epithelial height, and thickness of the lamina propria in each segment of the epididymis revealed some striking changes. There was a reduction in the luminal diameter, whereas a progressive thickening of the lamina propria in each segment of the epididymis was noted. The height of the epithelium was not affected by age in any region of the tissues except for the corpus epididymidis, where a marked increase in epithelial height was noted as animals aged (21).

Major segment-specific changes in the appearance of cells along the epididymis with age were noted. As early as 12 months, basal cells in the initial segment were found to emit pseudopods into the thickened basement membrane. By 18 months, clear cells in the caput epididymidis often showed bulging protrusions into the lumen; they were filled with lysosomes. In the corpus epididymidis, there was a remarkable increase in the number and size of lysosomes in the cytoplasm of principal cells. The percentage of cell surface occupied by lysosomes increased from less than 2% at 3 months to more than 15% by 15 months; these lysosomes were found both below and above the nucleus. There was also a striking increase in lipofuscin in these cells, as assessed by their autofluorescece when examined with a confocal microscope (Fig. 16.1). Apical cells, which are normally never seen beyond the caput epididymidis in young animals, were found in the corpus epididymidis of older animals; they were usually occupied by one giant membranous lysosome. In the proximal cauda epididymidis, clear cells became filled with dense lysosomes and princi-

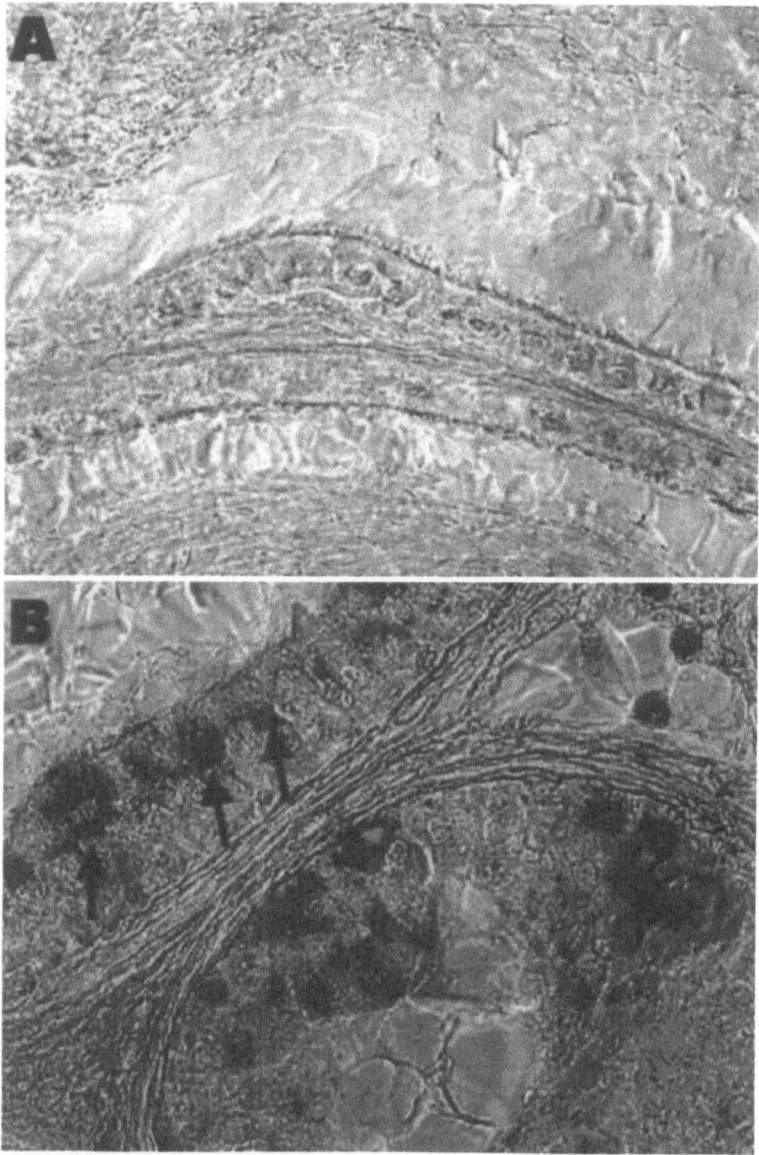

FIGURE 16.1. Confocal micrographs of the corpus epididymidis of young (3 months) (A) and old (24 months) (B) BN rats. These sections (5 μm) were not stained with a fluorescent antibody. The dark granules (arrows) observed in principal cells of old animals are autofluorescent lipofuscin. Magnification = 540×

pal cells presented with large clear vacuoles; debris from spermatozoa was found in these larger vacuoles. The number of halo cells, which are cells of the immune system, increased progressively with age in all segments of the epididymis. Thus, aging of the epididymis was accompanied by the emergence of characteristic features of aging as well as many cell- and segment-specific changes; these were not related to the presence of spermatozoa, and often preceded their disappearance, thus indicating that there may be an intrinsic mechanism of aging in the epididymal epithelial cells.

Cells of the Immune System

Because there was a dramatic increase in the number of halo cells present in the epididymal epithelium of the BN rat during aging, a more detailed study of these cells, postulated to be lymphocytes or monocytes, was undertaken (22). To identify the immunological origin of halo cells, markers for helper T lymphocytes, cytotoxic T lymphocytes, and monocytes-macrophages were investigated in epididymides of BN rats ranging in age from 3 to 24 months. A count of the number of immunocompetent cells in the epithelium and interstitial tissue of the epididymis was done in relation to age, epididymal segment, and luminal content. We found that monocytes-macrophages, helper T lymphocytes, and cytotoxic T lymphocytes all belong to the population of halo cells. Furthermore, there was an increase in the number of cytotoxic T helper cells and monocytes-macrophages recruited in the epididymal epithelium of aged rats in all segments of the epididymis with the exception of the cauda region. In older animals, this immune cell recruitment was markedly higher in animals that had few or no sperm in the lumen when compared with those that continued to have a large number of sperm in the lumen of the epididymis. It is of interest to note that the immunolocalization of all cells of the immune system (halo cells) differed markedly from that found for basal cells (22,23). In summary, the major increase in the concentration of immune cells in the epididymal epithelium was segment specific and luminal content dependent. Based on these results, it is interesting to speculate that the accumulation of damaged cells and antigens (of spermatozoal or postpubertal germ-cell origin) leak through a dysfunctional blood–epididymis barrier and contribute to the active recruitment of immune cells during aging.

Functional Changes in the Epididymis During Aging

Cell–Cell Interactions

The blood–epididymis barrier is formed by tight junctions in the apical region of adjoining principal cells (24). The barrier normally protects spermatozoa from immunological attack, which is necessary because spermatozoa are viewed by the organism as nonself as a result of novel antigenic proteins synthesized during spermacytogenesis and spermiogenesis. As a consequence of the alterations in epididymal epithelial histology and the increase in halo cells during aging, we hypothesized that there would be changes in the structure and function of the blood–epididymis barrier with age.

To test this hypothesis, the immunocytochemical localization of markers postulated to play key roles in tight junction formation (e.g., occludin, ZO-1, and E-cadherin), as well as lanthanum nitrate permeability of the blood–

epididymis barrier, were assessed in the epididymides of BN rats aged 3, 18, and 24 months (25). Occludin is responsible for sealing the adjacent plasma membranes of tight junctions together (26). ZO-1, a peripheral membrane protein, is directly associated with the carboxyl terminus of occludin in the tight junction (27). Together, occludin and ZO-1 have been postulated to maintain the structural integrity of the tight junction (27–29). The cadherins, a family of calcium-dependent cell adhesion glycoproteins joining together adjacent cells (30), play a role in the formation and maintenance of tight junctions between epithelial cells.

In the initial segment, occludin, ZO-1, an E-cadherin immunostaining was observed at the apico-lateral junction between principal cells in the 3-month-old animals. Occludin and ZO-1 reactivity decreased with increasing age, whereas E-cadherin staining increased along the lateral membrane between principal cells. In the caput, corpus, and cauda epididymidis, occludin, ZO-1, and E-cadherin immunostaining showed segment-specific and age-dependent differences in their staining patterns. The most dramatic changes with age were seen in the corpus epididymidis; the intense E-cadherin cytoplasmic staining that was observed at 3 months was absent by 24 months and no occludin or ZO-1 reactivity was observed in older animals. The greatest penetration of lanthanum nitrate across the blood–epididymis barrier and in the lumen was seen in the aging corpus epididymidis, whereas there was no barrier permeability in the initial segment or cauda epididymidis of the aged animals. A schematic representation of these findings is shown in Figure 16.2. Taken together, these data indicate that there are segment-specific decreases in the structural and functional integrity of the blood–epididymis barrier with age, most notably in the corpus epididymidis.

Androgen Responsiveness

The decrease in testosterone production along with the histological changes in the epididymis seen during aging in the BN rat suggested the possibility that the expression of key genes in this tissue would be affected by aging. BN rats ranging in age from 6 to 30 months were examined at 6-month intervals; epididymides were sectioned into caput-corpus and cauda regions. Relative mRNA concentrations were assessed using Northern blot analysis and specific cDNAs for the rat 5α-reductase isozymes, types 1 and 2, proenkephalin, the androgen receptor, epididymal proteins B/C and D/E, and clusterin (sulfated glycoprotein-2, SGP-2) (12).

In the caput-corpus epididymidis, 5α-reductase type 1 and type 2 mRNA concentrations decreased significantly by 43% and 33%, respectively, between 6 and 12 months, and by 64% and 40%, respectively, between 6 and 30 months. No significant change, however, was found in the expression of the 5α-reductase mRNAs in the cauda epididymidis. It is interesting that proenkephalin mRNA was only detected in the caput-corpus epididymidis of 6-month-old rats. In marked contrast to the 5α-reductase isozymes and proenkephalin, no significant age-related changes were observed in the mRNA concentrations for the

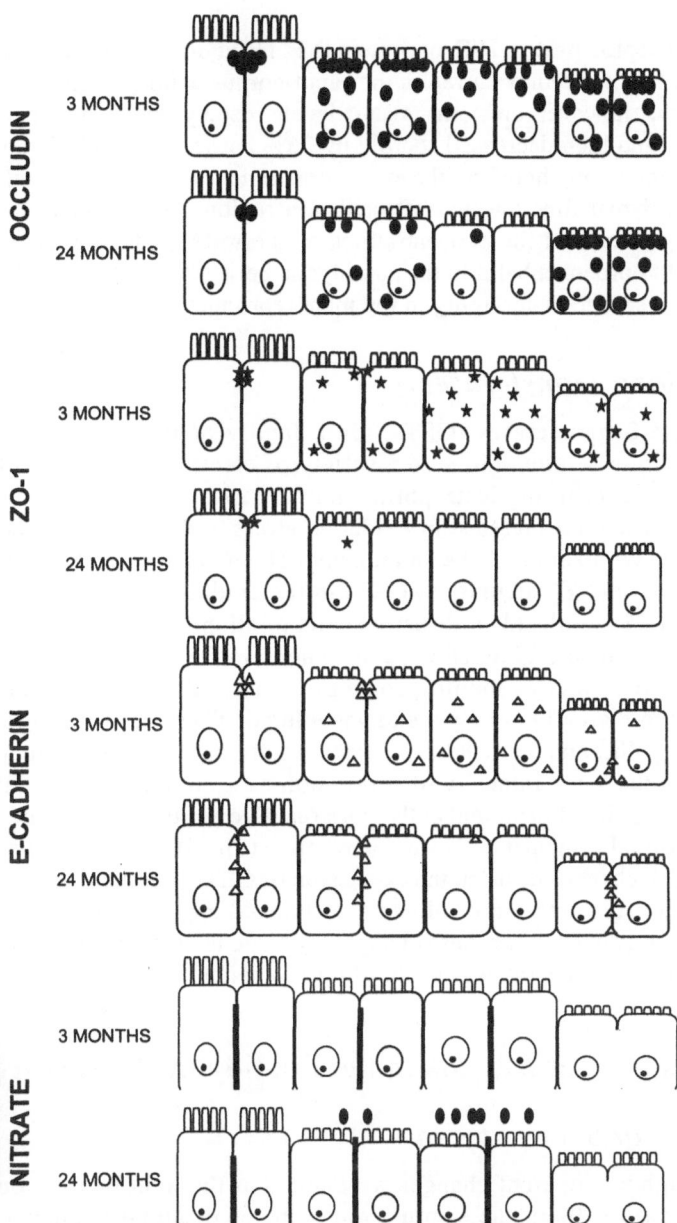

FIGURE 16.2. Diagrammatic representation of the relative expression of occludin (filled circles), ZO-1 (stars), E-cadherin (triangles), and lanthanum (black lines and black ovals) in principal cells along the epididymis of young (3 months) and old (24 months) BN rats. The relative size of cells along the epididymis and during aging are only an approximate representation of the changes observed. The intensity of immunohistochemical staining is represented by the density of the symbols used for each marker. Adapted from (25).

androgen receptor, protein B/C, or protein D/E. No age-related changes in mRNA expression for clusterin occurred in the caput-corpus epididymidis. In the cauda epididymidis, however, clusterin mRNA levels rose by two fold between 6 and 18 months, and then decreased sharply by 75% between 18 and 30 months. As the epididymis aged, therefore, the expression of genes for certain specific markers of epididymal function was affected in a region-specific manner. Furthermore, the decrease in the concentrations of the mRNAs for the 5α-reductase isozymes and proenkephalin in the epididymis between 6 and 12 months is thus far the earliest marker for aging in the male reproductive tract of the BN rat.

Glutathione Transferases

Glutathione S-transferases (GSTs) are a family of isozymes that catalyze the conjugation of glutathione to a variety of electrophiles, and protect cellular constituents from electrophilic and oxidative attack. Aging is associated with an overall increase in oxidative stress and, therefore, free radical production. We examined the immunocytochemical localization of Ya, Yc, Yb_1, Yb_2, Yo, and Yf subunits of GSTs in the epididymis of BN rats aged 3, 12, 18, and 24 months (31). Principal cells of all epididymal regions, except the proximal cauda region, showed no change in GST expression at any age examined. At 18 and 24 months, some principal cells of the proximal cauda region became greatly enlarged and vacuolated. These cells were unreactive for Yo, Yb_1, Yb_2, and Yc, whereas adjacent normal-appearing principal cells maintained the same intensity of expression as seen in 3-month controls. In contrast, vacuolated principal cells were reactive for the Ya subunit, whereas adjacent normal principal cells were unreactive (Fig. 16.3). These data indicate that selective changes occur in the expression of GSTs in principal cells of older animals that have both a normal and a vacuolated appearance. The underlying mechanism responsible for these changes with age is unresolved, but we speculate that this indicates the loss of the ability to handle oxidative stress.

Changes in Spermatozoa in the Epididymis During Aging

Structure of Spermatozoa

Even though no apparent changes were noted at the light or electron microscope in germ cells in the seminiferous tubules of aging animals (32), the appearance of spermatozoa and other components in the lumen of the epididymis in older animals showed some marked abnormalities. There was the appearance of a significant number of cells that appeared to be spermatocytes or round spermatids; many of these cells had pycnotic nuclei and appeared to undergo degradation. The proportion of spermatozoa that retained their cytoplasmic droplet was markedly elevated. Most striking, however, was the large number of spermatozoa that had abnormal axonemal strucures and multiple tails surrounded by a single outer membrane; examples of these abnormalities are shown in Figure 16.4.

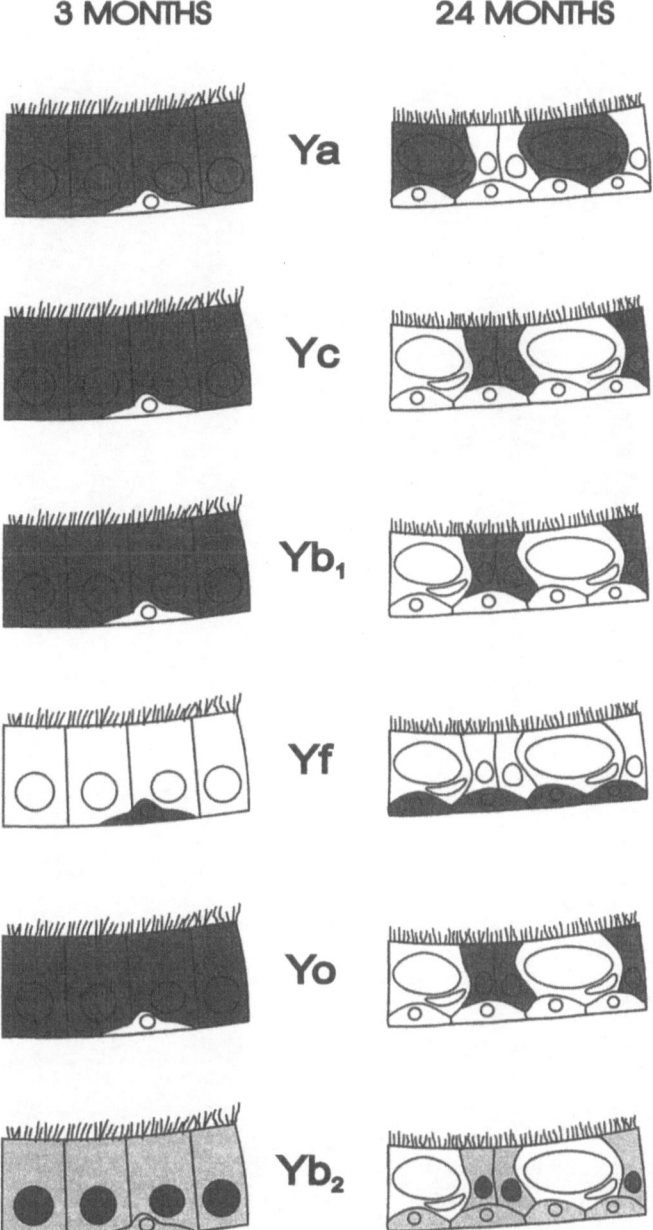

FIGURE 16.3. Schematic representation of the intensity of immunohistochemical staining for the Ya, Yc, Yb_1, Yf, Yo, and Yb_2 subunits of glutathione S-transferases in the proximal cauda epididymidis of young (3 months, left) and old (24 months, right) BN rats. Only principal and basal cells are represented.

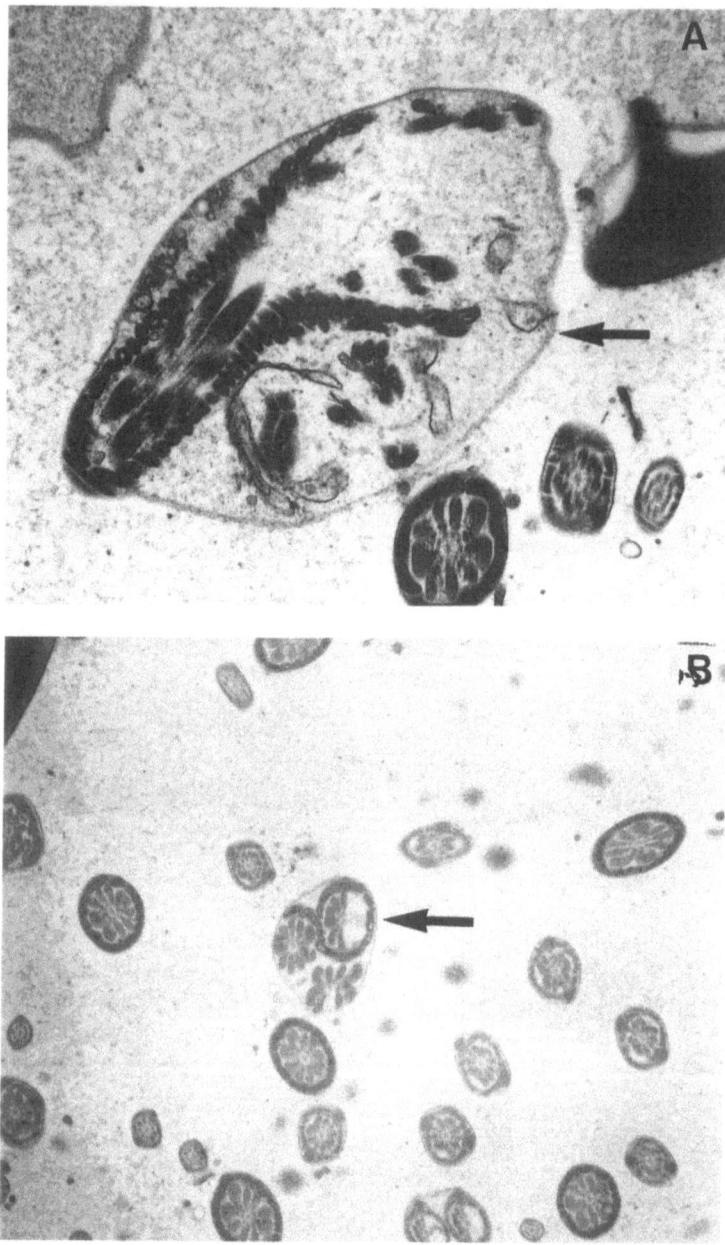

FIGURE 16.4. Electron micrographs of the luminal content of the cauda epididymidis of 18-month-old BN rats. The arrow in panel A points to a germ cell that has completed spermatogenesis. The arrow in panel B points to an abnormal sperm tail that has elements of at least two axonemes. Magnification = 6100×

Effects of Age on Fertility and Progeny Outcome

The dramatic effects on epididymal structure and function, along with the altered appearance of a high proportion of spermatozoa in the epididymis, led to the hypothesis that age may affect the quality of spermatozoa in such a way that either fertility or progeny outcome may be affected deleteriously.

Although the effects of maternal age on both fertility and progeny outcome have rendered genetic counseling routine, the effects of paternal age have been relatively neglected. It has been hypothesized that point mutations may be associated with the replication process and that such mutations may increase with increasing paternal age (33). Several studies have shown that paternal age can indeed increase the incidence of autosomal and X-linked hereditary diseases (34–36), with mutation rates several times higher in the older age groups (37). There are few well-controlled studies, however, on the relationship between aging and male fertility (38,39).

We undertook a study in which male rats of increasing age were mated to young females; pregnancy outcome was assessed by counting the numbers of corpora lutea, resorptions, and live fetuses on day 20 of gestation (40). To evaluate progeny outcome, pups were examined for external malformations and weighed daily for 2 months. There were no significant changes in the numbers of resorptions, live offspring, or the incidence of external malformations; however, there was an increase in pre-implantation loss (corpora lutea minus implantation sites) from less than 6% in litters fathered by young males to more than 20% in litters fathered by older males. There was, surprisingly, a significant decrease in the average fetal weight that was directly associated with increasing paternal age. In addition, a greater than threefold increase in neonatal deaths was noted for progeny fathered by older males. These results together clearly indicate that the quality of spermatozoa decreases as males age.

Summary

Remarkable changes take place in the epididymis of the BN rat during aging with respect to both the histological appearance and the expression of a number of genes. The underlying causes(s) for these changes is (are) unresolved. It is interesting to note, however, that several changes found during aging would be consistent with the hypothesis that increased oxidative stress is in part responsible for aging. Such changes include the increased number of lysosomes and the appearance of large amounts of lipofuscin (both point to the inability of principal cells to handle an increased load of oxidized lipids properly), and the decreased levels of glutathione S-transferases. The reasons for the region specificity of many of the age-dependent changes observed is also not clear, but the association between the site where there is the most dramatic breakdown of the blood–epididymis barrier, the decreased presence of proteins involved in the formation of this barrier, and the increased presence of macrophages all point to a complex dynamic interaction among the decreased quality of the content of the lumen of the epididymis (degenerating and abnormal spermatozoa), altered epididymal epithelium, and the immune system.

Acknowledgments. These studies were supported by a grant from the National Institute of Aging ((NIH AG08321).

References

1. Festing MFW. Inbred strains. In: Baker HJ, Lindsey JR, Weisbroth SH, eds. The laboratory rat. New York: Academic Press; 1979:55–72.
2. Zirkin BR, Santulli R, Strandberg JD, Wright WW, Ewing LL. Testicular steroidogenesis in the aging brown Norway rat. J Androl 1993;14:118–23.
3. Richardson LL, Kleinman HK, Dym M. The effects of aging on the basement membrane in the testis. J Androl 1995;16:118–26.
4. Wright WW, Fiore C, Zirkin BR. The effect of aging on the seminiferous epithelium of the brown Norway rat. J Androl 1993;14:110–17.
5. Wang C, Leung A, Sinha-Hikim AP. Reproductive aging in the male brown Norway rat: a model for the human. Endocrinology 1993;133:2773–81.
6. Bonavera JJ, Swerdloff RS, Leung A, Lue YH, Baravarian S, Superlano L, et al. In the male brown-Norway (BN) rat, reproductive aging is associated with decreased LH-pulse amplitude and area. J Androl 1997;18:359–65.
7. Zirkin BR, Santulli R, Strandberg JD, Wright WW, Ewing LL. Testicular steroidogenesis in the aging brown Norway rat. J Androl 1993;14:118–23.
8. Gruenewald DA, Naai MA, Hess DL, Matsumoto AM. The brown Norway rat as a model of male reproductive aging: evidence of both primary and secondary testicular failure. J Gerontol 1994;49:b42–50.
9. Chen H, Hardy MP, Huhtaniemi I, Zirkin BR. Age-related decreased Leydig cell testosterone production in the brown Norway rat. J Androl 1994;15:551–57.
10. Zirkin BR. Regulation of spermatogenesis in the adult mammal: gonadotropins and androgens. In: Desjardins L, Ewing LL, eds. Cell and molecular biology of the testis. New York: New York University Press, 1993:166–88.
11. Luo L, Chen H, Zirkin BR. Are Leydig cell steroidogenic enzymes differentially regulated with aging? J Androl 1996;17:509–15.
12. Viger RS, Robaire B. Gene expression in the aging brown Norway rat epididymis. J Androl 1995;16:108–17.
13. Cran DG, Jones R. Aging of male reproductive system: changes in the epididymis. Exp Gerontol 1980;15:93–101.
14. Markey CM, Meyer GT. A quantitative description of the epididymis and its microvasculature: an age-related study in the rat. J Anat 1992;180:255–62.
15. Taylor GT, Weiss J, Pitha J. Epididymal sperm profiles in young adult, middle-aged, and testosterone-supplemented old rats. Gamete Res 1988;110–17.
16. Regadera J, Nistal M, Paniagua R. Testis, epididymis, and spermatic cord in elderly men. Correlation of angiographic and histologic studies with systemic arteriosclerosis. Arch Pathol Lab Med 1985;109:663–67.
17. Oshima S, Okayasu I, Uchima H, Hatakeyama S. Histopathological and morphometrical study of the human epididymis and testis. Acta Pathol Jap 1984;34:1327–42.
18. Rumke P. Autoantikorperbildung gegen spermatozoa infolge extravasation von spermatozoen ins interstitium der epididymis alterer manner. Schweizerishe Med Wochenshr 1971;101:1439–41.

19. Mitchinson MJ, Sherman KP, Stainer-Smith AM. Brown patches in the epididymis. J Pathol 1975;115:57–62.
20. Baskerville A, Cook RW, Dennis MJ, Cranage MP, Greenaway PJ. Pathological changes in the reproductive tract of male rhesus monkeys associated with age and simian AIDS. J Comp Pathol 1992;107:49–57.
21. Serre V, Robaire B. Segment specific morphological changes in the aging brown Norway rat epididymis. Biol Reprod 1998;58:497–513.
22. Serre V, Robaire B. Distribution of immune cells in the epididymis of the aging brown Norway rat is segment-specific and related to the luminal content. Biol Reprod 1999;61:705–14.
23. Yeung CH, Cooper TG. Basal cells of the human epididymis: antigenic and ultrastructural similarities to tissues-fixed macrophages. Biol Reprod 1994;50:917–26.
24. Hoffer AP, Hinton BT. Morphological evidence for a blood–epididymis barrier and the effects of gossypol on its integrity. Biol Reprod 1984;30:991–1004.
25. Levy S, Robaire B. Segment-specific changes in the expression of junctional proteins and the permeability of the blood-epididymis barrier with age. Biol Reprod 1999;60:1392–401.
26. Furuse M, Hirase T, Itoh, M, Nagafuchi A, Yonemura, S, Tsukita S, et al. Occludin: a novel integral membrane protein localizing at tight junctions. J Cell Biol 1993;6:1777–88.
27. Furuse M, Itoh M, Hirase T, Nagafuchi A, Yonemura S, Tsukita S, et al. Direct association of occludin and ZO-1 and its possible involvement in the localization of occludin at tight junctions. J Cell Biol 1994;127:1617–26.
28. Citi S. The molecular organization of tight junctions. J Cell Biol 1993;121:485–89.
29. Tsukita S, Furuse M, Itoh M. Molecular architecture of tight junctions: occludin and ZO-1. Soc Gen Physiol Ser 1997;52:69–76.
30. Shapiro L, Fannon AM, Kwong PD, Thompson A, Lehmann MS, Grubel G, et al. Structural basis of cell–cell adhesion by cadherins. Nature 1995;372:327–37.
31. Mueller A, Hermo L, Robaire B. The effects of aging on the expression of glutathione S-transferases in the testis and epididymis of the brown Norway rat. J Androl 1998;19:450–65.
32. Levy S, Serre V, Hermo L, Robaire B. The effects of aging on the seminiferous epithelium and the blood-testis barrier of the brown Norway rat. J Androl 1999; 20:356–65.
33. Crow JF. The high spontaneous mutation rate: is it a health risk? Proc Natl Acad Sci USA 1997;94:8380–86.
34. Auroux M. The quality of conceptus as a function of father's age. La qualite du conceptus en fonction de l'age du pere. J Urol (Paris) 1993;99:29–34.
35. Friedman JM. Genetic disease in the offspring of older fathers. Obstet Gynecol 1981;57:745–49.
36. Jones KL, Smith DW, Segwick-Harvey MA, Hall BD, Quan L. Older paternal age and fresh gene mutation: data on additional disorders. J Pediatr 1975;86:84–88.
37. Vogel F, Motulsky AG. Mutation: spontaneous mutation in germ cells. In: Vogel F, Motulsky AG, eds. Human genetics, 3rd ed. Berlin: Springer; 1997:385–430.
38. Stene J, Stene E. On data and methods in investigations on parental-age effects. Ann Hum Gen 1978;41:465–68.
39. Mineau GP, Trussell J. A specification of marital fertility by parents' age, age at marriage and marital duration. Demography 1982;19:335–50.
40. Serre V, Robaire B. Paternal age affects fertility and progeny outcome in the brown Norway rat. Fertil Steril 1998;70:625–31.

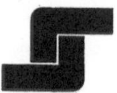

17

The Molecular Basis of
Sperm–Egg Interactions

DAVID L. GARBERS AND TIMOTHY A. QUILL

Introduction

The identification of receptors on spermatozoa for egg or other female-derived signals has proven particularly difficult in the mammal. Although various candidate receptors or cell-recognition proteins have been identified, amd some have stronger credentials than do others, a consensus model for the molecular basis of mammalian fertilization has not yet arisen. Arguments that each species possess a unique signaling paradigm are so antithetical that it can be dismissed outright. Technical limitations (e.g., the paucity of material in mammals relative to many invertebrates/lower vertebrates) and the asynchronous nature of the mammalian sperm population certainly represent significant barriers to discovery. New technological advances, however, as well as the EST, protein, and genome databases, however, offer substantial means by which to now overcome many of the limitations of the past. We will concentrate in this chapter on just a few topics associated with signaling in mammalian sperm cells.

Defining Signaling with Populations
of Mammalian Spermatozoa

The downstream signaling pathways utilized by germ cells appear to be similar or identical across the species, and also similar or identical to those of somatic cells. The cell and species specificity arises principally from the recognition/receptor molecules, and potentially to a few proteins immediately downstream of the receptors (e.g., cyclases, channels, and transporters). Whether studying germ or somatic cell signaling, we must often use these downstream signaling molecules (e.g., cyclic nucleotides, protein kinase activity, Ca^{2+}) as evidence the cell has detected an extracellular signal. It then becomes possible to define the extracellular signal as well as the receptor through the use of these intracellular signals as functional bioassays. Inherent in this process, however, is an assumption that a majority of cells both respond to a given signal and that such cells also respond within the same temporal time frame. Activation of spermatozoa, specific egg binding, and fertilization of a sea urchin egg occur within 1 minute after mixing the gametes. Activation also sets in motion a rapid loss of fertilization potential. Thus, within echinoderms, the behavior of individual sperm cells is adequately reflected in studies on the sperm population (assuming that a subsecond/second time frame of synchronization is acceptable). Thus, changes in signaling molecule concentrations or activities adequately serve as an indicator of individual cell behavior.

The mammal, however, is not particularly accommodating. If we analyze a rather typical series of experiments, using those of Lee et al. (1) as an example, 60% of mouse spermatozoa demonstrate an acrosome reaction between 150 and 180 minutes after binding to the zona pellucida (Fig. 17.1). This also means, however, that 40% (or nearly one half) either react outside this time frame or fail to display an acrosome reaction at all. Furthermore, if we were to assume that the percentage of cells undergoing the acrosome reaction was constant throughout the 150–180 minute time period, then only 2% of the entire population actually acrosome-reacts during each minute. If signaling events exhibit the same characteristics as the final morphological event in terms of a time frame, they become literally impossible to use as a means for reliable detection of receptor activation. Thus, many of the as-

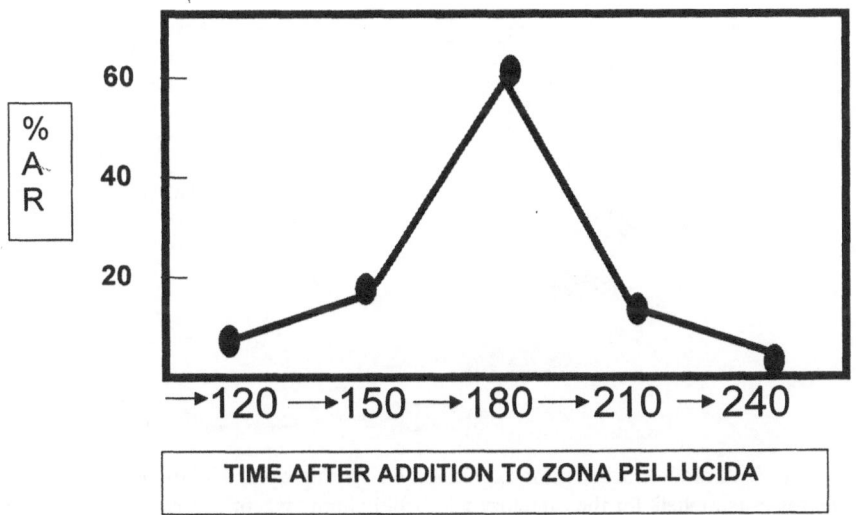

FIGURE 17.1. Percentage acrosome reactions as a function of time after addition of spermatozoa to the zona pellucida of the mouse. The data are modified from (1).

signments of signaling pathways in mammalian sperm cells have arisen through the use of inhibitors or activators, whether it be signaling molecule analogs, inhibitory drugs, inhibitory or activating antibodies, or gene disruption. The inherent problem with these approaches is they often do not facilitate the direct identification of the signaling pathway components, particularly the molecules most immediate to the primary extracellular signal.

"Leaky Transcription" and Diversity

Aside from the asynchronous nature of the sperm-cell population, the notion that a multiplicity of signaling pathways exist, any of which could initiate a behavioral change such as the acrosome reaction, represents an additional model that would necessarily interrupt the anticipation of establishing a consensus and unique signaling pathway for induction of the acrosome reaction or other behavioral responses (Fig. 17.2). For a given sperm cell, it is certainly conceivable that the acrosome reaction, for example, might be induced either by the cumulus cells, the zona pellucida, or through a variety of pathways, including inherent self-programming (which could appear spontaneous), all of which would ultimately result in a behavioral change. In such conceptual models of fertilization, a single signaling pathway for successful fertilization would not exist (although a given one may dominate); rather, a multitude of possibilities would present themselves, with the one ultimately utilized dependent on the status of

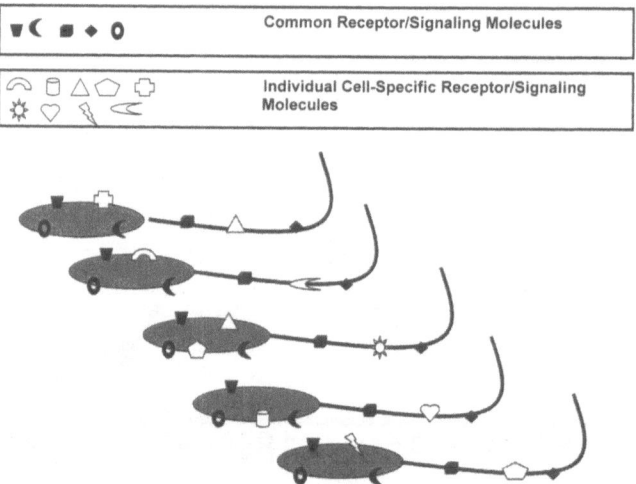

FIGURE 17.2. A model for receptor expression on spermatozoa. The model replicates in some respects models for the olfactory neuroepithelium, except expression of receptors that are not necessarily unique to spermatozoa are suggested to be expressed in a rather random manner. A given sperm cell would express a number of receptors/adhesion molecules common to all sperm cells within its own species, but would also express a unique combination of other potential receptor/adhesion molecules.

the sperm cell at any given moment. Convergence of signaling pathways, possibly at a very early step in the process (e.g., G-protein activation), could lead to false impressions that a singular pathway existed because of the use of inhibitors upstream or downstream of the convergence point.

This conceptual model of sperm cells yields magnificent diversity instead of conservative stagnation. It is easy to magnify this proposed diversity even further by a consideration of what has been referred to as "leaky transcription." Take, for example, the simple question: Given that spermatozoa are relatively small cells, is it better to build them all the same, or is it better to build each one somewhat differently, even though in both cases the numbers of proteins would necessarily be limited? Strong arguments can be made that in the latter case, successful fertilization would be more likely under a wide variety of environments, thus assuring that at least some sperm cells in any particular female environment would have the capacity to respond to signals and successfully fertilize the egg. That members of the seven-transmembrane odorant receptor family are found in germ cells may support this concept, in that multiple apparent receptors are expressed in the testis (2). In the olfactory epithelium, it is clear that most neurons express only a single seven-transmembrane receptor. Because each receptor presumably detects a different series of chemicals, that germ cells are expressing multiple genes suggests either that (1) all sperm cells contain each of the receptors (unlike the olfactory neurons), and a multitude of different signals are monitored at different times, or (2) different sperm cells express different receptors, possibly even in a mutually exclusive fashion. The latter would impose considerable diversity within the sperm cell population, and lead to the conclusion that high numbers of spermatozoa at ejaculation are important to exaggerate the diversity of cells and not to provide 1 million nearly identical cells, leading to an increased probability that a reasonable number of cells within the population would be perfectly suited to the environment they enter.

We could assume, for example, that 1000 genes would be expressed as common to all sperm cells, but that a significant number (e.g., 25% of the genome; those described as expressed due to leaky transcription) would be distributed to individual sperm cells as a protective mechanism. This would mean about 35,000 genes, and possibly those most directly involved with environmental detection (signaling), could be distributed to individual sperm cells in various combinations. A bias to express some genes in a larger proportion of sperm cells could occur. Because this would likely vary across the species, it could explain apparent species-specificity with respect to the effects of some common hormones (e.g., progesterone, prostaglandins).

The latter hypothesis would also explain a probable need for spermatozoa to be blocked from responding to any external signal for a considerable period of time, thus explaining a need for the process of capacitation. Although the process of capacitation could represent a means by which to stabilize sperm cells in the male reproductive tract in other manners, it could also "stabilize" by prevention of acrosome reactions and activations of other processes because of the diversity of signaling receptors within the sperm population.

What might we expect if the population is this diverse? If we consider the acrosome reaction as an example, then, first, a very low percentage of acrosome reactions would be expected to occur in response to a specific external signal and thus go unnoticed. Only a small fraction of the cells would respond to a given external signal except where a particular receptor/signaling molecule was common. Some common receptors would be expected to exist, however, and these could explain, for example, the ability of ZP3 to induce the acrosome reactions in a large percentage of the sperm population.

We will end with examples of three approaches we have used in attempts to define receptors/recognition/signaling molecules on sperm cells, where an initial criterion for us often has been that a molecule is expressed in a sperm-specific manner. Based on the preceding arguments, it could be contended that sperm specific is not a reliable indicator of importance, but this criterion at least suggests a protein with unique functions in spermatozoa.

A Sperm Plasma Membrane Protein That Binds to the Zona Pellucida

In the work of Dan Hardy and later Zeren Gao of our laboratory (3–5), a protein we named *zonadhesin* was identified based on its binding to the zona pellucida in a relative species-specific manner. A schematic of the domain structure of zonadhesin from pig and mouse is shown in Figure 17.3. The protein, first expressed by the haploid spermatid, is unique in nature. From the signal peptide toward the carboxyl end of the protein, the mouse contains three tandem repeats, and the pig contains one full and one partial MAM domain. MAM domains are about 160-amino acids in length and contain four conserved Cys residues, as well as a number of conserved hydrophobic and aromatic amino acids. MAM domains are present in various membrane proteins including meprins (6), A5 protein (7), and receptor protein tyrosine phosphatases (8–10). The meprins are Zn-metalloproteases that contain an α- and β-subunit (6,11), whereas the MAM domain has been suggested to mediate dimerization or oligomerization of these subunits (11). A5 protein is a developmentally regulated cell-surface molecule involved in neurite outgrowth and axonal guidance, whereas the MAM domain has been suggested important for cell–cell interactions (7). Various receptor protein tyrosine phosphatases (RPTP$_\mu$, RPTP$_\kappa$, RPTP$_\psi$, PCP-2) contain MAM domains that have been proposed as essential for homophilic cell–cell interactions (9,10). The function of the zonadhesin MAM domains is not known, but because this region can be eliminated without disruption of zona pellucida binding (3–5), it may function early during sperm development.

To the carboxyl side of the MAM domains is a mucinlike domain. The mouse zonadhesin domain is larger than that of the pig. It has been suggested that the core mucin domain protein exists in an extended form and serves as a scaffold for O-linked carbohydrate (12). Relatively short mucinlike

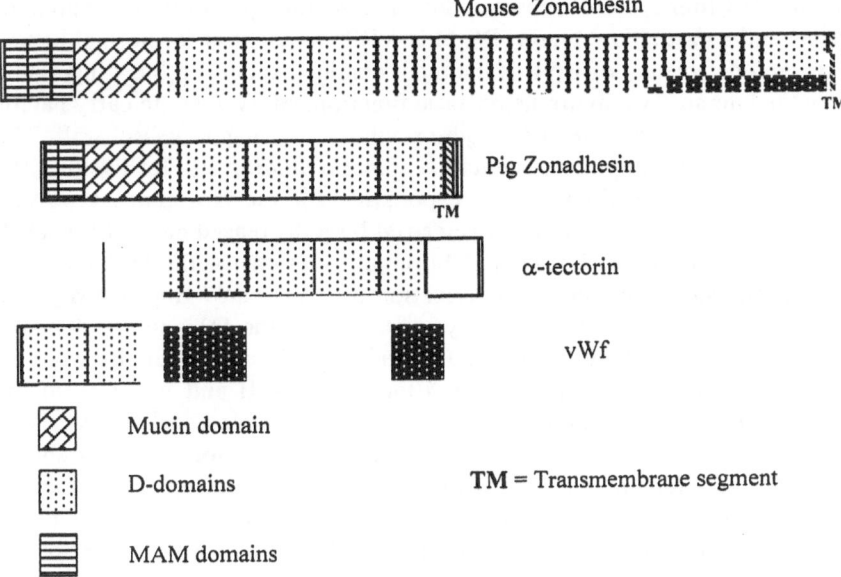

FIGURE 17.3. Comparison of pig and mouse zonadhesins with two proteins that contain homologous domains (α-tectorin and vWF).

domains present in some receptors have been suggested to lift the ligand-binding site above the glycocalyx (13). In addition, membrane associated mucins serve as ligands for cell surface receptor selectins (14). The mucin domain in zonadhesin, therefore could lift the MAM domain above the glycocalyx and thereby facilitate cell–cell interactions in the male reproductive tract, and/or act as a repulsive barrier to prevent nonspecific interactions between spermatozoa and other cells in the male or female reproductive tract, and/or promote adhesion of spermatozoa to the oviductal isthmus, a sperm reservoir.

Following the mucinlike domain is a partial D-domain (D0), three full D-domains (D1–D3), 20 tandem repeats of partial D3 domains (D3p1–20), and, finally, a D4 domain in the mouse. The pig contains only one partial D0 domain and four full D domains. The D1, D2, D3, and D4 domains of the mouse are highly identical to those of the pig (61, 68, 47, and 63%, respectively). Like the D0 domain, D3p1–20 are rich in Cys (18 Cys within each 120–amino acid repeat). Each Cys is conserved, suggesting that these residues are critical for the integrity of the protein structure. We designated these 120–amino acid repeats as D3 partial domains instead of as D0 domains because they have higher similarities to the C-terminus of the D3 domain (56–67%) than to the D0 domain (26–37%). Within the 21 partial D domains, D3p16 has the highest sequence similarity (28%) to D' of prepro von Willebrand factor (pp-vWF). vWF is a large multimeric plasma protein composed of four types of repeated domains, including four intact D domain repeats and a partial D domain (D′) (15). vWF is essential for normal hemostasis, and deficiency of vWF is the most common inherited bleeding disorder in the human. Two major hemostatic functions of vWF are to carry Factor VIII and to promote platelet interaction with the damaged vessel wall. The D′ domain of vWF appears to contain a specific binding site for Factor VIII, and mutations in D′ domain are responsible for the Normandy-type von Willebrand disease, which is characterized by a decreased capacity of vWF to interact with Factor VIII (15). Additional functions of the D domains in pp-vWF appear to include oligomerization of vWF, packaging of vWF into storage granules (15), and, via a Cys-rich area of the D1 and D2 domains interaction with collagen (16,17). It is of some interest that the work of Ensslin et al. (18) has not considered the Factor VIII and V nature of the sperm protein p47 in the context of zonadhesin. As noted earlier vWF is an important carrier of Factor VIII via D-domain interaction as noted above. Given the apparent identical distribution of p47 on the apical surface of spermatozoa, it is quite reasonable to assume that this protein is actually binding to zonadhesin in the same manner that Factor VIII binds to von Willebrand factor.

D domains also have been found in several functionally diverse extracellular proteins, including secreted intestinal mucins of human, mouse, and rat (MUC2 orthologs) (12,19,20), *Xenopus laevis* integumentary mucin FIM-B.1 (21), insect humoral lectin hemocytin (22), and mouse inner ear matrix protein α-tectorin (23). The arrangement of D domains can be divided into at least two groups with zonadhesin and α-tectorin in one group, and vWF, MUC2, and hemocytin in another. Mouse α-tectorin has been cloned from a cochlea cDNA library (23), where it is one of two major noncollagenous proteins of the mouse inner ear tectorial membrane. It interacts with another noncollagenous protein, β-tectorin. α-tectorin contains the D domain repeats in the same order as that of pig zonadhesin. Both α-tectorin and β-tectorin contain a ZP domain (24). The ZP domain is a conserved sequence found in zona pellucida glycoproteins ZP1, ZP2, and ZP3 and various other proteins (e.g., uromodulin). In the tectorial membrane, two distinct filament types exist—a light and a dark staining filament—which suggests that the α- and β-tectorins form homomeric filaments *via* the ZP domain, whereas the two filament types interact with each other to form a striated sheet matrix through D domain interactions. D domains in α-tectorin may also interact with other collagenlike proteins in the tectorial membrane.

Regarding the binding of zonadhesin to the zona pellucida, it is intriguing that the D-domain region of zonadhesin, which is responsible for this interaction, is quite different between the mouse and pig orthologs. The tandem D-domains of zonadhesin have the potential to evolve species-specific interactions by concerted evolution, as has been proposed for a species-specific recognition protein found in abalone (25). Thus, this difference could represent a molecular basis accounting for the observed species specificity of this interaction.

A Unique Sperm Protein Identified Though the Sceening of Testis cDNA Expression Libraries with Antibodies to Sperm Plasma Membranes

A second unique sperm-specific plasma membrane protein from guinea pig, named *sperad*, was identified by expression cloning with sperm membrane antibodies produced in females (26). Sperad is a transmembrane glycoprotein that consists of two extracellular immunoglobulin domains and a repetitive proline-rich intracellular domain. The extracellular domains are related to a group of apparent cell adhesion molecules known as *biliary glycoproteins* (27). The domain organization of this widely expressed group of proteins, including sperad, is highly conserved, consisting of an amino terminal immunoglobulin variable-type domain followed by between 0 and 3 immunoglobulin C2-type domains (27,28). Each of the immunoglobulin domains corresponds to a single exon with differential splicing of the C2 domain exons producing multiple forms of a biliary glycoprotein.

In vitro expression experiments indicate that biliary glycoproteins (BGP) and other carcinoembryonic antigen (CEA) family members mediate intercellular adhesion primarily through a homotypic reciprocal interaction of the amino terminal domains (29). Alternative interactions of these proteins, however, have been reported, including heterotypic amino terminal immunoglobulin domain binding among family members (30), and CEA amino terminal binding to a membrane proximal C2 domain of an apposed CEA molecule (31). In addition, the initial binding of human granulocytes to cytokine-activated endothelium is mediated by oligosaccharides present on BGP and endothlial cell expressed E-selectin (32). Heterologous expression of sperad in Sf9 cells did not cause cellular aggregation either among the transfected cells or with spermatozoa despite apparent glycosylation and cell plasma membrane association (26). Thus, combined with the spatiotemporal expression pattern, sperad may mediate heterotypic interactions of extratesticular spermatozoa with other cell types encountered in the male or female reproductive tract.

The intracellular region of sperad is unique compared with those found in the biliary glycoproteins. The site of divergence is located just to the carboxy-terminal side of the transmembrane segment corresponding to a conserved intron/exon boundary (33). The intracellular region of sperad consists primarily of a short repetitive proline-rich sequence (PPQPEQ). Such sequences can mediate low affinity protein–protein binding, which suggests a potential signaling role (34). It is also possible that sperad could regulate a signaling event independent of the intracellular domain through association with another transmembrane protein, as has been reported for GPI-anchored members of the human CEA family (27).

Establishing Libraries of Sperm Membrane Proteins

To identify virtually all membrane and secretory proteins synthesized by spermatozoa, we have initiated studies using the novel signal peptide trapping method (35,36). Signal peptide trapping is a potentially powerful method by which to define important signaling molecules on the sperm surface when used in conjunction with the EST, genomic, and protein databases. This approach relies on the inability of some yeast strains that do not express invertase to grow in the presence of sucrose as the sole carbon source. Both the synthesis and secretion of invertase are required to hydrolyze extracellular sucrose into fructose and glucose that the yeast can then import as energy sources. These yeast strains are transformed with a cDNA library subcloned in a yeast expression vector that contains a selectable metabolic marker, the native invertase promoter, and immediately 3' of the plasmid cloning site, a mutated form of the invertase coding sequence lacking the initiating methionines and the signal peptide. Following selection of transformed yeast on an appropriate medium, the transformants are replica plated and subjected to a second selection for growth on sucrose medium. Only transformants containing cDNAs that encode a methionine followed by a functional signal peptide cloned in-frame with the invertase coding sequence produce and secrete invertase, and therefore grow on the sucrose medium.

The combined results from both studies using several independent cDNA libraries indicate that 80% of the identified positive clones appear to encode eukaryotic proteins targeted to the secretory pathway (35,36). Of the known and homologous sequences, 97% possessed the natural start methionine and signal peptide. Thus, the signal peptide selection strategy is particularly efficient. For signal peptide trap screening, we have transformed *S. cerevisiae* strain YT455 (suc2Δ9, ade 2-101, ura 3-52) (37,38) with a random-primed cDNA plasmid library prepared from an enriched round and elongating spermatid fraction isolated from adult mouse testis spermatogenic cells (26,39). In order to enrich for sperm-specific transcripts and reduce the inherent library redundancy resulting from the natural variability of gene expression, we used the suppression subtractive hybridization PCR method to produce the cDNA library (40). The spermatid cDNA was subtracted using a pool of cDNAs made from from brain, heart, intestine, kidney, liver, lung, ovary, skeletal muscle, spleen, and stomach. Positive clones are currently being analyzed by reverse transcriptase–PCR and in situ hybridization for specific expression in haploid stage spermatogenic cells.

References

1. Lee MA, Kopf GS, Storey BT. Effects of phorbol esters and a diacylglycerol on the mouse sperm acrosome reaction induced by the zona pellucida. Biol Reprod 1987;36:617–27.

2. Vanderhaeghen P, Schurmans S, Vassart G, Parmentier M. Specific repertoire of olfactory receptor genes in the male germ cells of several mammalian species. Genomics 1997;39:239–46.

3. Hardy DM, Garbers DL. Species-specific binding of sperm proteins to the extracellular matrix (zona pellucida) of the egg. J Biol Chem 1994;269:19000–4.

4. Hardy DM, Garbers DL. A sperm membrane protein that binds in a species-specific manner to the egg extracellular matrix is homologous to von Willebrand factor. J Biol Chem 1995;270:26025–28.

5. Gao Z, Garbers DL. Species diversity in the structure of zonadhesin, a sperm-specific membrane protein containing multiple cell adhesion molecule-like domains. J Biol Chem 1998;273:3415–21.

6. Jiang W, Gorbea CM, Flannery AV, Beynon RJ, Grant GA, Bond JS. The alpha subunit of meprin A. Molecular cloning and sequencing, differential expression in inbred mouse strains, and evidence for divergent evolution of the alpha and beta subunits [published erratum appears in J Biol Chem 1992 ;267:13779]. J Biol Chem 1992;267:9185–93.

7. Takagi S, Hirata T, Agata K, Mochii M, Eguchi G, Fujisawa H. The A5 antigen, a candidate for the neuronal recognition molecule, has homologies to complement components and coagulation factors. Neuron 1991;7:295–307.

8. Jiang YP, Wang H, D'Eustachio P, Musacchio JM, Schlessinger J, Sap J. Cloning and characterization of R-PTP-kappa, a new member of the receptor protein tyrosine phosphatase family with a proteolytically cleaved cellular adhesion molecule-like extracellular region. Mol Cell Biol 1993;13:2942–51.

9. Wang H, Lian Z, Lerch MM, Chen Z, Xie W, Ullrich A. Characterization of PCP-2, a novel receptor protein tyrosine phosphatase of the MAM domain family. Oncogene 1996;12:2555–62.

10. Zondag GC, Koningstein GM, Jiang YP, Sap J, Moolenaar WH, Gebbink MF. Homophilic interactions mediated by receptor tyrosine phosphatases mu and kappa. A critical role for the novel extracellular MAM domain [published erratum appears in J Biol Chem 1995;270:24621]. J Biol Chem 1995;270:14247–50.

11. Dumermuth E, Sterchi EE, Jiang WP, Wolz RL, Bond JS, Flannery AV, et al. The astacin family of metalloendopeptidases. J Biol Chem 1991;266:21381–85.

12. Gendler SJ, Spicer AP. Epithelial mucin genes. Annu Rev Physiol 1995;57:607–34.

13. Hilkens J, Ligtenberg MJ, Vos HL, Litvinov SV. Cell membrane-associated mucins and their adhesion-modulating property. Trend Biochem Sci 1992;17:359–63.

14. Shimizu Y, Shaw S. Cell adhesion. Mucins in the mainstream. Nature 1993;366:630–31.

15. Meyer D, Girma JP. von Willebrand factor: structure and function. Thromb Haemost 1993;70:99–104.

16. Fujisawa T, Takagi J, Sekiya F, Goto A, Miake F, Saito Y. Monoclonal antibodies that inhibit binding of propolypeptide of von Willebrand factor to collagen. Localization of epitopes. Eur J Biochem 1991;196:673–77.

17. Takagi J, Fujisawa T, Sekiya F, Saito Y. Collagen-binding domain within bovine propolypeptide of von Willebrand factor. J Biol Chem 1991;266:5575–79.

18. Ensslin M, Vogel T, Calvete JJ, Thole HH, Schmidtke J, Matsuda T, et al. Molecular cloning and characterization of P47, a novel boar sperm-associated zona pellucida-binding protein homologous to a family of mammalian secretory proteins. Biol Reprod 1998;58:1057–64.

19. Ohmori H, Dohrman AF, Gallup M, Tsuda T, Kai H, Gum JR, et al. Molecular cloning of the amino-terminal region of a rat MUC 2 mucin gene homologue. Evidence for expression in both intestine and airway. J Biol Chem 1994;269: 17833–40.
20. Gum JR, Hicks JW, Toribara NW, Siddiki B, Kim, YS. Molecular cloning of human intestinal mucin (MUC2) cDNA. Identification of the amino terminus and overall sequence similarity to prepro-von Willebrand factor. J Biol Chem 1994;269:2440–46.
21. Joba W, Hoffmann W. Similarities of integumentary mucin B.1 from *Xenopus laevis* and prepro-von Willebrand factor at their amino-terminal regions. J Biol Chem 1992;272:1805–10.
22. Kotani E, Yamakawa M, Iwamoto S, Tashiro M, Mori H, Sumida M, et al. Cloning and expression of the gene of hemocytin, an insect humoral lectin which is homologous with the mammalian von Willebrand factor. Biochim Biophys Acta 1995;1260:245–58.
23. Legan PK, Rau A, Keen JN, Richardson GP. The mouse tectorins—modular matrix proteins of the inner ear homologous to components of the sperm-egg adhesion system. J Biol Chem 1997; 272:8791–801.
24. Bork P, Sander C. A large domain common to sperm receptors (Zp2 and Zp3) and TGF-beta type III receptor. FEBS Lett 1992;300:237–40.
25. Swanson WJ, Vacquier VD. Concerted evolution in an egg receptor for a rapidly evolving abalone sperm protein. Science 1998; 281:710–72.
26. Quill TA, Garbers DL. Sperad is a novel sperm-specific plasma membrane protein homologous to a family of cell adhesion proteins. J Biol Chem 1996;271: 33509–14.
27. Obrink B. CEA adhesion molecules: multifunctional proteins with signal-regulatory properties. Curr Opin Cell Biol 1997;9:616–26.
28. Prall F, Nollau P, Neumaier M, Haubeck HD, Drzeniek Z, Helmchen U, et al. CD66a (BGP), an adhesion molecule of the carcinoembryonic antigen family, is expressed in epithelium, endothelium, and myeloid cells in a wide range of normal human tissues. J Histochem Cytochem 1996;44:35–41.
29. Teixeira AM, Fawcett J, Simmons DL, Watt SM. The N-domain of the biliary glycoprotein (BGP) adhesion molecule mediates homotypic binding: domain interactions and epitope analysis of BGPc. Blood 1994;84:211–19.
30. Oikawa S, Kuroki M, Matsuoka Y, Kosaki G, Nakazato H. Homotypic and heterotypic Ca(++)-independent cell adhesion activities of biliary glycoprotein, a member of carcinoembryonic antigen family, expressed on CHO cell surface. Biochem Biophys Res Commun 1992;186:881–87.
31. Zhou H, Fuks A, Alcaraz G, Bolling TJ, Stanners CP. Homophilic adhesion between Ig superfamily carcinoembryonic antigen molecules involves double reciprocal bonds. J Cell Biol 1993;122:951–60.
32. Stocks SC, Kerr MA, Haslett C, Dransfield I. CD66-dependent neutrophil activation: a possible mechanism for vascular selectin-mediated regulation of neutrophil adhesion. J Leukoc Biol 1995;58:40–48.
33. McCuaig K, Rosenberg M, Nedellec P, Turbide C, Beauchemin N. Expression of the Bgp gene and characterization of mouse colon biliary glycoprotein isoforms. Gene 1993;127:173–83.
34. Williamson MP. The structure and function of proline-rich regions in proteins. Biochem J 1994;297:249–60.

35. Klein RD, Gu Q, Goddard A, Rosenthal A. Selection for genes encoding secreted proteins and receptors. Proc Natl Acad Sci USA 1996;93:7108–13.
36. Jacobs KA, Collins-Racie LA, Colbert M, Duckett M, Golden-Fleet M, Kelleher K, et al. A genetic selection for isolating cDNAs encoding secreted proteins. Gene 1997;198:289–96.
37. Kaiser CA, Botstein D. Secretion-defective mutations in the signal sequence for *Saccharomyces cerevisiae* invertase. Mol Cell Biol 1986;6:2382–91.
38. Becker DM, Guarente L. High-efficiency transformation of yeast by electroporation. Meth Enzymol 1991;194:182–87.
39. Bellve AR. Purification, culture, and fractionation of spermatogenic cells. Meth Enzymol 1993;225:84–113.
40. Diatchenko L, Lau YF, Campbell AP, Chenchik A, Moqadam F, Huang B, et al. Suppression subtractive hybridization: a method for generating differentially regulated or tissue-specific cDNA probes and libraries. Proc Natl Acad Sci USA 1996;93:6025–30.

Part V

Genetic Defects
and Remedies

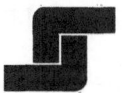

18

Heritable Sperm Degeneration in the Domestic Fowl

JOHN D. KIRBY, DAVID P. FROMAN, AND DOUGLAS D. RHOADS

Overview of Reproduction in the Fowl

The domestic fowl is among the most fecund of all terrestrial vertebrates. This tremendous capacity is suggested by the fact that a single female may produce as many as 300 progeny in a single year. This ability is due to several factors, including oviparity, selection for uninterrupted egg production; and artificial incubation. Oviparity has facilitated the production of numerous progeny by allowing females to produce up to one egg per day in the absence of pregnancy and its concomitant pause in egg production.

One consequence of oviparity in terrestrial vertebrates is that the developing embryo must be provided with all of the nutrients it requires for development in a carefully protected, aqueous environment at oviposition. This has resulted in the formation of large, yolky oocytes that can represent from 0.5 to 2.0 % of the female's body weight. These large oocytes are then sequentially invested with a proteinaceous covering (the albumen), membranes, and a calcified shell. This process takes about 25 hours in the domestic hen. Upon completion of egg formation, oviposition takes place and the next oocyte is ovulated approximately 30 minutes later. Thus, the single functional oviduct of the hen is occluded for approximately 98% of the ovulatory cycle by the nascent egg (reviewed in Ref. 1).

In the domestic fowl fertilization occurs in the infundibulum within 10 minutes of ovulation, immediately before the deposition of the first proteinaceous layer (i.e., the outer perivitelline layer). The short interval between ovulation and fertilization, coupled with the long period of oviducal obstruction, requires the capacity for sperm storage at one or more sites in the oviduct. The fowl's highly specialized sperm storage tubules are located at the juncture of the shell gland and the vagina (uterovaginal junction; reviewed in Ref. 2). Sperm may remain sequestered within the sperm storage tubules for periods ranging from a few hours to 1 or more weeks: As a result of this phenomenon there is no need for the domestic fowl to coordinate copulation with ovulation and sperm may be available to traverse the patent oviduct prior to ovulation.

Fowl spermatozoa are small, vermiform cells, approximately 0.5 μm in diameter at the nucleus and range from 80 to 100 μm in length. These cells appear to require progressive forward motility only to reach and become sequestered within the sperm storage tubules. Any subsequent movement up to the site of fertilization (infundibulum) results from antiperistaltic contractions of the oviduct. Once sperm reach the infundibulum they may become sequestered within epithelial folds, where they may continue to reside for a period ranging from minutes to several days (reviewed in Refs. 1,3).

Fertilization in the domestic fowl appears to be relatively simple when compared with eutherian mammals. First, the hen's oocyte is not invested with a complex structure that is equivalent to either the cumulus or the zona pellucida. Second, fowl sperm are not required to capacitate; thus, little if any postejaculation modification of the sperm cell is required for fertilization (reviewed in Ref. 1). Sperm receptors appear to be concentrated over the germinal portion of the highly polarized oocyte. Once sperm–egg binding occurs, an acrosome reaction follows and the sperm can pass through the inner-perivitelline layer and fuse with the oocyte plasma membrane in proximity of the female pronucleus. Sperm–egg fusions cease only upon the deposition of the outer-perivitelline layer; thus, unlike most mammals physiological polyspermy appears to be the rule rather than the exception during most fertilizations in the domestic fowl (reviewed in Refs. 1, 3).

Spermatogenesis and Sperm Maturation in the Fowl

Spermatogenesis occurs at core body temperature within testes located proximal to the heart and lungs of the male fowl (4). The fowl produces sperm that are capable of fertilization immediately upon spermiation (5). In order for fertilization to occur, however, the nonmotile testicular sperm must be placed in the oviduct beyond the uterovaginal junction. Testicular sperm must be placed well within the oviduct, beyond the uterovaginal junction, due to the requirement for sperm to be mobile to traverse the vagina and become sequestered within the sperm storage tubules (5,6). Thus, due to this ability and the relatively simple nonprotein-secreting epithelium of the epididymis, epididymal function in the fowl was long thought to be of minimal importance to sperm maturation. Bedford and co-workers (7,8) demonstrated that several proteins, probably less than 10, were attached to maturing sperm as they transited the excurrent ducts of the testis. Although none of these proteins were found to be associated with fertilization per se, at least one was associated with the sperm's ability to become sequestered within the uterovaginal sperm storage tubules. Due to the organization of the excurrent ducts, those proteins that become associated with sperm are most likely to be produced and secreted by the efferent ducts, which are the only highly differentiated and metabolically active region of the excurrent ducts. Furthermore, the efferent ducts comprise the largest portion (>70%) and the site of longest occupancy within the epididymal region in birds (see Ref. 3). For these reasons, the excurrent ducts of the fowl's testis have received little attention from researchers in the past.

Identification of Subfertile Males

Genetic models of poor fertility in male domestic fowl are limited to very few examples. The most widely studied model has been the poor fertilizing ability of sperm from roosters who are homozygous for the rose comb allele (RR) originally described by Cochez (9). This defect has subsequently been shown to be due to poor sperm motility as a result of reduced metabolic capacity (10–12). The second, a genetic model for sperm degeneration within the ductus deferens originally characterized by Froman and Bernier (13) is the basis for the work presented here.

Froman and Bernier (13) identified a population of subfertile Delaware roosters that were characterized by large proportions of dead sperm within their ejaculates following a week of sexual rest. They also determined that collecting ejaculates on five to seven consecutive days resulted in a profound improvement in the proportion of live sperm (>99% live sperm) in the ejaculates of affected males that was rapidly reversed with 5–7 days of sexual rest. The authors then evaluated the proportion of dead cells observed along the length of the ductus deferens, determining that sperm death and degeneration was observed initially at about the midpoint of the ductus deferens, and then became progressively worse the more distal the point of sampling. Froman and Bernier (13) postulated that premature sperm death could be due to one of the following causes: (1) abnormal spermatogenesis or sperm formation resulting in an inherent sperm defect; (2) aberrant epididymal function resulting in abnormal posttesticular sperm maturation; (3) abnormal excurrent duct sperm storage that resulted in premature sperm death within the ductus deferens.

Evaluation of Sperm Function
in Subfertile Delaware Males

To determine if there was an inherent defect in the sperm of affected Delaware males, as had been previously observed in RR males, a series of experiments was conducted. First, because abnormal organization of axonemal, mitochondrial, and nuclear structures was a common feature in the dead sperm found within the ductus deferens of affected males, the seminiferous epithelium was evaluated by both electron and light microscopy [Fig. 18.1 (cells 1–8); Kirby and Sogut, unpublished). Observations and measurements of many sperm nuclei, axonemes, and mitochondria revealed no observable

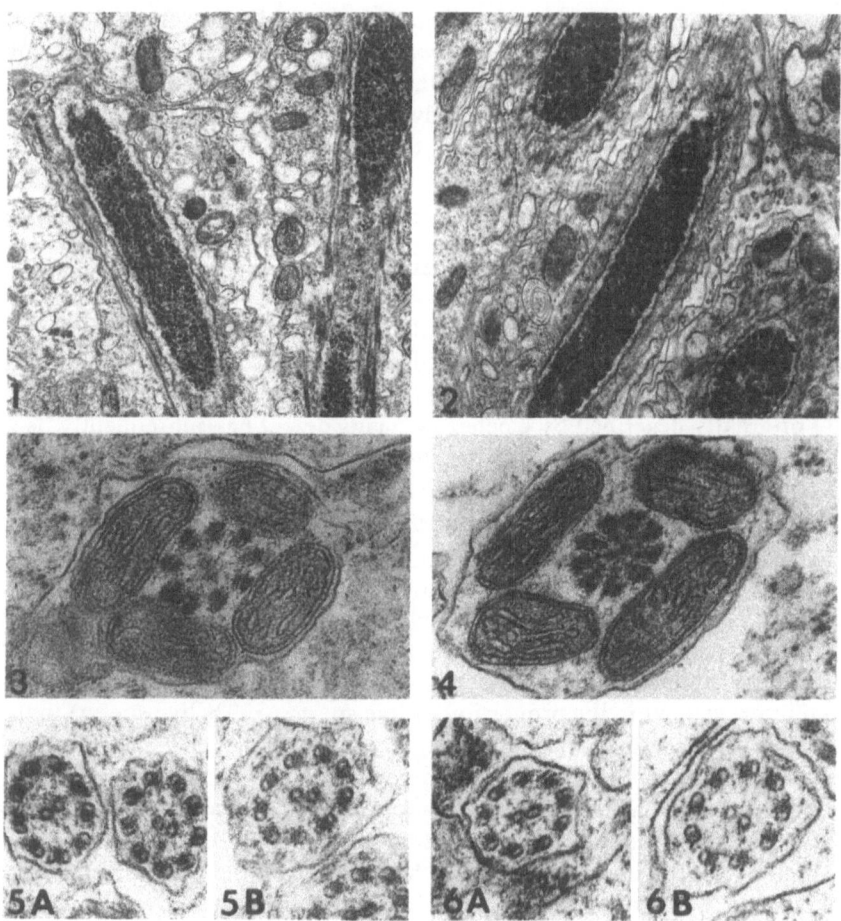

FIGURE 18.1. Electron (Cells 1–6) and light micrographs (Cells 7–8) of the seminiferous epithelium, maturing germinal cells, or organelles—including elongated spermatid nuclei, mitochondria, and axonemes within the testes of affected and nonaffected Delaware cross-bred males. (Cells 1 and 2): Representative nuclei and mitochondria from elongated spermatids of nonaffected and affected Delaware cross-bred males, respectively. Notice the similarity in the degree of compaction and overall structure in the nuclei of both males, demonstrating no apparent decondensation within the testis. (× 20 k). (Cells 3 and 4): Representative elongated spermatid midpiece cross-sections from nonaffected and affected males, respectively. Notice that the mitochondria surrounding the normal axonemes of both males appear to have no unusual vacuolization or lack of organization as reported for such structures in the midductus deferens by Froman and Bernier (13). (3- × 80 k; 4- × 75 k).

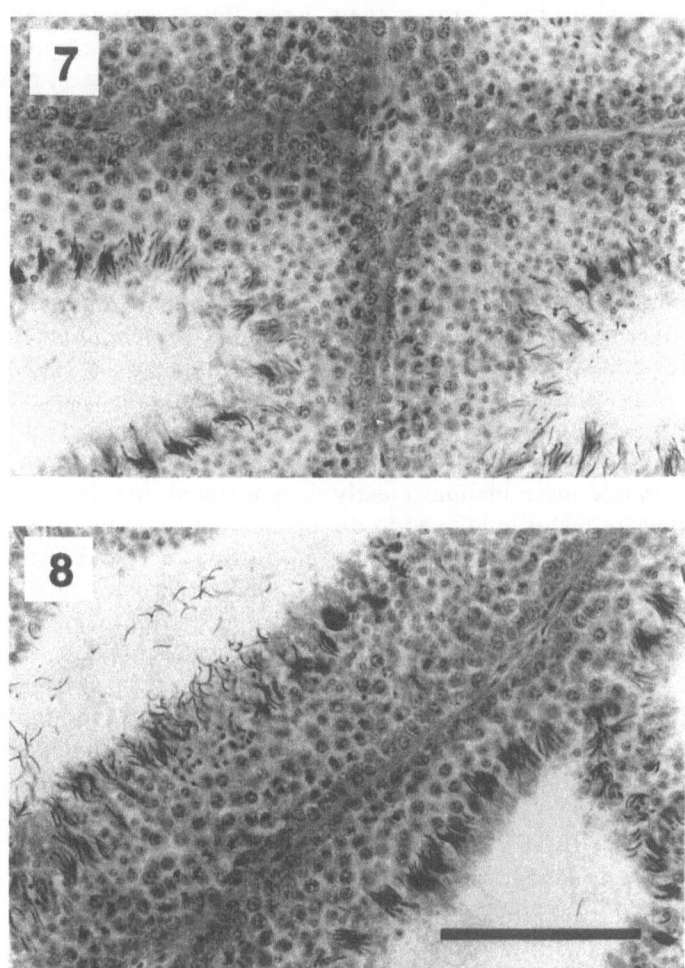

Figure 18.1. (*Continued*). (Cells 5a–6b): Depict representative cross-sections through the axonemes within the tails of elongated spermatids distal to the midpiece. These micrographs clearly show the normal doublet structure of the axoneme in the sperm of both nonaffected (5a–b) and affected (6a–b), with no missing elements as described by Froman and Bernier (13) (5a&6a, × 80 k; 5b&6b, × 95 k). (Cells 7 and 8): Representative sections through the seminiferous tubules of nonaffected (7) and affected Delaware cross-bred males at 36 weeks of age. Observations of numerous cross-sections from each of a large number of males has revealed no consistent differences in testicular histology between nonaffected and affected males. Coupled with studies on testicular sperm function, this suggests that sperm are normal when they leave the testes of affected males (Bar = 100 µm).

differences between the sperm or their organelles in affected and control males [Fig. 18.1 (cells 1–6)]. Evaluation of the seminiferous epithelium at the light microscope level further supported the idea that sperm maturation in the testes of affected males was not different than that observed in nonaffected control males [Fig. 18.1 (cells 7 and 8)].

A subsequent series of experiments was completed to determine if postejaculation sperm function was impaired in affected males (as in RR males). These tests evaluated the ability of sperm from affected males to survive within the oviduct, measured competitive sperm fertilizing ability, and determined the relative metabolic rate of ejaculated sperm. The first two objectives were accomplished by heterospermic inseminations of pooled semen to evaluate sperm competition and were completed by exploiting the ability of surgical inseminations reliably to place sperm deep within the oviduct (14) to minimize the effects of motility and sperm sequestration within sperm storage tubules on apparent sperm fertilizing ability.

Heterospermic inseminations clearly demonstrated that the sperm of affected Delaware males continued to die in the oviduct of the hen at a relatively rapid rate (Table 18.1; 15). The proportion of chicks produced by ejaculated sperm from affected males declined at similar rates following both intramagnal and intravaginal inseminations. In the next experiment, hens were either intravaginally or intramagnally inseminated with ejaculated sperm from either highly fertile males, poorly fertile RR males (poor motility), or affected Delaware males. Even though both the highly fertile and RR males showed increased 21-day fertility as well as increased duration of fertility following intramagnal insemination, and relative to the intravaginal inseminations, there were no differences observed in affected males (Table 18.2; 15,16). These results further strengthened the concept that the primary defect in the sperm of affected males was a decreased duration of survivability, within either the oviduct or ductus deferens, and not due to poor motility or fertilizing ability. That aberrant sperm metabolism was not involved in the abnormal rate of sperm loss in affected males, the relative metabolic rate of sperm from highly fertile, poorly fertile (RR), and affected males was studied using a dye reduction assay (17). In these experiments it was further confirmed that, even though sperm from RR males had significantly lower metabolic rates relative to those from highly fertile males the sperm from affected Delaware males had similar metabolic rates at both 25 and 40° C (Table 18.3; 11).

To determine directly if the rate of sperm loss from the oviduct was due to an inherent defect in the sperm cell that occurs during spermatogenesis, testicular sperm from affected Delaware cross-bred males, their nonaffected siblings or subfertile RR males were used to surgically inseminate hens. In Figure 18.2 (11,16), the testicular sperm of affected males were at least comparable to those of their nonaffected siblings or the homozygous RR males. Thus, based on this sequence of experiments we concluded that the sperm of affected males are normal when they leave the testis, but that some maturational defect occurs in the excurrent ducts that results in a decreased period of survival in either the ductus deferens or in the oviduct.

TABLE 18.1. Percentages of chicks sired by subfertile Delaware roosters following either intravaginal or intramagnal inseminations of New Hampshire[a] hens with equal numbers of live sperm mixed from Delaware and Brown Leghorn males.

Insemination route	Total # chicks	Fertility (%)	Chicks sired by Delaware (%)			
			Day 1	Day 7	Day 14	Overall
Intravaginal	199	69	36	38	0	36
Intramagnal	192	70	67	28	0	33

Adapted from 15.
[a]The use of New Hampshire hens was dictated by the ability to identify the progeny of Delaware (yellow at hatch) and Brown Leghorn (brown at hatch) males at hatch.

TABLE 18.2. Effects of insemination route and rooster type on 21-day fertility and the duration of fertility following a single intravaginal or intramagnal insemination of sperm from highly fertile Leghorn, subfertile RR males with known poor motility, or subfertile Delaware males.

Insemination route	Rooster type	Eggs (#)	Fertility[1] (%)	Calculated[2] initial fertility (%)	Fertility[2] duration (days)
Intravaginal	Leghorn	1366	51±1.2 [a,*]	97	11.8*
	RR	1348	26±1.4 [c,*]	94	6.0*
	Delaware	1295	42±1.3 [b]	100	9.1
Intramagnal	Leghorn	161	64±1.2 [a,*]	94	15.2*
	RR	176	57±1.0 [b,*]	97	13.9*
	Delaware	202	41±0.4 [c]	100	9.6

[a,b,c]Denotes significant differences within an insemination route between rooster types at $p < 0.0001$.
*Denotes significant differences within a rooster type between insemination routes at $p < 0.001$.
[1]Mean + SEM.
[2]Values calculated from the model $y(x)=(\gamma/(1+e^{\beta*(\tau-x)}))$, where β is "slope" term, γ is the calculated fertility (%) at time 0, and τ is the half-maximal duration of fertility in days, estimated by iterative least squares nonlinear regression (22).

TABLE 18.3. Formazan formation as an indicator of relative metabolic rate of sperm from three lines of male domestic fowl: high fertility leghorns, subfertile RR males with known poor sperm motility, and subfertile Delaware males.

Male Line	n	Formazan formation (picomoles/10^6 sperm)[1]			
		25°C	Rank	40°C	Rank
High fertility Leghorn	6	204.2±2.7[a]	4.8	81.9±2.5[a]	6.5
Subfertile RR	6	129.7±5.0[c]	15.5	54.7±2.4[b]	15.0
Subfertile Delaware	6	183.6±5.0[b]	8.0	82.8±2.5[a]	6.8

[a,b,c]Means in a column with a different superscript are significantly different at $p < 0.0001$.
[1]Values are presented as mean ± SEM for triplicate samples of each male at each temperature. Assay conditions atm 25°C included calcium (required for motility at temperatures < 37°C) and cyanide in order to maximize the apparent metabolic activity of sperm in this solution. At 40°C calcium and cyanide were removed from the buffer in order to evaluate metabolic activity under near physiological conditions.

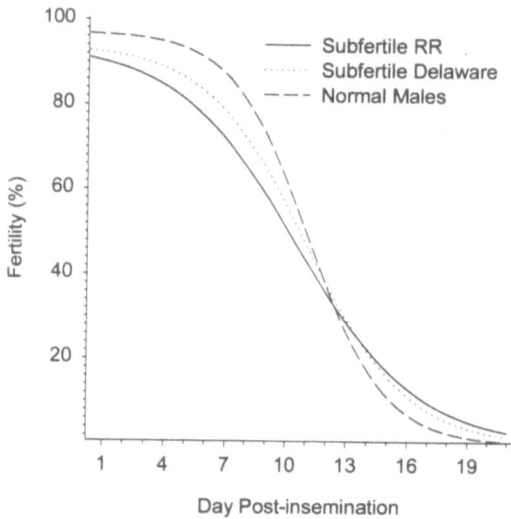

FIGURE 18.2. Duration of fertility following a single intramagnal insemination of Leghorn hens with testicular sperm from subfertile RR, high fertility Leghorns or, subfertile Delaware males. The subfertile Delaware males produced ejaculates containing from 40 to 60% dead sperm when collected weekly prior to sacrifice. Each hen was inseminated surgically with 7×10^7 testicular sperm in a volume of 300 µl. The lines represent the functions $y(x)=(94/(1+e^{-.3314*(10.5-x)})$, $y(x)=(94/(1+e^{-.4007*(11.0-x)})$, and $y(x)=(94/(1+e^{-.5256*(11.1-x)})$, for subfertile RR, subfertile Delaware and high fertility Leghorn males, respectively. Adapted from (12,16).

Analysis of the Excurrent Ducts of Affected Males

The observations that seminiferous tubule morphology and the pattern of germ-cell maturation appear normal in affected males, coupled with the observation that testicular germ cells of affected males survived in the oviduct for at least as long as those of normal males, strongly suggested that sperm leave the testis of affected males with no apparent defect. The next experiments evaluated whether or not there was an age-related effect on sperm quality in affected males. We started by looking at males at the onset of semen production and over the first 12 weeks following the initial collection of an ejaculate (18). It was apparent from this work that the initial ejaculates of affected males were of higher quality and that the proportion of degenerate sperm increased steadily until the maximal level of sperm production was reached by 28–30 weeks of age (Table 18.4; 18). This study also demonstrated that there was little, certainly not any abnormal level of, immune system interaction with the reproductive tract of affected males (18). Unlike subsequent studies that immunized males with sperm cell suspensions (19), there were few detectable antisperm antibodies in the reproductive tracts of affected males. Those cells that were immunoglobulin positive were primarily mast cells. As might be expected, however, the excurrent ducts of affected males contained significantly more macrophages than did those from

TABLE 18.4. Percentages (mean ± SEM) of viable spermatozoa produced by affected (subfertile) and nonaffected (normal fertility) cross-bred Delaware roosters over a 12-week period beginning with their first collectable ejaculate.

Male type	n	Sampling (week)			
		1	4	8	12
Nonaffected	25	$98 \pm 0.3^{a,x}$	$99 \pm 0.1^{a,x}$	$99 \pm 0.1^{a,x}$	$99 \pm 0.1^{a,x}$
Affected	86	$91 \pm 1.2^{b,x}$	$70 \pm 2.5^{b,y}$	$53 \pm 1.8^{b,x}$	$51 \pm 0.9^{b,x}$

[a,b]Denotes that means within a column are significantly different at $p < 0.0001$.
[x,y,z]Denotes that means within a row are significantly different at $p < 0.0001$.

nonaffected males (18). One unexpected observation arising from this study was the loss of symmetry and apparent disorganization in the pattern of folding of the ductus deferens of affected males. That is, the normally tightly folded excurrent ducts were loosely folded and appeared to be lacking the typical level of organization, even if this was only superficial.

A histological evaluation of the excurrent ducts of affected and normal Delaware cross-bred males followed. The entire excurrent ductal system, from the paracloacal receptaculum to the rete testis was dissected in toto. The ductal system was then fixed and serially sectioned, and the resultant cross sections were then evaluated for general morphology. In addition, volume estimates and peripheral epithelial characteristics were determined. At the completion of the histological evaluation only one region, the proximal efferent ducts, appeared to be grossly abnormal (Fig. 18.3; 16). In affected males, the luminal cross-section area was approximately twofold greater ($233,421 \pm 19,751$ vs. $110,923 \pm 9,118$ μ^2) than what was observed in control males. This observed increase in cross-sectional area (and implied increase in volume) was associated with a 40% reduction in luminal periphery, primarily because of the loss of the highly folded epithelium with its numerous associated crypts. The only apparent defect to date is organization loss of the highly folded epithelium of the proximal efferent ducts; however, the timing and cause of this developmental anomaly has yet to be determined.

Genetic Basis for Heritable Sperm Degeneration

The production of cross-bred males assisted in the identification of the mode of inheritance of sperm degeneration in the domestic fowl. The population of Delaware males used in prior experiments had been closed between 1947 and 1989, approximately 43 generations, with a base population size of 10 males and 45–50 females. In order to remove any effects of inbreeding on sperm quality, cross-bred progeny were produced by mating affected (>40% dead sperm in ejaculates) and nonaffected (>99% live sperm in ejaculates) with unrelated Leghorn females of an extremely high-fertility line (16). The F_1 male progeny were evaluated for semen quality and were subsequently mated to a new population of Leghorn females of the same high-fertility line. The F_2 male progeny were then evaluated for semen quality and classified as either affected (>10% dead sperm in ejaculates) or nonaffected

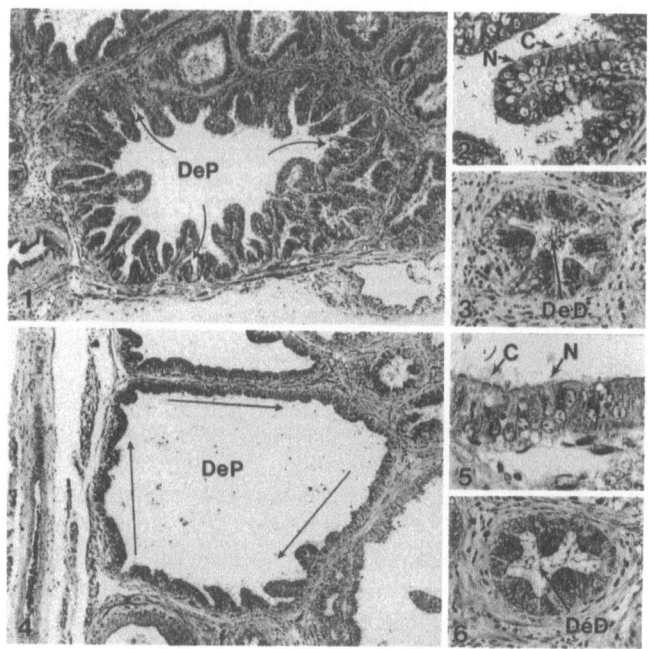

FIGURE 18.3. (Cell 1): Ductulus efferens proximales (DeP) from a nonaffected rooster. The cross-section (× 95) is characterized by a highly folded epithelium with numerous crypts. (Cell 2): Epithelial fold (× 385) within the proximal efferent ductule from a nonaffected rooster. Both ciliated (C) and nonciliated (N) cells are evident. (Cell 3): Ductulus efferens distalis (DeD) from a nonaffected rooster. The cross-section (× 220) is characterized by low epithelial folds containing numerous ciliated cells. (Cell 4): Ductulus efferens proximales (DeP) from an affected rooster. The cross-section (× 95) is characterized by a relatively even epithelial surface (arrows) with some low folds. Increased luminal area is proportional to decreased epithelial folding. (Cell 5): Epithelial cells (× 500) adjoining the lumen of a proximal efferent duct from an affected rooster. The cellular composition of the epithelium appears normal, containing both ciliated (C) and nonciliated (N) cells. (Cell 6): Ductulus efferens distalis (DeD) from an affected rooster. The cross-section (× 220) is characterized by low epithelial folds containing numerous ciliated cells similar to those of nonaffected roosters. This plate is reprinted with the permission of the Society for the Study of Reproduction. Reprinted from 16.

(≥99% live sperm in ejaculates). The nonaffected males never produced progeny with either large proportions of dead sperm in their ejaculates or with aberrant efferent ductule morphology. In contrast, approximately one half of the male progeny sired by affected cross-bred males (F_2 and beyond), or by nonaffected males mated to the female sibs of affected males, produced ejaculates that contained large proportions of dead sperm and had aberrant proximal efferent duct morphology (Kirby, Froman, and Bernier, unpublished observations). In a subsequent series of experiments using males from nonrelated flocks of commercial meat-type males, the pattern of inheritance has proven to be similar (20,21). Thus in two genetically isolated populations of domestic fowl, heritable sperm degeneration has appeared as an autosomal dominant trait. Evidence using a PCR-based assay for this trait suggests that we will be able to identify males in ovo in order to evaluate efferent duct growth and differentiation in affected males to better identify the mechanisms through which heritable sperm degeneration functions to affect sperm survival.

Summary

A dominant allele associated with heritable subfertility and sperm degeneration has been identified in the domestic fowl. Because of morphological and functional analyses of testicular sperm, it seems that sperm cells of affected males are normal when they leave the testis. On transit through the excurrent ducts of the testis, however, the sperm of affected males have a reduced functional life span. To date, the only apparent anomaly in the excurrent ducts of affected males is in the proximal efferent ducts, which are highly distended and have reduced epithelial folding compared with nonaffected males. As the efferent ducts are the principle site for posttesticular modifications, reduced or altered function of the proximal efferent ducts seems to result in abnormal sperm maturation and premature death. In a series of breeding experiments, we determined this trait is inherited due to a single autosomal dominant allele. The development of a PCR-based test for the trait is promising for the determination of the biological basis for heritable sperm degeneration in the domestic fowl.

Acknowledgments. The authors thank Drs. Paul Bernier, Hal Engel, Jr., Rita Lawler, and Rex Hess for their work in characterizing this trait. Butch Sizemore, Fawzi Alqubiel, Idri Csiki, Bunjamin Sogut, and Marsha Rhoads are thanked for their ongoing work in the molecular characterization and analysis of the sperm degeneration allele. This work has been supported by the Arkansas and Oregon Agricultural Experiment Stations and grants from the United States Department of Agriculture.

References

1. Perrault SD, Kirby JD. Internal fertilization in birds. In: Knobil E, Neill JD, ed. *The encyclopedia of reproduction.* New York: Academic Press, 1999:856–66.
2. Bakst MR, Wishart G, Brillard J-P. Oviducal sperm selection, transport and storage in poultry. Poul Sci Rev 1994;5:117–43.
3. Kirby JD, Froman DP. Reproduction in male birds. In: Whittow GC, ed. *Sturkie's Avian Physiology,* Fifth ed. New York: Academic Press, 2000:597–615

4. Beaupre CE, Tressler CJ, Beaupre SJ, Morgan JLM, Bottje WB, Kirby JD. Determination of testis temperature rhythms and effects of constant light on testicular function in the domestic fowl (*Gallus domesticus*). Biol Reprod 1997;56:1570–75.
5. Howarth B. Fertilizing ability of cock spermatozoa from testis, epididymis, and vas deferens following intramagnal insemination. Biol Reprod 1983;28:586–90.
6. Froman DP, Feltman A, Rhoads ML, Kirby JD. Sperm mobility: a primary determinant of fertility in the domestic fowl (*Gallus domesticus*). Biol Reprod 1999; 61:400–5.
7. Esponda P, Bedford JM. Surface of the rooster spermatozoon changes in passing through the Wolffian duct. J Exp Zool 1985;234:441–49.
8. Morris SA, Howarth B, Crim JW, Rodriguez de Cordoba S, Esponda P, Bedford JM. Specificity of sperm-binding proteins and their persistence on spermatozoa in the female host glands. J EXP Zool 1987;242:189–98.
9. Cochez LP. An infertility factor balanced by breeding in White Wyandottes. Proc Ninth World's Poultry Congress I 1951; I:122–28.
10. Buckland RB, Wilcox FH, Shaffner, CS. Influence of homozygosity for rose comb on fumarase, aconitase, isocitric dehydrogenase and malic dehydrogenase activity in spermatozoa of the domestic fowl (*Gallus domesticus*). J Reprod Fertil 1969; 18:89–95.
11. Kirby JD, Froman DP. Comparative metabolism of spermatozoa from subfertile Delaware and Wyandotte roosters. J Reprod Fert 1991;91:125–30.
12. Kirby JD, Engel HN, Froman DP. Analysis of subfertility associated with homozygosity of the rose comb allele in the male domestic fowl. Poul Sci 1994;74: 871–78.
13. Froman DP, Bernier PE. Identification of heritable spermatozoal degeneration within the ductus deferens of the chicken (*Gallus domesticus*). Biol Reprod 1987;37: 969–77.
14. Engel HN, Jr, Froman DP, Kirby JD. An improved procedure for intramagnal insemination of the chicken. Poul Sci 1991;70:1965–69.
15. Kirby JD, Froman DP, Engel HN Jr., Bernier PE. Decreased sperm survivability in subfertile Delaware roosters as indicated by comparative and competitive fertilization. J Reprod Fertil 1989;86:671–77.
16. Kirby JD, Froman DP, Engel HN Jr., Bernier PE, Hess RA. Decreased spermatozoal survivability associated with aberrant morphology of the ductuli efferentes proximales of the chicken. Biol Reprod 1990;42:383–89.
17. Chaudhari D, Wishart GJ. Predicting the fertilising ability of avian semen: the development of a simple colourimetric method for determining the metabolic activity of fowl spermatozoa. Br Poul Sci 1987;29:837–45.
18. Froman DP, Kirby JD, Lawler RM, Bernier PE. Onset of spermatozoal degeneration in low-fertility Delaware roosters and test for autoimmune basis. J Androl 1990;11:113–19.
19. Kirby JD, Classen HL, Smyth JR, Jr, Froman DP. Induction of immunity to spermatozoa in male domestic fowl and effects on fertility. J Reprod Fert 1992;95: 79–86.
20. Kirby JD, Tressler CJ, Rhoads ML. Evaluation of the duration of sperm fertilizing ability in five lines of commercial broiler breeder and Delaware cross males. Poul Sci 1998;77:1688–94.
21. Kirby YK, Sizemore FG, Rhoads DD, Kirby JD. Excurrent duct dysfunction due to SDD allele alters sperm survival and fertilizing ability in domestic fowl. Proc Boden Conference on the Epididymis: Cellular and Molecular Aspects, 1998:31 (Abstr.).
22. Kirby JD, Froman DP. Analysis of poultry fertility data. Poul Sci 1990;69: 1764–68.

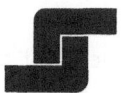

19

The *DAZ* Gene Family and Germ-Cell Development

Renee A. Reijo Pera

Introduction

Many genes that are required for fertility have been identified in model organisms (1–3). Mutations in these genes cause infertility due to defects in development of the germ-cell lineage, but the organism is otherwise healthy. Although human reproduction is undoubtedly as complex as that of other organisms, very few fertility loci have been mapped (4–6). This is in spite of the prevalence of human infertility, the lack of effective treatments to remedy germ-cell defects, and the cost to couples and society of assisted reproductive techniques. Fifteen percent of couples are infertile, and half of all cases can be traced to the male partner. Aside from defects in sperm production, most infertile men are otherwise healthy. This chapter will discuss work that has led to the identification of several genes on the Y chromosome that likely function in sperm production.

The Y Chromosome and the Origin of the *AZF* Hypothesis

The idea that the Y chromosome might be important for sperm production is relatively recent. In 1976, Tiepolo and Zuffardi used karyotyping to demonstrate that 6 azoospermic men had deletions of the long arm of the Y chromosome. In two cases, they found that the fathers of these men had the whole Y chromosome, as expected, if the deletions had caused azoospermia. Based on these findings, they hypothesized that a fertility gene(s) was present on the Y chromosome and that in its absence, men would make no sperm (7). This hypothesis later was termed the *azoospermia factor* or *AZF* hypothesis. Since then, many papers have reported long-arm deletions in azoospermic men (8,9). In fact, the existence of smaller interstitial deletions in azoospermic men was demonstrated shortly thereafter (10,11).

Despite the bulk of this work, however, several observations deserved more attention. First, the possibility that deletions that remove large segments of the Y chromosome might cause azoospermia by disrupting the X and Y pairing regions had not yet been explored (12). Thus, the existence of *AZF* was questionable if based solely on large deletions of an entire arm of the Y chromosome. Second, in most cases, the interstitial deletions that were reported had not been shown to be de novo. They may well be polymorphisms of a normal Y chromosome. It is well known that the heterochromatic half of the Y chromosome is polymorphic; men are fertile with or without this region (13). Third, there were no cellular phenotypes associated with potentially interesting deletions of the Y chromosome. Finally, no genes had been mapped indisputably to any deleted intervals. In summary, no defined phenotype was associated with deletions in infertile men, a reproducible map of the deleted regions had not been constructed, and specific genes within the regions had not yet been identified.

Azoospermia and Overlapping, De Novo, Interstitial Deletions of the Y Chromosome

In the early 1990s, several authors published deletion maps of the Y chromosome that used Southern blotting markers to detect deletions in infertile but not fertile men (14–17). In these studies, most of the deletions were shown to be interstitial. This effort led to increased interest in the role of the Y chromosome in determining male fertility and culminated in efforts that led to the identification of many genes on the Y chromosome, including the *RBM* and *DAZ* genes.

The RBM *Genes*

The *RBM* genes, *RBM1* and *RBM2,* were identified in 1993 (15). Approximately 15–30 copies of these genes are dispersed to the short and long arms of the Y chromosome (18). It is likely that many copies are functional (19) and that many are nonfunctional (20). Some authors report that the *RBM2* gene is polymorphic (in that both fertile and infertile men of Japanese ancestry frequently have no *RBM2* genes (21), whereas others report that Japanese men also have *RBM2* genes (19).

   Deletions of the *AZFb* region of the Y chromosome encompass at least one functional copy of the *RBM1* gene. This *RBM* gene is translated and produces a protein that localizes to the nucleus of all spermatogenic cell types (22,23). It is probable that the *RBM1* genes are required for normal fertility in men; however, it is not clear whether the loss of the *RBM1* genes in men with *AZFb* deletions causes infertility. Deletions of the gene(s) have been reported using Southern blotting and PCR (15,17,24–26); however, because *RBM1* and *RBM2* genes are dispersed across the short and long arms of the Y chromosome, it is unclear how a negative PCR result should be interpreted. In other words, how does the loss of a subset of the *RBM* genes lead to a negative PCR result when other family members, presumably with the same or similar sequence, remain on the Y chromosome? To overcome this ambiguity, Vogt et al. (1996) used both PCR and Southern blotting with the *RBM1* cDNA to ascertain *RBM1* deletions.

The DAZ Genes

In 1995, a study was published that included the analysis of leukocyte DNA samples from four populations of men obtained from the urological practice of Dr. Sherman Silber. Azoospermic men who had undergone testicular biopsies and had cellular phenotypes characterized either as (1) no germ cells or (2) meiotic arrest, (3) the paternal relatives of affected individuals, and (4) a panel of fertile men who reported fathering children. Eighty-nine azoospermic men who had testicular biopsies were included in this work (4).

The DNA samples were analyzed for the presence or absence of 113 PCR markers that had previously been ordered and covered the entire Y chromosome (27,28). Thirteen percent of azoospermic men had overlapping deletions of the Y chromosome that together defined an *AZF* region (4). No deletions were found in DNA samples from paternal relatives, and no deletions were detected in DNA samples from 90 fertile controls. The deletions were strongly correlated with azoospermia. This region, flanked by markers sY142 and sY143 and markers sY158, sY159, and sY160, is now termed the *Deleted in AZoospermia* or *DAZ* region. The term *AZF-c* has also been applied to the region, although the boundaries referred to by that term are unclear (5). Deletion analysis using these marker sets on DNA from several thousand infertile and fertile men have now been published and three regions that are required for normal fertility have been identified as shown in Figure 19.1 (5,24,26,29–36). Markers which are particularly informative are listed in Table 19.1.

Analysis of Phenotypes Associated with
Y Chromosome Deletions of the *DAZ* Gene Cluster

It is interesting that it was found that in initial studies to determine what phenotypes mapped to the *DAZ* region, there was no apparent correlation between the extent of the deletion in an azoospermic man and the severity of the phenotype. Some men with no germ cells had equivalent deletions to those who had meiotic arrest. In fact, when the biopsies of men with deletions were reexamined, it was found that in one azoospermic man, WHT2376,

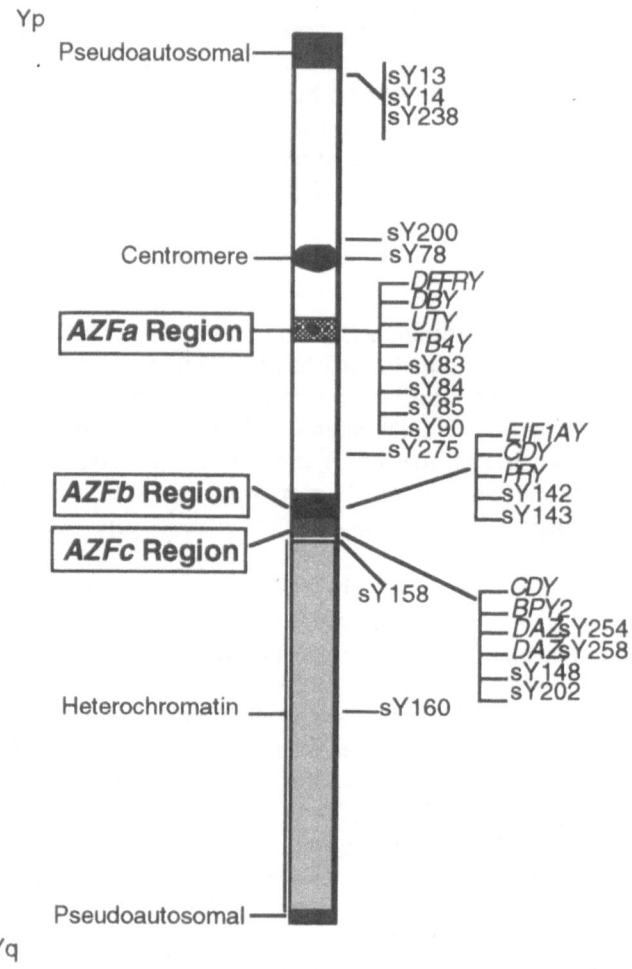

FIGURE 19.1. Overlapping deletions of the distal long arm of the Y chromosome are found in 13% of azoospermic men, but not in fertile men. Deletions may involve any one or more of three regions termed the *AZFa, AZFb,* and *AZFc* regions.

TABLE 19.1. STS and gene sequence for deletion analysis.

sY Number (gene)	Left primer sequence	Right primer sequence	Size (BP)
sY13	GTGACACACAGACTATGCTTC	TCAAGGTTGTTGTTTAAGCT	178
sY14 (*SRY*)	GAATATTCCCGCTCTCCGGA	GCTGGTGCTCCATTCTTGAG	472
sY238 (*ZFY*)	AACAAGTGAGTTCCACAGGG	GCAAAGCAGCATTCAAAACA	350
sY200 (*TSPY*)	CGGGGAAGTGTAAGTGACCGATGGG	CTGCTCTTCAAAAAGATGCCCCAAA	189
sY78	TCCTTTTCCACAATAGACGTCA	CCAAGTATCTTCCCTTAAAAGCTATG	180
DFFRY	GAGCCCATCTTTGTCAGTTTAC	CTGCCAATTTTCCACATCAACC	111
DBY	CATTCGGTTTTACCAGCCAG	CAGTGACTCGAGGTTCAATG	83
TB4Y	CAAAGACCTGCTGACAATGG	CTCCGCTAAGTCTTTCACC	102
sY83	CTTGAAATCAAAGAAGGCCCT	CAATTTGGTTTGGCTGACAT	275
sY85	TGGCAATTTGCCTATGAAGT	ACAGGCTATTTGACTGGCAG	369
sY90	CAGTGCCCCATAACACTTTC	ATGGTAATACAGCAGCTCGC	176
E1F1AY	CTCTGTAGCCAGCCTCTTC	GACTCCTTTCTGGCGGTTAC	84
sY142	AGCTTCTATTCGAGGGCTTC	CTCTCTGCAATCCCTGACAT	196
sY143	GCAGGATGAGAAGCAGGTAG	CCGTGTGCTGGAGACTAATC	311
sY254 (*DAZ*)	GGGTGTTACCAGAAGGCAAA	GAACCGTRATCTACCAAAGCAGC	350
sY283 (*DAZ*)	CAGTGATACACTCGGACTTGTGTA	GTTATTTGAAAAGCTACACGGG	375
sY202	ACAGTTTGAAATGAAATTTAAATGTGTT	TGACAAAGTGAGACCCTACTACTA	121
sY158	CTCAGAAGTCCTCCTAATAGTTCC	ACAGTGGTTTGTAGCGGGTA	231
sY160	TACGGGTCTCGAATGGAATA	TCATTGCATTCCTTTCCATT	236

STS and gene primer sequences are from Foote et al., 1992; Vollrath et al., 1992; Reijo et al., 1995; Vogt et al. 1996, and Lahn and Page, 1997.

some spermatogenic tubules contained mature sperm (4). This meant that the *DAZ* region is not absolutely required to complete spermatogenesis. In addition, the phenotypic diversity associated with essentially equivalent deletions could be due to differences in genetic background or to differences in the environmental impacts each man has encountered.

Y Chromosome Deletions of the *DAZ* Gene Cluster in Oligospermic Men

Oligospermia is a leading cause of infertility. Because spermatogenesis can be completed in some tubules of azoospermic men with deletions, we wondered whether deletions of the *DAZ*-region lead to oligospermia. Thus, blood DNA samples were collected from 35 oligospermic men in order to analyze their Y chromosome content. Two men with sperm counts of 40,000–100,000/ ml had deletions that overlapped those previously reported in azoospermic individuals. Y deletions were not detected in their fathers. Thus, the deletions were de novo mutations, demonstrating conclusively that Y deletions can cause oligospermia (33). The frequency of deletions in men presenting with moderate or mild oligospermia, teratozoospermia, and asthenospermia is not yet known.

Deletions of the *DAZ* Region Are Carried in Sperm DNA and Are Compatible with Fertilization, Embryonic Activation, and Pregnancy When Used in ICSI

Because oligospermia is a common reason for using ICSI, it was conceivable that oligospermic men with *DAZ* deletions produced sperm with deletions. One of the oligospermic men that had a deletion in original studies provided a sperm sample. PCR analysis of sperm DNA indicated that he carried the same Y deletion in sperm DNA as observed in leukocyte DNA (33).

Did this mean that *DAZ* deletions can be passed from father to son via ICSI? Were the sperm produced by men with *DAZ* deletions functional in ICSI? After examination of the Y chromosomes of men preparing to undergo ICSI, it was found that indeed ICSI with sperm from men with Y chromosome deletions could result in pregnancy (37). Several other reports have documented male births in couples where the male partner carries a *DAZ*-deletion (5,30). In addition, the first demonstration of inheritance of *DAZ* deletions in boys conceived via assisted reproduction has more recently been reported (38).

Note that nearly all of the deletion analysis performed to date has been done with DNA samples derived from patient leukocytes. One report indicates, however, that as many as 7% of oligospermic men with normal, intact Y chromosomes in leukocyte DNA may father children with deleted Y chromosomes through assisted reproductive techniques such as intracytoplasmic sperm injection (ICSI) (39). This simple observation suggests that some oligospermic fathers are "mosaic" for Y chromosome deletions. Although the leukocytes contain intact Y chromosomes, the germ cells harbor deleted Y chromosomes. The likelihood that mosaicism in Y-chromosome deletions exists within individuals implies that the sole use of blood DNA tests to detect deletions may underestimate the frequency of Y chromosomal abnormalities in the germline. This has important implications for counseling patients considering ICSI to overcome infertility problems because the real risk of an oligospermic or azoospermic man transmitting a Y-chromosome deletion to male offspring is unknown.

Isolation of the *DAZ* Gene Cluster That Maps to the *DAZ* Region

To identify genes that map to the *DAZ* region, cosmids were captured from a Y-specific cosmid library using the pooled subtraction material as a probe. In addition, some of the YACs in the distal *DAZ* region were subcloned to obtain coverage of this end of the deleted interval. Exon-trapping was then used to search for genes in these subclones (40). For this procedure, each human Y cosmid was subcloned into a vector containing a splice donor and an acceptor. A pool of subclones was transfected into COS7 cells, RNA was isolated, reverse-transcribed, and "mini" cDNA libraries were constructed and probed for the presence of introns derived from the human Y clones. Northern blot analysis of one exon, 325.7, revealed a 3.5 kb testis-specific band. Thus, 325.7 became a candidate for the *AZF* proposed by Tiepolo and Zuffardi (1976). Its candidacy was verified further when it was found to map to the deleted region. Infertile men with *DAZ* region deletions were missing the exon, whereas their fathers and fertile controls were not. Thus, the gene that encodes 325.7 was named the *DAZ* gene. Note that the use of exon trapping in these studies precluded the identification of genes that lack exon–intron structure, the bulk of the genes found on the Y chromosome!

Nucleotide Sequence of the *DAZ* Genes

Sequencing of a *DAZ* cDNA revealed that the predicted amino acid sequence contains a single RNA-binding domain and a series of repeated 24 amino acid motifs, called *DAZ* repeats (4). The *DAZ* RNA-binding domain contains an RNP (RNA-binding Protein) consensus sequence that is found in many RNPs in diverse organisms (41).

It was originally thought that the *DAZ* gene was present in a single copy because Southern blots yield a single hybridizable band when probed with 325.7 (4). We now know, however, that there are several, perhaps as many as seven, tandem copies of *DAZ* on the Y chromosome, all deleted in infertile men containing *DAZ*-region deletions (42). In addition, there is a more divergent copy of *DAZ*, called *DAZL* on chromosome 3. The *DAZ* genes arose from the autosomal *DAZL* gene during primate evolution (43–45). RNA substrate(s) of the proteins have not yet been identified.

Is the *DAZ* Gene Family a Candidate for *AZF*?

The discovery of a point mutation within the *DAZ* genes of an oligospermic or azoospermic man would be ultimate proof of *DAZ* being required for fertility, yet this proof has not come. One problem in obtaining such proof is inability to distinguish the copies of the *DAZ* genes within the *DAZ* region. Their remarkable conservation makes it difficult to examine each copy for point mutations (43), so the evidence that *DAZ* plays a role in spermatogenesis has come from model organisms.

Loss of Function of *DAZ* Homologs in Flies or Mice Causes Infertility

A fly homolog of *DAZ*, *Boule*, has been identified (46). Loss of function of the fly *DAZ* homolog leads to male sterility characterized by meiotic arrest in pachytene I.

A mouse homolog of *DAZ*, *Dazl*, has also been identified (47–49). Its disruption leads to prenatal loss of all germ cells in both sexes during prenatal germ-cell development (50). The loss of germ cells is dosage dependent. Mice with no functional *Dazl* genes are sterile, whereas mice with one intact *Dazl* gene have reduced numbers of germ cells with many immobile, abnormally shaped sperm. This indicates that the copy number of *DAZ* genes may decide germ-cell number and acquisition of morphology and mobility.

Infertility in men with deletions of the *DAZ* gene cluster resembles that of both flies and mice that lack *DAZ* homologs. Men lacking the *DAZ* gene cluster may present with no germ cells, meiotic arrest, or simply fewer sperm (4,29,33). These observations are strong indicators that *DAZ* is a fertility factor whose deletion could lead to infertility in men. Organisms other than primates, however (e.g., flies or mice), have autosomal *DAZ* homologs but no Y chromosome gene cluster. Can we rightly infer from "knockout" phenotypes that *DAZ* is required for fertility in men? The best proof that Y chromosome *DAZ* functions, just as mouse *Dazl*, to determine fertility would be obtained if the human Y chromosome *DAZ* gene cluster were to complement a *Dazl1* deletion.

DAZ Proteins: Expressed Pre- and Postnatally

Antibodies have been developed that recognize an epitope specific to Y-chromosome encoded DAZ, an epitope specific to autosomal DAZL, and an epitope common to both proteins to determine when and where DAZ and DAZL proteins are expressed (51). Using these antibodies, we have found that both proteins are present in the nucleus and cytoplasm of fetal gonocytes. In adult testis, both proteins are abundant in the nucleus of spermatogonia, but transit to the cytoplasm of primary spermatocytes at meiosis. This is in contrast to other reports (52). In this report, authors suggest that the DAZ protein is restricted to postmeiotic cells. This may be because they used a single antibody; the antibodies developed earlier were prepared in duplicate and three different isotopes were used. In addition, we have found that mouse *Dazl* protein is not restricted to the cytoplasm of adult germ cells, rather, it is also expressed during fetal germ-cell development and transits at meiosis just as human *DAZL* (51,53). This suggests that human and mouse genes of the *DAZ* family likely function in the nucleus of premeiotic germ cells and in the cytoplasm of meiotic germ cells. RT-PCR analysis of mRNA expression from the *DAZL* gene also demonstrated that *DAZL* message is confined to the germ lineage (within the testis and ovary), and, in addition, the embryonic stem cells (Fig. 19.2). Because these cells are progenitors of the germ-cell lineage, perhaps, the *Dazl* gene is required to allocate cells to the germ-cell lineage or to maintain the totipotency of cells in the germ lineage. This is further suggested by the observation that in frogs, *X-Dazl* is expressed in the germ plasm, that region of the frog oocyte that ultimately gives rise to the germ lineage (54).

The *AZF* Debate: Which Genes Are Bona Fide Fertility Factors?

The identity of the critical fertility gene(s) within the *DAZ* region has been the subject of considerable debate. Several genes map within or near the *DAZ* region (4,15,55). As I have described earlier, there is increasing evidence that indicates that infertility is caused by loss of one or more of the *DAZ* genes. In fact, the evidence linking the *DAZ* gene deletions to infertility in men surpasses that of any other Y chromosome gene family; however, the role of other genes that map in or near the *DAZ* genes in determining fertility is not yet known. This issue is being actively researched and we should soon more clearly understand the role of other genes in the intervals deleted from the Y chromosomes of infertile men.

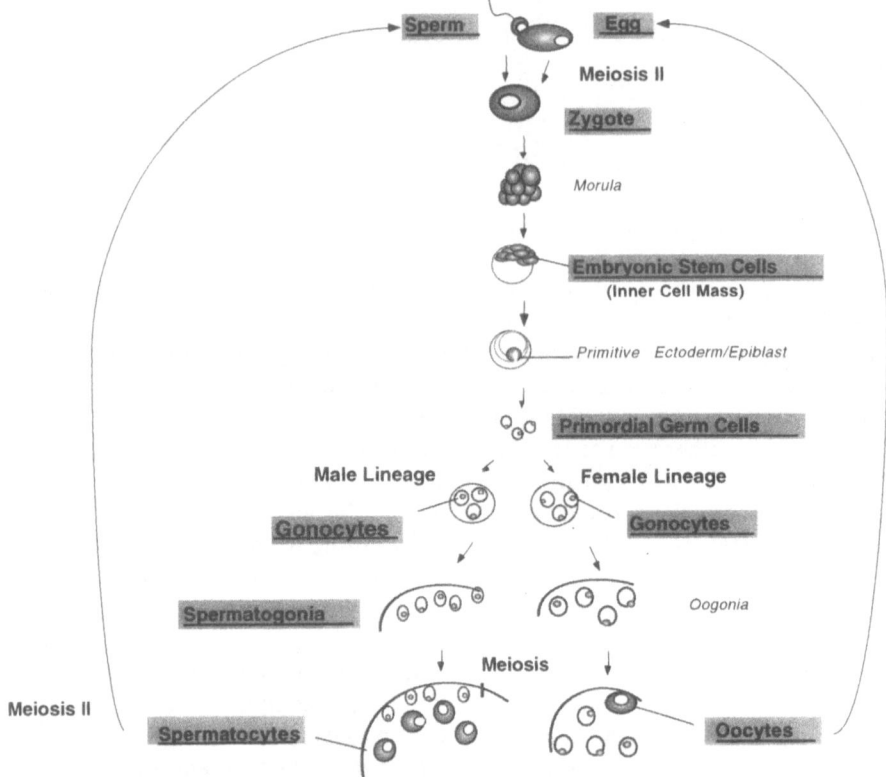

FIGURE 19.2. The *DAZ/DAZL* family of proteins is expressed in germ cells in the male and female lineages. In this figure, cells that have been shown to express DAZ/DAZL proteins are shown in bold and underlined; cells in italics have not been tested. Many cells of the female and male germ-cell lineage express DAZ/DAZL protein (Reijo et al., in press; Dorfman et al., 1999). In addition, expression of *DAZL* message was also demonstrated in embryonic stem cells.

References

1. Castrillon DH, Gonczy P, Alexander S, Rawson R, Eberhart CG, Viswanathan S, et al. Toward a molecular genetic analysis of spermatogenesis in *Drosophila melanogaster*: characterization of male-sterile mutants generated by single P element mutagenesis. Genetics 1993;135:489–505.
2. Chubb C. Genetic control of spermatogenesis and steroidogenesis. In: Desjardins C, Ewing LL, eds. Cell and molecular biology of the testis. New York: Oxford University Press, 1993:90–107.
3. Mello CC, Draper BW, Krause M, Weintraub H, Priess JR. The *pie-1* and *mex-1* genes and maternal control of blastomere identity in early *C. elegans* embryos. Cell 1992;70:163–76.
4. Reijo R, Lee TY, Salo P, Alagappan R, Brown LG, Rosenberg M, et al. Diverse spermatogenic defects in humans caused by Y chromosome deletions encompassing a novel RNA-binding protein gene. Nat Genet 1995;10:383–93.

5. Vogt PH, Edelmann A, Kirsch S, Henegariu O, Hirschmann P, Kiesewetter F, et al. Human Y chromosome *azoospermia factors* (*AZF*) mapped to different subregions in Yq11. Hum Mol Genet 1996;5:933–43.
6. Aittomaki K, Lucena JL, Pakarinen P, Sistonen P, Tapanainen J, Gromoll J, et al. Mutation in the follicle-stimulating hormone receptor gene causes hereditary hypergonadotropic ovarian failure. Cell 1995;82:959–68.
7. Tiepolo L, Zuffardi O. Localization of factors controlling spermatogenesis in the nonfluorescent portion of the human Y chromosome long arm. Hum Genet 1976;34:119–24.
8. Fitch N, Richer C-L, Pinsky L, Kahn A. Deletion of the long arm of the Y chromosome and review of Y chromosome abnormalities. Am J Med Genet 1985;20: 31–42.
9. Hartung M, Devictor M, Codaccioni JL, Stahl A. Yq deletion and failure of spermatogenesis. Ann Genet 1988;31:21–26.
10. Johnson MD, Tho SPT, Behzadian Z, McDonough PG. Molecular scanning of Yq11 (interval 6) in men with Sertoli-cell-only syndrome. Am J Obstet Gynecol 1989;161:1732–37.
11. Skare J, Drwinga H, Wyandt H, vanderSpek J, Troxler R, Milunsky A. Interstitial deletion involving most of Yq. Am J Med Genet 1990;36:394–97.
12. Burgoyne PS, Mahadevaiah SK, Sutcliffe MJ, Palmer SJ. Fertility in mice requires X-Y pairing and a Y-chromosomal "spermiogenesis" gene mapping to the long arm. Cell 1992;71:391–98.
13. Borgaonkar DS, Hollander DH. Quinacrine fluorescence of the human Y chromosome. Nature 1971;230:52.
14. Ma K, Sharkey A, Kirsch S, Vogt P, Keil R, Hargreave TB, et al. Towards the molecular localisation of the AZF locus: mapping of microdeletions in azoospermic men within 14 subintervals of interval 6 of the human Y chromosome. Hum Mol Genet 1992;1:29–33.
15. Ma K, Inglis JD, Sharkey A, Bickmore WA, Hill RE, Prosser EJ, et al. A Y chromosome gene family with RNA-binding protein homology: Candidates for the azoospermia factor AZF controlling human spermatogenesis gene. Cell 1993;75:1287–95.
16. Vogt P, Chandley AC, Hargreave TB, Keil R, Ma K, Sharkey A. Microdeletions in interval 6 of the Y chromosome of males with idiopathic sterility point to disruption of AZF, a human spermatogenesis gene. Hum Genet 1992;89:491–96.
17. Kobayashi K, Mizuno K, Hida A, Komaki R, Tomita K, Matsushita I, et al. PCR analysis of the Y chromosome long arm in azoospermic patients: evidence for a second locus required for spermatogenesis. Hum Mol Genet 1994;3:1965–67.
18. Delbridge ML, Harry JL, Toder R, O'Neill RJ, Ma K, Chandley AC, et al. A human candidate spermatogenesis gene, *RBM1*, is conserved and amplified on the marsupial Y chromosome. Nat Genet 1997;15:131–36.
19. Chai NN, Salido EC, Yen PH. Multiple functional copies of the *RBM* gene family, a spermatogenesis candidate of the human Y chromosome. Genomics 1997;45: 355–61.
20. Prosser J, Inglis JD, Condie A, Ma K, Kerr S, Thakrar R, et al. Degeneracy in human multicopy *RBM* (*YRRM*), a candidate spermatogenesis gene. Mamm Genome 1996;7:835–42.
21. Nakahori Y, Kobayashi K, Komaki R, Matsushita I, Nakagome Y. A locus of the candidate gene family for azoospermia factor (*YRRM2*) is polymorphic with a null allele in Japanese males. Hum Mol Genet 1994;3:1709.

22. Elliot DJ, Millar MR, Oghene K, Ross A, Kiesewetter F, Pryor J, et al. Expression of *RBM* in the nuclei of human germ cells is dependent on a critical region of the Y chromosome long arm. Proc Natl Acad Sci USA 1997;94:3848–53.

23. Elliot DJ, Ma K, Kerr SM, Thakrar R, Speed R, Chandley AC, et al. An *RBM* homologue maps to the mouse Y chromosome and is expressed in germ cells. Hum Mol Genet 1996;5:869–74.

24. Foresta C, Ferlin A, Garolla A, Rossato M, Barbaux S, De Bortoli A. Y-chromosome deletions in idiopathic severe testiculopathies. J Clin Endocrinol Metab 1997;82:1075–80.

25. Nakahori Y, Kuroki Y, Komaki R, Kondoh N, Namiki M, Iwamoto T, et al. The Y chromosome region essential for spermatogenesis. Horm Res 1996;46:20–23.

26. Pryor JL, Kent-First M, Muallem A, Van Bergen AH, Holten WE, Meisner L, et al. Microdeletions in the Y chromosome of infertile men. N Engl J Med 1997;336:534–39.

27. Foote S, Vollrath D, Hilton A, Page DC. The human Y chromosome: overlapping DNA clones spanning the euchromatic region. Science 1992;258:60–66.

28. Vollrath D, Foote S, Hilton A, Brown LG, Beer-Romero P, Bogan JS, et al. The human Y chromosome: a 43-interval map based on naturally occurring deletions. Science 1992;258:52–59.

29. Girardi SK, Mielnik A, Schlegel PN. Submicroscopic deletions in the Y chromosome of infertile men. Hum Reprod 1997;12:1635–41.

30. Kent-First MG, Kol S, Muallem A, Ofir R, Manor D, Blazer S, et al. The incidence and possible relevance of Y-linked microdeletions in babies born after intracytoplasmic sperm injection and their infertile fathers. Mol Hum Reprod 1996;2:943–50.

31. Simoni M, Gromoll J, Dworniczak B, Rolf C, Abshagen K, Kamischke A, et al. Screening for deletions of the Y chromosome involving the DAZ (Deleted in AZoospermia) gene in azoospermia and severe oliogozoospermia. Fertil Steril 1997;67:542–47.

32. Stuppia L, Mastroprimiano G, Calabrese G, Peila R, Tenaglis R, Palka G. Microdeletions in interval 6 of the Y chromosome detected by STS-PCR in 6 of 33 patients with idiopathic oligo- or azoospermia. Cytogenet Cell Genet 1996;72:155–58.

33. Reijo R, Alagappan RK, Patrizio P, Page DC. Severe oligospermia resulting from deletions of the *Azoospermia Factor* gene of the Y chromosome. Lancet 1996;347:1290–93.

34. Vereb M, Agulnik AI, Houston JT, Lipschultz LI, Lamb DJ, Bishop CE. Absence of DAZ gene mutations in cases of non-obstructed azoospermia. Mol Hum Reprod 1997;3:55–59.

35. Yoshida A, Nakahori Y, Kuroki Y, Motoyama M, Araki Y, Miura K, et al. Dicentric Y chromosome in an azoospermic male. Mol Hum Reprod 1997;3:709–12.

36. Kremer JAM, Tuerlings JHAM, Meuleman EJH, Schoute F, Mariman E, Smeets DFCM, et al. Microdeletions of the Y chromosome and intracytoplasmic sperm injection: from gene to clinic. Hum Reprod 1997;12:687–91.

37. Mulhall JP, Reijo R, Alagappan R, Brown L, Page D, Carson R, et al. Azoospermic men with deletion of the *DAZ* gene cluster are capable of completing spermatogenesis: fertilization, normal embryonic development and pregnancy occur when retrieved testicular spermatozoa are used for intracytoplasmic sperm injection. Hum Reprod 1997;12:503–8.

38. Page DC, Silber S, Brown LG. Men with infertility caused by *AZFc* deletion can produce sons by intracytoplasmic sperm injection, but are likely to transmit the deletion and infertility. Hum Reprod 1999;14:1722–26.
39. Kent-First MG, Kol S, Muallem A, Blazer S, Itskovitz-Eldor J. Infertility in intra-cytoplasmic-sperm-injection-derived sons. Lancet 1996;348:332.
40. Duyk GM, Kim S, Meyers RM, Cox DR. Exon trapping: a genetic screen to identify candidate transcribed sequences in cloned mammalian genomic DNA. Proc Natl Acad Sci USA 1990;87:8995–99.
41. Burd CG, Dreyfuss G. Conserved structures and diversity of functions on RNA-binding proteins. Science 1994;265:615–21.
42. Gläser B, Yen PH, Schempp W. Fibre-fluorescence in situ hybridization unravels apparently seven *DAZ* genes or pseudogenes clustered within a Y-chromosome region frequently deleted in azoospermic males. Chromosome Res 1998;6:481–86.
43. Saxena R, Brown LG, Hawkins T, Alagappan RK, Skaletsky H, Reeve MP, et al. The DAZ gene cluster of the human Y chromosome arose from an autosomal gene that was transposed, repeatedly amplifed and pruned. Nat Genet 1996;14:292–99.
44. Yen PH, Chai NN, Salido EC. The human autosomal gene DAZLA: testis specificity and a candidate for male infertility. Hum Mol Genet 1996;5:2013–17.
45. Yen PH, Chai NN, Salido EC. The human *DAZ* genes, a putative male infertility factor on the Y chromosome, are highly polymorphic in the DAZ repeat regions. Mamm Genome 1997;8:756–59.
46. Eberhart CG, Maines JZ, Wasserman SA. Meiotic cell cycle requirement for a fly homologue of human *Deleted in AZoospermia*. Nature 1996;381:783–85.
47. Reijo R. Seligman J, Dinulos MD, Jaffe T, Brown LG, Disteche CM, et al. Mouse autosomal homolog of DAZ, a candidate male sterility gene in humans, is expressed in male germ cells before and after puberty. Genomics 1996;35:346–52.
48. Cooke HJ, Lee M, Kerr S, Ruggiu M. A murine homologue of the human DAZ gene is autosomal and expressed only in male and female gonads. Hum Mol Genet 1996;5:513–16.
49. Maiwald R, Luche RM, Epstein CJ. Isolation of a mouse homolog of the human *DAZ* (*Deleted in AZoospermia*) gene. Mamm Genome 1996;7:628.
50. Ruggiu M, Speed R, Taggart M, McKay SJ, Kilanowski F, Saunders P, et al. The mouse *Dazla* gene encodes a cytoplasmic protein essential for gametogenesis. Nature 1997;389:73–77.
51. Reijo RA, Dorfman D, Renshaw A, Loughlin K, Page DC. *DAZ* family proteins, fertility factor candidates, are present throughout male germ cell development and transit from nucleus to cytoplasma at meiosis. Biol Reprod (in press).
52. Habermann B, Mi HF, Edelmann A, Bohring C, Backert IT, Kiesewetter F, et al. *DAZ* (*Deleted in AZoospermia*) genes encode proteins located in human late spermatids and in sperm tails. Hum Reprod 1998;13:363–69.
53. Dorfman DM, Genest DR, Reijo Pera RA. Human *DAZL1* encodes a candidate fertility factor in women that localizes to the prenatal and postnatal germ cells. Hum Reprod 1999;14:2531–36.
54. Houston DW, Zhang J, Maines JZ, Wasserman SA, King ML. A *Xenopus DAZ-like* gene encodes an RNA component of germ plasm and is a functional homologue of *Drosophila boule*. Development 1998;125:171–80.
55. Lahn BT, Page DC. Functional coherence of the human Y chromosome. Science 1997;278:675–80.

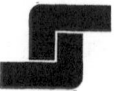

20

Genetic Defects of
Male Infertility and ICSI

JAN A.M. KREMER, JOEP H.A.M. TUERLINGS,
RON VAN GOLDE, ERIC J.H. MEULEMAN,
AND DIDI D.M. BRAAT

Intracytoplasmic sperm injection (ICSI) has caused a revolution in the treatment of severe male infertility. The direct injection of a single spermatozoon into the oocyte enables pregnancies in couples of whom the man has severe oligozoospermia or even azoospermia. This therapeutic revolution has unfortunately not been accompanied by a revolution in the knowledge of the etiology of the underlying problem. There are indications that genetic factors play a major role, and this may have serious consequences for the offspring.

ICSI

In the case of ICSI the process of fertilization is dramatically changed. Fertilization takes place outside the body, and physiological sperm selection and sperm penetration are bypassed. A micropipette is used to inject a single sperm cell into the cytoplasm of the oocyte, which is fixed by a holding pipette with the polar body at 6 or 12 o'clock.

The first report of ICSI resulting in a human pregnancy appeared in 1992 (1). Today, more than 10,000 children have been born after ICSI treatment, and pregnancy rates of 35% per cycle have been reported (2). The interactive IVF-registration on the Web site of the Dutch Society of Gynecologists (NVOG-net) mentioned 3062 started ICSI cycles in 1997 (3). These cycles resulted in 2805 ovum pickups (92%), 2635 embryo transfers (86%), 771 pregnancies (25%) and 644 ongoing pregnancies (21%), and, based on a multiple pregnancy rate of 25%, about 800 ICSI babies. In the Netherlands almost 200,000 babies were born in 1997, so it can be estimated that one of every 250 Dutch babies is an ICSI child.

ICSI Procedure

An ICSI cycle starts with the downregulation of pituitary gonadotropins by gonadotropin releasing hormone (GnRH) analogues, which prevents premature luteinizing hormone (LH) surges before the ovum pickup. Ovarian stimulation is performed by daily injections of urinary or recombinant follicle stimulating hormone (FSH). Follicular growth is monitored by vaginal ultrasound. If the follicles are big enough, an injection of human chorionic gonadotropin (hCG) is given, and the ovum pickup is scheduled about 36 hours later. The follicles are punctured under ultrasound guidance. The oocyte/granulosa cell complexes are cleaned with hyaluronidase and an ICSI procedure is performed the same day. If fertilization took place, embryo transfer is performed 2–3 days after the ovum pickup. Progesterone or hCG is given as luteal support. After 2 weeks the couple will know whether the treatment was successful or not.

Surgical Retrieved Sperm

Only sperm retrieved from the ejaculate was initially used for ICSI. Soon after the introduction of ICSI it became evident that epididymal sperm or even testicular retrieved sperm could also be used successfully (4). It was later shown that pregnancies can be achieved using spermatids (5). Thus, spermatozoa do not have to go through the full length of the genital tract before they are able to achieve fertilization. Because the effects of ICSI with surgically retrieved sperm for the offspring are not clear, the professional organizations in The Netherlands announced a moratorium in 1996 on ICSI with surgically retrieved sperm.

Risks of ICSI

Because ICSI bypasses part of the natural selection mechanism, concerns have been expressed on the possible risk(s) for the offspring. Patrizio divided these risks into two groups (6): Problems related to the ICSI technique (i.e., bypassing the nature of sperm selection, mechanical sperm introduction, injection of foreign material, medium, and other chemical contaminants into the oocyte, physical disturbance of the ooplasm, mechanical oocyte activation, and damage to the meiotic spindle) and problems not directly related to the ICSI technique (i.e., transmission of genetic anomalies, gametes carrying structural defects, and sperm activation defects). The conditions in this latter group mainly concern the use of ICSI without understanding the precise etiology of the fertility problem.

The introduction of ICSI in 1992 was embraced as a major breakthrough for the "treatment" of male factor infertility. It should be noted that the rapid introduction of ICSI was not accompanied by randomized clinical trials or studies on the effect of ICSI on the offspring. It has been observed that there are no increased risks for congenital anomalies. Bonduelle presented the follow-up of 1987 children born after ICSI, including 209 children resulting from ICSI with surgically retrieved sperm (7). The number of congenital abnormalities in their cohort of children did not seem to differ from the expected number in the normal newborn population; however, they found an increased frequency of sex chromosome aberrations (0.9% compared with 0.5% in the normal newborn population). Furthermore, two reports on the developmental outcome of a small group of young children conceived by ICSI have been published (8,9). Bowen showed an increased risk of developmental delay in 100 ICSI children at the age of 1 year (8). This increased risk, however, was not found by Bonduelle who studied 200 ICSI children at the age of 2 years (9). Data on long-term follow-up of the "ICSI children" are not yet available.

Genetics of Male Infertility

Male infertility can occur either as an isolated disorder or within the framework of a known complex disorder or syndrome. Due to the stormy developments in molecular genetics over the past decade, a significant proportion of idiopathic male infertility in healthy males is now known to be of genetic origin. Genetic factors involved in male infertility comprise chromosomal disorders, monogenic disorders, and multifactorial disorders. Much research is currently focused on microdeletions of the Y chromosome and the genes involved as a cause of male infertility.

The list of genetic disorders that may cause male infertility is far from complete. Lilford showed that 12% of men with oligozoospermia have male relatives with a fertility problem (10). Spermatogenesis is a complex process, and hundreds or thousands of genes may be involved. At present, despite the interest in the processes involved in this pathway, only a few human "spermatogenic genes" have been identified without knowing their precise function.

Chromosomal Abnormalities

It has been known for a long time that chromosomal abnormalities are found more frequently in men with severe fertility problems. Tuerlings (11) conducted a nationwide study of 1792 male ICSI candidates and found that 72 of these men (4.0%) have a chromosomal abnormality: 1.7% sex-chromosomal abnormalities (especially Klinefelter's syndrome) and 2.4% autosomal abnormalities (especially Robertsonian translocations).

In men with these chromosomal abnormalities genetic counseling is important. There is a risk on transmission of the chromosomal abnormality and associated problems. Giltay (12) analyzed the decisions of these couples after counseling: 56% of them decided to go on with ICSI, 31% decided to refrain from ICSI, and 13% did not make a decision before the end of the study.

Microdeletions of the Y Chromosome

Microdeletions in the azoospermia factor (AZF) region of the Y chromosome have been described in infertile men. We studied the frequency of these deletions in ICSI men with severe oligozoospermia (13). Seven of the 111 men appeared to have a microdeletion in the AZFc region (6.3%). Finding a microdeletion is important for couples who want ICSI because their sons will have the same genotype and probably the same phenotype. Testing for microdeletions should be offered to all ICSI men. After knowing the results the couple can make their own, well-informed decision.

These de novo mutations create a unique situation from a population-genetic point of view: They are Y-linked and were genetically lethal before the ICSI era. We developed a mathematical model to estimate the frequency of microdeletions in future generations after the introduction of ICSI (14). We made several scenarios for the two variables in this model (spontaneous mutation frequency and reproductive fitness). It seemed that the rise in this frequency of microdeletions remains limited as long as the fitness remains limited. Based on a realistic scenario (fitness of 0.5), the frequency rises in five generations from 1 in 10,000 to 2 in 10,000. After these five generations a plateau is reached and there is no further increase in frequency. Hence, the rise in frequency remains limited as long as the fitness remains limited. As long as we make ICSI not as successful as normal reproduction, we should not be too worried about an increase of the frequency of microdeletions.

Couples dealing with microdeletions should be counseled before they can make a decision about ICSI or no ICSI. We analyzed the counseling and the decision of 28 couples in six fertility centers. Eighty percent of the couples decided to go on with ICSI and 20% chose its alternatives (e.g., artificial insemination with donor semen) or refrained from further treatment (unpublished data). The final decision of the couple was related to several aspects of the process of counseling. The possibility of performing ICSI in the department of the counselor was especially important. Most couples chose ICSI if it was available.

CFTR Mutations

Mutations in the cystic fibrosis transmembrane regulator (CFTR) gene are found frequently in men with azoospermia based on congenital absence of the vas. In general men with an absence of the vas are tested for CFTR mutations before entering an ICSI program. If mutations are present their wives must be tested. If they are carriers, too, then genetic counseling should be offered.

It has been suggested by van der Ven that CFTR mutations may play a role in the etiology of oligozoospermia (15). She found that 18% of men with idiopathic oligozoospermia had at least one CFTR mutation. This finding has not been confirmed by others. Tuerlings did a complete mutation analysis of the CFTR gene in 75 male ICSI candidates with severe oligozoospermia (16). CFTR mutations have been found in only 3% of these men (6% in the normal population). Thus, at this time routine screening of CFTR mutations in idiopathic oligozoospermia is not indicated.

Other Genetic Factors

Mutations in the FSH receptor have been described in infertile men, but we did not detect FSH receptor mutations in 28 ICSI men with high FSH levels (17). The clinical relevance of these mutations, therefore, is not yet clear.

There will be more genetic factors related to severe male infertility. A lot of current research is done to reveal these factors. Despite this we do not know what they are and we do not know their frequency. We are obligated to tell the ICSI couples that there may be genetic causes of the male infertility, which are unknown until now and which may be transmitted to the offspring.

Clinical Consequences

The current genetic knowledge must have consequences for the clinical ICSI practice. We have to inform our patients what we know and what we do not know about the chance of transmission of fertility problems or associated problems to the offspring. Male ICSI candidates should be offered a genetic workup, consisting of a detailed family history, chromosomal analysis and specific molecular analysis (18).

The family history is an easy and important tool. The family history may reveal other genetic problems associated with the fertility problem. Furthermore, it may give answers about heredity and variability in cases of male infertility of unknown origin with a familiar pattern. Finally, the family history may be the starting point of clinical and molecular research. In our center we use an extensive questionnaire, which is sent to the couple before the first visit.

Chromosomal analysis must be offered to all ICSI candidates with severe oligozoospermia or azoospermia. Specific molecular diagnostic tests should be limited to the analysis of microdeletions in the AZF region. CFTR mutation analysis is only necessary in the case of congenital absence of the vas.

If abnormalities are found during this genetic screening, the couple should be counseled by a clinical geneticist. After optimal information the couple can make their own, well-informed choice about their reproductive future (18).

The Future

The knowledge of the genetics of male infertility is expanding rapidly. New spermatogenesis genes will be discovered (Human Genome Project), and testing of mutations will become easier (DNA chips). This causes new questions concerning the clinical impact and significance of the findings. The gap between diagnostic possibilities and therapeutic options will be larger and larger, which will lead to more ethical questions being asked by society.

One of the major problems for the next decade is the increasing gap between the molecular scientists and reproductive clinicians. Molecular scientists are learning more and more, and this increasing knowledge has to be translated to society. This is a task for the reproductive clinicians, who have to inform their patients about all possibilities. Clinicians, however, know little about molecular science, and molecular scientists know little about clinical practice. This has to change, especially in light of the rapid developments in this field. Both groups—clinicians and scientists—have the task to speak the language of the other party. More interaction is necessary. Only then will it be possible to implement the increasing molecular knowledge in the clinical practice.

References

1. Palermo G, Joris H, Devroey P, Van Steirteghem AC. Pregnancies after intracytoplasmic injection of single spermatozoon into an oocyte. Lancet 1992;340:17–18.
2. Van Steirteghem AC, Nagy Z, Joris H, Liu J, Staessen C, Smitz J, et al. High fertilization and implantation rates after intracytoplasmic sperm injection. Hum Reprod 1993;8:1061–66.
3. Anonymus. IVF resultaten over 1997 cumulatief. NVOG-net: http://www.nvog.nl
4. Tournaye H, Devroey P, Liu J, Nagy Z, Lissens W, Van Steirteghem A. Microsurgical epididymal sperm aspiration and intracytoplasmic sperm injection: a new effective approach to infertility as a result of congenital bilateral absence of the vas deferens. Fertil Steril 1994;61:1045–51.
5. Tesarik J, Mendoza C, Testart J. Viable embryos from injection of round spermatids into oocytes. N Engl J Med 1995;333:525.
6. Patrizio P. Intracytoplasmic sperm injection (ICSI): potential genetic concerns. Hum Reprod 1995;10:2520–23.
7. Bonduelle M, Aytoz A, Wilikens A, Buysse A, Van Assche E, Devroey P, et al. Genetic problems and congenital malformations in 1987 ICSI children. Hum Reprod 1998;13 (Abstract book):108–9 (O-211).
8. Bowen JR, Gibson FL, Garth LI, Saunders DM. Medical and developmental outcome at 1 year for children conceived by intracytoplasmic sperm injection. Lancet 1998;351:1529–31.
9. Bonduelle M, Joris H, Hofmans K, Liebaers I, Van Steirteghem AC. Mental development of 201 ICSI children at 2 years of age. Lancet 1998;351:1553.
10. Lilford R, Jones AM, Bishop DT, Thornton J, Mueller R. Case-control study of whether subfertility in men is familial. Br Med J 1994;309:570–73.

11. Tuerlings JH, de France HF, Hamers A, Hordijk R, Van Hemel JO, Hansson K, et al. Chromosome studies in 1792 males prior to intra-cytoplasmic sperm injection: the Dutch experience. Eur J Hum Genet 1998;6:194–200.
12. Giltay JC, Kastrop PMM, Tuerlings JHAM, Kremer JAM, Tiemessen CHJ, Gerssen-Schoorl KBJ, et al. The majority of subfertile men with constitutive chromosome abnormalities do not refrain from ICSI treatment. A follow-up study on 75 Dutch patients. Hum Reprod 1999;14:318–20.
13. Kremer JA, Tuerlings JH, Meuleman EJ, Schoute F, Mariman E, Smeets DF, et al. Microdeletions of the Y chromosome and intracytoplasmic sperm injection: from gene to clinic. Hum Reprod 1997;12:687–91.
14. Kremer JA, Tuerlings JH, Borm G, Hoefsloot LH, Meuleman EJ, Braat DD, et al. Does intracytoplasmic sperm injection lead to a rise in the frequency of microdeletions in the AZFc region of the Y chromosome in future generations? Hum Reprod 1998;13:2808–11.
15. van der Ven K, Messer L, van der Ven H, Jeyendran RS, Ober C. Cystic fibrosis mutation screening in healthy men with reduced sperm quality. Hum Reprod 1996;11: 513–17.
16. Tuerlings JH, Mol B, Kremer JA, Looman M, Meuleman EJ, te Meerman GJ, et al. Mutation frequency of cystic fibrosis transmembrane regulator is not increased in oligozoospermic male candidates for intracytoplasmic sperm injection. Fertil Steril 1998;69:899–903.
17. Tuerlings JH, Ligtenberg MJ, Kremer JA, Siers M, Meuleman EJ, Braat DD, et al. Screening male intracytoplasmic sperm injection candidates for mutations of the follicle stimulating hormone receptor gene. Hum Reprod 1998;13:2098–101.
18. Tuerlings JH, Kremer JA, Meuleman EJ. The practical application of genetics in the male infertility clinic. J Androl 1997;18:576–81.

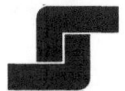

21

Spermatids: Clinically Useful Gametes?

Fay L. Shamanski, Paul J. Turek, and Roger A. Pedersen

Without doubt, the impact of intracytoplasmic sperm injection (ICSI) on the treatment of male infertility has been revolutionary. In most major fertility centers, close to half of in vitro fertilization (IVF) cases now involve ICSI, and the majority of these cases are performed for male factor infertility. To overcome either obstructive or nonobstructive problems in the male, it is routine to use mature spermatozoa retrieved from the ejaculate, vas deferens, epididymis, and testicle for ICSI. Fertilization and pregnancy rates with the use of spermatozoa aspirated from the reproductive tract are excellent, virtually approximating those observed with ejaculated sperm. ICSI is associated with normal embryo and early postnatal outcomes among offspring so conceived (1). Reports indicate, however, that an increased incidence of sex chromosomal abnormalities is observed with the use of testicular sperm from azoospermic men (2) and that developmental delays have been noted in ICSI children (3).

Despite this tremendous success with ICSI, men with testicular failure remain who may not possess mature sperm for use with this technique. The number of men so afflicted is not clinically insignificant: Consider that 5–10% of infertile men present with azoospermia and that 60% of this subset has testis failure. Among a consecutive series of azoospermic infertile men who presented to the UCSF Male Infertility Clinic, approximately 18% exhibited early maturation arrest (primary spermatocyte) and 7% showed late maturation arrest (spermatid stage) patterns of spermatogenic failure on testis biopsy. Although these patients may have no available spermatozoa for ICSI, they may be excellent candidates for technologies that enables the use of earlier germ cell forms for fertilization.

Driven by a demand for such technology, the use of round spermatid injection (ROSI) or round spermatid nuclear injection (ROSNI) progressed very quickly into the clinical arena, well in advance of adequate scientific study in animal models. Upon introduction into the human literature, ROSI and ROSNI met squarely with two major criticisms: How can spermatids be reliably recognized in fresh, unstained preparations, and how can we be sure that spermatids have undergone the appropriate epigenetic modifications to ensure that, like mature sperm, they are genetically ready for embryonic development? The ethical, medical, and legal implications of these criticisms are quite real and are only now beginning to be investigated. In the meantime, clinicians have been encouraged to exhaust all available technological options that can identify mature spermatozoa (4,5) rather than simply acquiesce to clinical spermatid injections, about which our understanding is incomplete.

Success with ROSI in fertility clinics has been low; perhaps related to an inability to identify this cell type reliably or a limitation in the capacity of spermatids to act as competent gametes. A concern with the clinical use of spermatids for ICSI is whether the genetic material within this cell is correctly "packaged" for use as a gamete. This concern certainly warrants extensive scientific testing before simply "seeing what happens" clinically, as some clinicians have suggested be done. Changes to the chromatin during germ cell development or gametogenesis differentially mark chromosomes contributed by the sperm and egg. This imprinting of the chromosomes results in unique expression patterns of some genes contributed by the sperm. This chapter will review the current state of research and understanding of the use of spermatids as gametes, specifically concentrating on the role of imprinting in late germ cells.

History of Spermatid Use

The first ROSI experiments in mammals were conducted in rabbit, hamster, and mouse. Experiments with rabbits reported in 1994 showed that ROSI-derived embryos could complete gestation and result in live births (6). The efficiency was low: Only three offspring were born out of 121 two-to-four cell embryos transferred back to the oviducts of foster mothers. In hamster experiments, a species in which oocytes more closely resemble human oocytes (7), the events involved in pronuclear formation in spermatid-injected embryos were described. In both hamster and mouse, spermatid fusion resulted in normal male pronuclei in less than 10% of the zygotes. More often smaller-than-normal pronuclei appeared. These small pronuclei were able to replicate their DNA and to participate in the first mitotic division (7). Though hamster oocytes and zygotes were more easily manipulated than mice, hamster embryos were difficult to culture and most resulting embryos did not grow beyond the two-cell stage. The culture and transfer of mouse embryos is now well established, but mouse oocytes are quite fragile and easily lyse if touched incorrectly with an injection needle. The fragility of mouse oocytes thus proved to be the limiting factor in early spermatid injection experiments.

In order to minimize oocyte damage, early ROSI experiments switched from injection to an electric pulse to fuse spermatids to oocytes. The spermatid is injected into the perivitelline space of the oocyte and then subjected to an electrical pulse (8). The effectiveness of electrical fusion is inversely related to the size difference of the cells being fused. The high voltages needed to fuse a 10 μm diameter spermatid to a 100 μm diameter oocyte are also high enough to lyse the oocyte, so a balance is necessary between the voltage needed for fusion and the voltage that would burst the oocytes. In addition to fusing the two gametes, the electric pulse also activates the oocyte. When fusion fails, activation may still occur that can result in oocyte cleavage and parthenogenetic development (9). Because electrical pulse technology often results in the fusion of the male and female pronuclei, it may be difficult to differentiate successfully fertilized oocytes from abnormal parthenogenetic oocytes as is the case in humans (10). Using fusion technology, successful births from ROSI in mice have been inefficient, with fusion rates of less than 10% (7) and 1% of oocytes injected resulting in live pups (8). This technical problem was overcome with the introduction of the piezoelectric drilling device (11,12). This technique is far less destructive to the mouse oocyte: In one study the efficiency increased to 28% (12). The success of these techniques has led to the theory that spermiogenesis, epididymal maturation, capacitation, and the acrosome reaction exist solely to deliver the haploid sperm cell to the oocyte (8).

It is significant that ROSI was being used in human infertility clinics at the same time that its safety and efficacy were being studied in model organisms. Successful fertilization of a human oocyte by round spermatid injection was reported in 1995 (13). In the same year the reports of the first pregnancy (14) and first birth (15) were published. Table 21.1 summarizes the published data on the clinical use of spermatids (15–20). One striking feature of these data is that oocyte fertilization and pregnancy rates are extremely low. The low fertilization rates in human ROSI may be explained by the timing of activation that is coincident with injection. In mice, higher fertilization rates were achieved when activation preceded injection by 30–60 minutes. It is also not clear whether the spermatids remain intact upon injection, whether this is important and if so, how the oocyte responds to the spermatid cell membrane. The feasibility of this technology is also limited because, clinically, most azoospermic patients have arrest prior to completion of meiosis (primary spermatocyte stage), which suggests that most patients who completely lack mature sperm on testicular biopsy also lack spermatids (21).

Identification of Spermatids

As mentioned earlier, the first and most obvious problem is the correct identification and selection of round spermatids. Spermatids are usually identified by their size and nuclear morphology. Several identification methods have been proposed, including classic histology (17), gradient separation and enrichment of germ cells (22), confocal microscopy (23), transmission electron microscopy (23), and image analysis (24). Most of these methods

TABLE 21.1. Summary of ROSI and ELSI data.

References	Gametes/ Source	Cycles (C) or Patients (P)	# Oocytes Injected	# Fertilized 2PN (inject.)	1 PN (% inject.)	# Patients with Pregnancy
Antinori	RS	19 P	135	75 (55)	19 (14)	2
1997 [19]	ELS	17 P	123	71 (58)	16 (13)	3
Vanderzwalmen 1997 [16]	RS	32 P	260	57 (22)	44 (17)	1*
	ELS	8 P	36	23 (57)	1 (3)	4
Yamanaka 1997 [20]	RS	9 P	53	34 (64)	13 (25)	0
Tesarik 1995 [15]	RS	12 P	39	14 (36)	—	2*
Ghazzawi 1999 [18]	RS	87 P	574	126 (22)	—	0
Sousa 1999 [17]	ERS	29 C	262	31 (12)	78 (30)	0
	TRS	21 C	132	12 (9)	42 (32)	0
	ELS	20 C	166	78 (47)	17 (10)	7*
Total	RS	209	1455	349 (24)		5
Total	ELS	45	325	172 (53)		14

RS = round spermatid, ELS = elongated spermatid, ERS = ejaculated round spermatid, TRS = testicular round spermatid. * At least one live birth at the time of reporting.

unfortunately rely on subtle morphological characteristics of spermatids for selection, making the development of rigorous and reliable identification criteria quite difficult. Moreover, most of the technologies used to identify spermatids accurately either kill the cell or render it clinically unusable. Two developments show promise in this regard, however. Spermatid identification based on size and nuclear complexity using a fluorescence-activated cell sorter (FACS) with light in the visible range may simplify the enrichment of spermatids within a heterogeneous population (22). These approaches need further verification, including cytogenetic studies. In addition, in vitro culture of round spermatids to more advanced spermatogenic stages may have potential in presperm cell identification and selection (25). From our experience in the mouse model, spermatid identification appears straightforward in a normal testes because samples have little blood and spermatids are an abundant cell type. In humans, the implications of incorrect identification of spermatids have far greater practical and ethical importance; therefore, definite identification for their use in clinical treatment of infertility is critical.

Round spermatids are incapable of activating eggs, most likely due to the absence of oocyte activating protein (12). The oocyte, therefore, must be artificially activated. The electrical pulse used with the fusion technique is sufficient to activate the oocyte, but when direct spermatid injection is used, an additional stimulus must be included to activate the oocyte. Several methods have been applied to achieve activation: electrical stimuli alone, electrical stimuli and cycloheximide treatment, injection of oscillogen (9), ethanol (26), and SrCl2 treatment (27). The temporal separation of injection and activation can lead to problems in timing for the female and male pronuclei: If a spermatid is placed in an unactivated oocyte, it will often result in premature chromosome condensation (12). For mouse oocytes, electroactivation approximately 1 hour prior to injection or fusion is most effective (12). If the oocyte is activated long before injection, the paternal chromosomes will not have time to fully decondense.

Imprinting in Spermatids

Another concern with spermatid use, noted in early ROSI experiments, was the state of genomic imprinting in these germ cells. Genomic imprinting is a phenomenon in which only one allele of a gene is expressed, depending on its parent of origin (28). An embryo with two maternal genomes or two paternal genomes will fail to develop properly. Approximately 25 imprinted genes have now been identified (29). A prerequisite for imprinting is that maternal and paternal genes become differentially marked before fertilization so that they are epigenetically distinct in the developing embryo. The mark must be placed on the chromosomes at a time when they are separated, either during germ-cell development or gametogenesis. The mark must be heritable, but must also be erased and reset in the germline of the next generation (Fig. 21.1). Imprinting also requires that embryos have a mechanism to interpret the mark. Differential CpG methylation has been seen in or near imprinted genes (29) and methylation has been shown to be essential for maintenance of imprinting (30). Because it is still not known exactly what the imprinting mechanism is or how and when marks are placed on chromosomes, we cannot be sure a priori that imprinting is complete by the spermatid stage. The fact that mice and babies have been born and appear normal after ROSI does not necessarily mean that imprinting is normal. Chimeric mice have shown extensive contribution of hybrid mouse embryonic stem (ES) cells to all tissues, but erasure of imprinting has been observed in the ES-derived cells within these normal-appearing mice (Villar, Gold, Mate, Meneses, McLaughlin, Pedersen, unpublished observations). In addition, methyltransferase-deficient ES cells that had lost their imprints also are able to contribute extensively to normal chimeras (31). Improper imprinting could result in several genetic diseases, including Prader-Willi, Angelmann, Jervell and Lange-Nielsen, Beckwith-Wiedemann, and Silver-Russel syndromes (32–34). In addition, relaxation of imprinting is seen in some tumor cells, such as adrenocortical carcinomas, bladder tumors and Wilms' tumour (35).

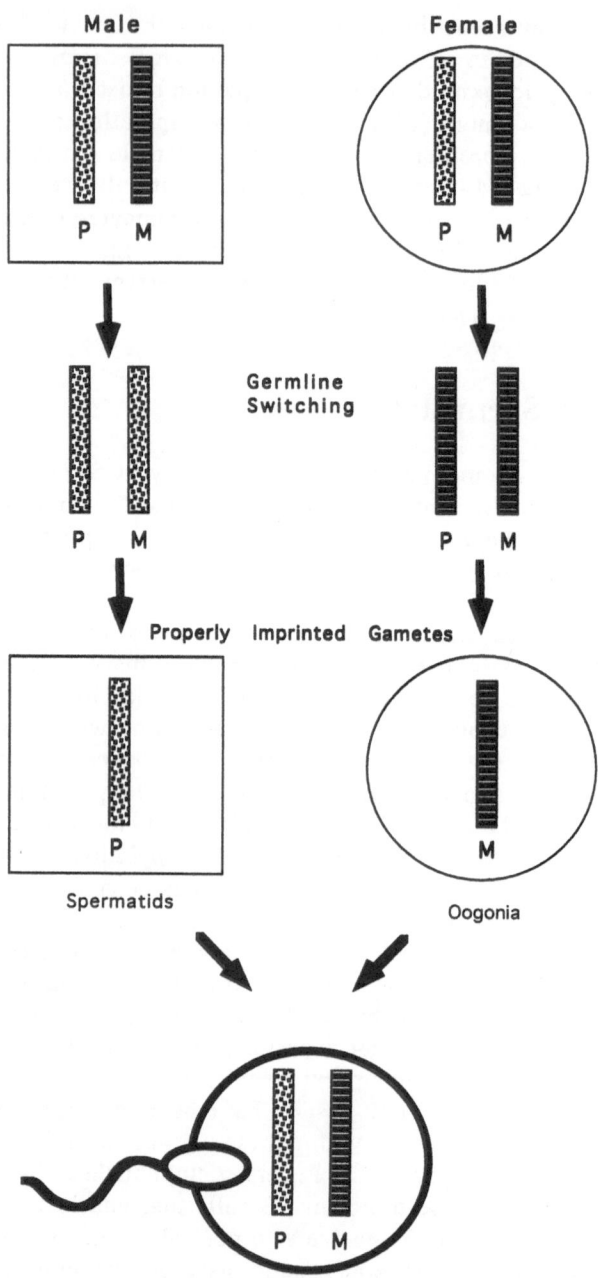

FIGURE 21.1. The imprint that differentiates the parental chromosomes must be switched in the germline of each generation.

Prior to offering ROSI treatment in infertility clinics, it is important to clarify the status of imprinting in spermatids because the absence of imprinting may pose serious health risks to offspring. During spermiogenesis, the haploid gamete reorganizes its chromatin structure and the effects of these nuclear protein changes on imprinting is unknown. To test whether imprinting is normal in mice spermatids, we investigated the offspring derived from ROSI. Throughout germ-cell development and gametogenesis, imprinted genes are bi-allelically expressed (36,37), which indicates either that the imprint is absent or that germ cells cannot interpret the imprint. In either case, analysis of expression of imprinted genes in spermatids does not reveal the status of the imprint. Because the identity of the critical methylation sites is also unknown, the investigation of methylation in spermatids does not reveal the status of the imprint. Because of these limitations, we sought to investigate ROSI-derived mouse embryos to learn the status of imprinted genes in spermatids (38).

The mouse model system is appropriate to study this question because many imprinted genes have been identified and cloned. Most of these genes have homologs in humans. We chose to study six imprinted genes: the maternally expressed genes, *H19* (39), *Mash-2* (40), and *Igf-2r* (41), and the paternally expressed genes, *Snrpn* (42), *Igf-2* (43), and *Peg-1* (44). To quantitate parental expresssion of imprinted genes, we selected genes that have polymorphisms between the *Mus musculus* alleles and *Mus castaneus* alleles for analysis. Using the Single Nucleotide Primer Extension (SNuPE) Assay (Fig. 21.2), we could distinguish the alleles of a gene based on a single base pair change. Polymorphisms in the maternal genes *H19*, *Igf-2r*, and *Mash-2* and the paternal genes, *Igf-2* and *Snrpn* had previously been identified (36,45). We were also able to identify an additional polymorphism in the Peg1 paternally expressed gene. Three stages of mouse embryonic development were studied: day 10 (by which time androgenetic and parthenogenetic embryos die) and days 12 and 13 (when many imprinted genes are expressed). The expression of each allele of the imprinted genes expressed in ROSI-derived embryos was compared with expression in embryos from natural matings or ICSI. No expression of the paternally expressed genes in either our experimental spermatid-injected embryos or naturally mated or ICSI control embryos, was seen from the maternal alleles. The maternally expressed genes, *Igf-2r* and *Mash-2*, had some expression (5–20%) from the paternal allele; however, the same levels of paternal expression were seen in the ROSI embryos and natural mating controls. The situation for *H19* was slightly different. No expression of the paternal allele of *H19* was seen in the embryos from natural matings; however, a low level of paternal expression was seen in both ROSI and ICSI derived embryos (38). Though the expression from the paternal *H19* allele was higher in ROSI embryos than in ICSI embryos, the fact that relaxation of the imprint was seen in both cases indicates that this most likely resulted from the injection or culture conditions.

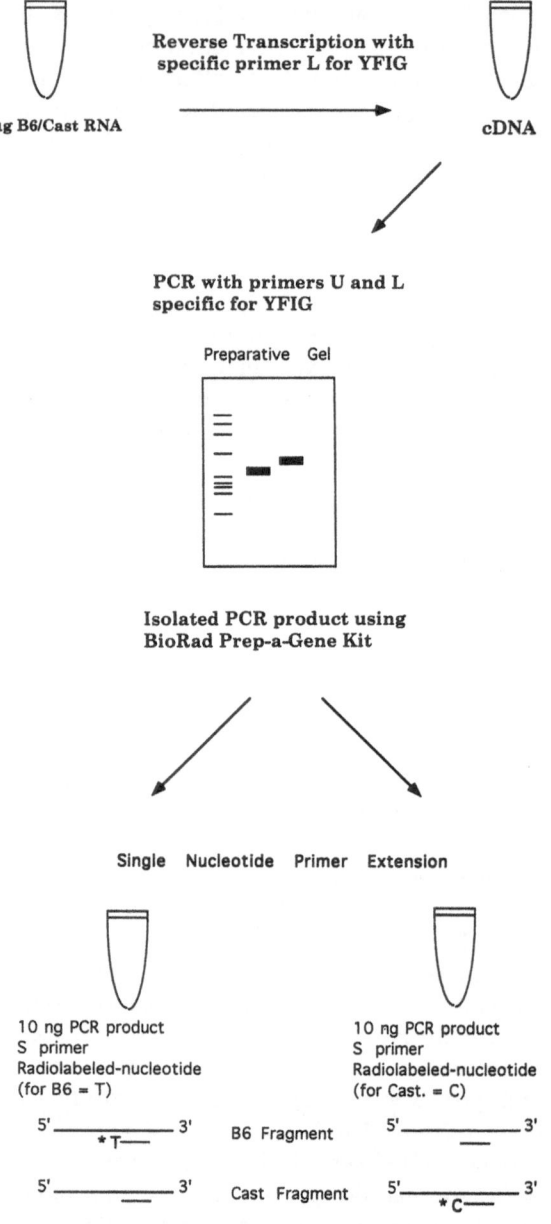

FIGURE 21.2. The SNuPE assay (36,49) uses single base pair changes to quantitate expression levels. cDNAs of your favorite imprinted genes (YFIG) are purified. Equal amounts of purified fragment and a single radiolabeled nucleotide are added to a reaction with a small primer that is adjacent to the known polymorphism. A single PCR cycle will add the labeled nucleotide only to primers annealed to the specific allele. The primers are electrophoresed through an acrylamide gel, and then relative amounts of radiolabeling are measured with a PhosphorImager.

TABLE 21.2. Summary of SNuPE assay of paternally expressed genes.

	Normal matings		Spermatid injections		Sperm injections	
	Maternal allele	Paternal allele	Maternal allele	Paternal allele	Maternal allele	Paternal allele
Igf-2	—	+++	—	+++		
Snrpn	—	+++	—	+++		
Peg-1			—	+++	—	+++

It has previously been reported that *H19* expression is labile in cultured embryos (46). Our results, summarized in Tables 21.2 and 21.3, indicate that imprinting is completed in spermatids. Our finding that *H19* imprinting is relaxed in ROSI and ICSI embryos, however, may raise some concern about prolonged culturing of human embryos in IVF clinics.

Normal healthy male mice were used as sperm or spermatid donors in our experiments; therefore, the status of imprinting in the case of incomplete spermatogenic maturation is not addressed by these studies. Two mouse models provide some answers to this question. ROSI using spermatids from hybrid sterile mice were able to produce offspring with similar efficiencies to normal males (47). Additional experiments using spermatids from artificially induced cryptorchid mice produced offspring at the same frequency as controls (48). These experiments using sterile mice with two different etiologies support the hypothesis that normal imprinting will be seen in offspring derived from males with defective spermiogenesis, although the expression of imprinted genes has not been studied in an infertile model.

The use of round spermatid injections has been investigated in the laboratory and tested in humans in quick succession. The studies on imprinting in ROSI-derived embryos begin to address an important question in the debate over spermatid injection, namely, whether spermatids have undergone proper epigenetic maturation. Our experiments indicate that imprinting is normal in embryos derived from spermatids of healthy fertile mice. Before the technique should be used for cases of abnormal spermiogenesis, however, further information from experiments in infertile model animals is needed.

TABLE 21.3. Summary of SNuPE assay of maternally expressed genes.

	Normal matings		Spermatid injections		Sperm injections	
	Maternal allele	Paternal allele	Maternal allele	Paternal allele	Maternal allele	Paternal allele
Igf-2r	+++	+	+++	+		
Mash-2	+++	+	+++	+		
H19	+++	—	+++	+	+++	+

Continued research should answer the remaining questions on the safety of ROSI for the treatment of male infertility.

References

1. Bonduelle M, Aytoz A, Wilikens A, Buysse A, Van Assche E, Devroey P, et al., Prospective follow-up study of 1,987 children born after intracytoplasmic sperm injection (ICSI). In: Treatment of infertility: the new frontiers. Princeton Junction, NJ: Communications Media for Education, Inc., 1998:445–61.
2. Liebaers I, Bonduelle M, Van Assche E, Devroey P, Van Steirteghem A. Sex chromosome abnormalities after intracytoplasmic sperm injection. Lancet, 1995; 346:1095.
3. Bowen JR, Gibson FL, Leslie GI, Saunderss DM. Medical and developmental outcome at 1 year for children conceived by intracytoplasmic sperm injection. Lancet 1998;351:1529–34.
4. Schlegel PN, Palermo GD, Goldstein M, Menendez S, Zaninovic N, Veeck L, et al. Testicular sperm extraction with intracytoplasmic sperm injection for nonobstructive azoospermia. Urology 1997;49(3):435–40.
5. Turek PJ, Givens C, Schriok ED, Meng M, Pedersen RA; Conaghans J. Testis sperm extraction and intracytoplasmic sperm injection guided by prior fine needle aspiration mapping in nonobstructive azoospermia. Fertil Steril 1999;71:552–58.
6. Sofikitis NV, Miyagawa I, Agapitos E, Pasyianos P, Toda T, Hellstrom WJ, et al. Reproductive capacity of the nucleus of the male gamete after completion of meiosis. J Assist Reprod Genet, 1994;11(7):335–41.
7. Ogura A, Yanagamachi R, Usuis N. Behavior of hamster and mouse round spermatid nuclei incorporated into mature oocytes by electrofusion. Zygote 1993;1:1–8.
8. Ogura A, Matsuda J, Yanagamachi R. Birth of normal young after electrofusion of mouse oocytes with round spermatids. Proc Natl Acad Sci USA 1994;91(16): 7460–62.
9. Sasagawa I, Yanagamachi R. Comparison of methods for activating mouse oocytes for spermatid nucleus transfer. Zygote 1996;4(4):269–74.
10. Tesarik J, Mendozas C. Spermatid injection into human oocytes. I. Laboratory techniques and special features of zygote development. Hum Reprod 1996; 11(4):772–79.
11. Huang T, Kimura Y, Yanagamachi R. The use of piezo micromanipulation for intracytoplasmic sperm injection of human oocytes. J Assist Reprod Genet 1996;13(4): 320–28.
12. Kimura Y, Yanagamachi R. Mouse oocytes injected with testicular spermatozoa or round spermatids can develop into normal offspring. Development 1995;121(8): 2397–405.
13. Vanderzwalmen P, Lejeune B, Nijs M, Segal-Bertin G, Vandemme B, Schoysmans R. Fertilization of an oocyte microinseminated with a spermatid in an in-vitro fertilization programme. Hum Reprod 1995;10:502–3.
14. Fishel S, Green S, Bishop M, Thornton S, Hunter A, Fleming S, et al. Pregnancy after intracytoplasmic injection of spermatid. Lancet 1995;345:1641–42.
15. Tesarik J, Mendoza C, Testarts J. Viable embryos from injection of round spermatids into oocytes. N Engl J Med 1995;333:525.
16. Vanderzwalmen P, Zech H, Birkenfeld A, Yemini M, Betin G, Lejeune B, et al.

Intracytoplasmic injection of spermatids retrieved from testicular tissue: influence of testicular pathology, type of selected spermatid and oocyte activation. Hum Reprod 1997;12(6):1203–13.

17. Sousa M, Barros A, Takahashi K, Oliveira C, Silva J, Tesariks J. Clinical efficacy of spermatid conception: analysis using a new spermatid classification scheme. Hum Reprod 1999;14(5):1279–86.

18. Ghazzawi IM, Alhasani S, Taher M, Sousos S. Reproductive capacity of round spermatids compared with mature spermatozoa in a population of azoospermic men. Hum Reprod 1999;14(3):736–40.

19. Antinori S, Versaci C, Dani G, Antinori M, Selmans HA. Successful fertilization and pregnancy after injection of frozen-thawed round spermatids into human oocytes. Hum Reprod 1997;12(3):554–56.

20. Yamanaka K, Sofikitis NV, Miyagawa I, Yamamoto Y, Toda T, Antypas S, et al. Ooplasmic round spermatid injection procedurres as an experimental treatment for nonobstructive azoospermia. J Assist Reprod Genet 1997;14(1):55–62.

21. Silber SJ, van Steirteghem A, Nagy Z, Liu J, Tournaye H, Devroeys P. Normal pregnancies resulting from testicular sperm extraction and intracytoplasmic sperm injection for azoospermia due to maturation arrest [see comments]. Fertil Steril 1996;66(1):110–17.

22. Aslam I, Robins A, Dowell K, Fishels S. Isolation, purification and assessment of viability of spermatogenic cells from testicular biopsies of azoospermic men. Hum Reprod 1998;13:639–45.

23. Sofikitis NV, Toda T, Miyagawa I, Zavos PM, Pasyianos P, Mastelous E. Beneficial effects of electrical stimulation before round spermatid nuclei injections into rabbit oocytes on fertilization and subsequent embryonic development. Fertil Steril 1996;65(1):176–85.

24. Sofikitis NV, Miyagawa I, Zavos PM, Yamamoto Y, Loutradis D, Mantzavinos T, et al. Micro- and macro-consequences of ooplasmic injections of early haploid male gametes. Hum Reprod Update 1998;4(3):197–212.

25. Cremades N, Bernabeu R, Barros A, Sousas M. In-vitro maturation of round spermatids using co-culture on Vero cells. Hum Reprod 1999;14:1287–93.

26. Wassarman PM, DePamphilis ML, eds. Guide to techniques in mouse development. In: Abelson JN, Simon MI, eds. Methods in enzymology, Vol. 225. San Diego: Academic Press, Inc. 1993:1019.

27. Wakayama T, Perry ACF, Zuccotti M, Johnson KR, Yanagamachi R. Full-term development of mice from enucleated oocytes injected with cumulus cell nuclei. Nature 1998;394:369–74.

28. Stewart CL, Pedersen R, Rotwein P, Bestor T, Rastan S, Hastie N, et al. Genomic imprinting. Reprod Toxicol 1997;11(2/3):309–16.

29. John RM, Suranis MA. Imprinted genes and regulation of gene expression by epigenetic inheritance. Curr Opin Cell Biol 1996;8(3):348–53.

30. Li E, Beard C, Jaenischs R. Role of DNA methylation in genomic imprinting. Nature 1993;366:362–65.

31. Tucker KL, Talbot D, Lee MA, Leonhardt H, Jaenischs R. Complementation of methylation deficiency in embryonic stem cells by a DNA methyltransferase minigene. Proc Natl Acad Sci USA 1996;93(23):12920–25.

32. Cassidy SB. Uniparental disomy and genomic imprinting as causes of human genetic disease. Environ Mol Mut 1995;25(Supplement 26):13–20.

33. Neyroud N, Tesson F, Denjoy I, Leibovici M, Donger C, Barhanin J, et al. A novel

mutation in the potassium channel gene KVLQT1 causes the Jervell and Lange-Nielsen cardioauditory syndrome. Nat Genet 1997;15:186–89.

34. Tesarik J, Sousa M, Greco E, Mendozas C. Spermatids as gametes: indications and limitations. Hum Reprod Suppl 1998;13(3):89–111.

35. Brenton JD, Viville S, Suranis MA. Genomic imprinting and cancer. Cancer Surv 1995;25:161–71.

36. Szabo PE, Manns JR. Biallelic expression of imprinted genes in the mouse germ line: implications for erasure, establishment, and mechanisms of genomic imprinting. Genes Dev 1995;9(15):1857–68.

37. Villar AJ, Eddy EM, Pedersens RA. Developmental regulation of genomic imprinting during gametogenesis. Dev Biol 1995;172:264–71.

38. Shamanski FL, Kimura Y, Lavoir M-C, Pedersen RA, Yanagamachi R. Status of genomic imprinting in mouse spermatids. Hum Reprod 1999;14(4):1050–56.

39. Bartolomei MS, Zemel S, Tilghmans SM. Parental imprinting of the mouse H19 gene. Nature 1991;351:153–55.

40. Guillemot F, Caspary T, Tilghman SM, Copeland NG, Gilbert DJ, Jenkins NA, et al. Genomic imprinting of Mash2, a mouse gene required for trophoblast development. Nat Genet 1995;9(3):235–42.

41. Barlow DP, Stoger R, Herrmann BG, Saito K, Schweifers N. The mouse insulin-like growth factor type-2 receptor is imprinted and closely linked to the *Tme* locus. Nature 1991;349:84–87.

42. Leff SE, Brannan CI, Reed ML, Ozcelik T, Francke U, Copeland NG, et al. Maternal imprinting of the mouse Snrpn gene and conserved linkage homology with the human Prader-Willi syndrome region. Nat Genet 1992;2(4):259–64.

43. DeChiara TM, Robertson EJ, Efstratiadiss A. Parental imprinting of the mouse insulin-like growth factor II gene. Cell 1991;64:849–59.

44. Kaneko-Ishino T, Kuroiwa Y, Miyoshi N, Kohda T, Suzuki R, Yokoyama M, et al. Peg1/Mest imprinted gene on chromosome 6 identified by cDNA subtraction hybridization. Nat Genet 1995;11(1):52–59.

45. Szabo PE, Manns JR. Allele-specific expression and total expression levels of imprinted genes during early mouse development: implications for imprinting mechanisms. Genes Dev 1995;9(24):3097–108.

46. Sasaki H, Ferguson-Smith AC, Shum ASW, Barton SC, Suranis MA. Temporal and spatial regulation of H19 imprinting in normal and uniparental mouse embryos. Development 1995;121:4195–202.

47. Sasagawa I, Tateno T, Yazawa H, Ichiyanagi O, Ishigooka M, Nakadas T. Round spermatids from hybrid sterile mice can initiate normal embryo development. Hum Reprod 1998;13(11):3099–102.

48. Sasagawa I, Yanagamachi R. Spermatids from mice after cryptorchid and reversal operations can initiate normal embryo development. J Andrology 1997;18(2):203–9.

49. Singer-Sam J, LeBon JM, Dai A, Riggs AD. A sensitive, quantitative assay for measurement of allele-specific transcripts differing by a single nucleotide. PCR Meth Appl 1992;1(3):160–63.

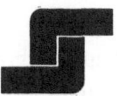

22

Effect of Embryo Culture on Imprinted Gene Expression in the Preimplantation Mouse Embryo

RICHARD M. SCHULTZ, KIMBERLY D. TREMBLAY,
ADAM S. DOHERTY, AND MARISA S. BARTOLOMEI

Genomic Imprinting: Definition, Evidence, and Genes

A small number of autosomal genes in mammals are expressed exclusively from a single parental allele. These genes are subjected to genomic imprinting. For example, in mice, the *H19, IGF-2/cation-independent mannose-6-phosphate receptor Igf2r, p57^{KIP2}*, and *Mash-2* genes are expressed from the maternally inherited chromosomes, whereas the (*insulinlike growth factor 2*) (*Igf2*) and *small nucleoprotein polypeptide N* (*Snrpn*) genes are expressed from the paternally inherited chromosomes (1). One consequence of imprinted genes is that both the maternal and paternal genomes are required for normal embryonic development. Another consequence is that for those genes that are imprinted only a single event (e.g., a somatic mutation deleteriously affecting the expressed allele) would result in the absence of a gene product.

Prior to the identification of imprinted genes in mammals, the existence of imprinted genes in mice was suggested by two main lines of evidence. First, in nuclear transplantation experiments embryos containing either two female pronuclei (gynogenones) or two male pronuclei (androgenones) failed to develop to term (2). Furthermore, the phenotypes of these uniparental embryos were somewhat complementary in that the gynogenetic embryos formed tissues of mostly embryonic origin, whereas androgenetic embryos formed tissues of mostly extraembryonic origin. It was therefore proposed that the maternal and paternal genomes were providing unique products that were essential to the embryos, and that these products were derived from imprinted genes. The second line of evidence derived from genetic studies using mice that contained translocated chromosome (3). Intercrosses of mice heterozygous for the translocation results in a small percentage of the progeny that inherit both copies of the translocated region from a single parent (i.e., uniparental disomy). Although mice harboring uniparental disomies for most regions developed normally (i.e., both parental chromosomes are not required), mice containing uniparental disomies for a few regions exhibited abnormal phenotypes, ranging from prenatal lethality to growth defects. It is in these regions that imprinted genes were proposed to reside. Identification of imprinted genes has shown this to be the case for a majority of the genes. The developmental failures observed in the absence of parental genomes or segments of genomes highlight the important role that imprinted genes play in development.

In the past 8 years more than 25 imprinted genes have been identified in mice and humans. These genes encode products with a wide range of functions including growth factors (i.e., *Igf2*), growth repressors (*Igf2r* and *p57^{KIP2}*), and splicing factors (*Snrpn*). It is interesting that a subset of imprinted genes encode conserved RNAs that are not translated (e.g., *H19*, *Ipw*, and *Xist*). A simple inspection of the genes does not reveal either the type of gene that has been chosen for imprinting or the reason why genes, in general, are imprinted. It is striking that a majority of imprinted genes identified thus far are located in two large clusters on mouse chromosome 7, with conserved clusters found in humans as well.

Allelic DNA Methylation as the Mechanism to Generate the Imprinting Mark

A central question in imprinting is how the two parental alleles of imprinted genes are differentiated or marked so that their appropriate expression pattern is assumed in the developing organism. The imprint or mark must be stable, heritable, and erasable so that the imprint is appropriately maintained in a given individual and correctly transmitted to subsequent generations. The substantial number of characterized imprinted genes allows the investigation of imprinting mechanism(s) because it is likely that multiple genes will share a common mechanism. Although a preliminary examination of the sequences within and around imprinted gene loci has not revealed common sequence motifs, analysis of other aspects of these loci will enable us to understand how imprinting is established and maintained. Experiments indicate accordingly that these genes do in fact share a common set of properties. First, as described in greater detail later, most imprinted genes are differentially methylated on the two parental alleles. Second, repetitive sequences have been identified at a large number of imprinted loci (4). Third, the parental alleles of loci containing imprinted genes replicate asynchronously (5). Although these latter two properties, as well as others not described here, are likely to contribute significantly to the process of genomic imprinting, differential DNA methylation is emerging as a central candidate for controlling imprinted expression.

Several properties of DNA methylation render it an excellent candidate for the imprinting mark. First, this covalent modification of the cytosine residue in CpG dinucleotides is stable and heritable because DNA methyl-transferase 1 (Dnmt1), the enzyme that catalyzes the majority of DNA methylation in mammalian embryos, prefers hemimethylated DNA as a substrate (6). Second, DNA methylation patterns can be erased either by an active or passive activity and re-established by a de novo methyltransferase activity. Third, in addition to marking an allele stably, DNA methylation can also serve to inhibit gene activity because hypermethylated DNA is typically transcriptionally repressed. Investigators have determined that the transcriptional repression associated with hypermethylated DNA is through the methyl-CpG-binding protein MeCP2 that interacts with a histone deacetylase complex (7). Histone hyperacetylation is highly correlated with transcriptionally permissive chromatin, and histone hypoacetylation is linked with transcriptionally repressed chromatin (8).

Evidence supporting a role for DNA methylation in allelic marking derives from the finding that most imprinted genes that have been examined exhibit parental-specific methylation. The most compelling evidence demonstrating the importance of allelic methylation comes from the analysis of mice in which *Dnmt1* was deleted. This gene is essential for development because mice deficient for *Dnmt1* die around the eight-somite stage of development (9). When analyzed prior to their death, *Dnmt1*-deficient mice exhibited perturbations in imprinted expression; *H19*, *Snrpn*, and *Xist*, which are methylated on the inactive allele, were biallelically expressed, and *Igf2* and *Igf2r*, which are methylated on the active alleles, were repressed (e.g., 10).

H19: A Model System to Study the Role of DNA in Genomic Imprinting

H19, which is located on mouse chromosome 7, is abundantly expressed in the developing mouse embryo (11). In situ hybridization studies indicate that transcripts are first detected in the trophectoderm of the day 4.5 blastocyst and accumulate in extraembryonic tissues following implantation transcripts (11). By day 8.5 postcoitum transcripts are detected in the embryo proper and are most abundant in tissues of endodermal and mesodermal origin. Following birth, however, the gene is repressed in essentially all tissues except for skeletal muscle. The gene encodes for a polyadenylated RNA that apparently does not direct the synthesis of a protein.

Although it is clear from the *Dnmt1*-null mice that DNA methylation is required to maintain a difference between the parental alleles in somatic cells, this experiment provides no insight as to whether DNA methylation is the initial gametic imprint. For this to be the case, the methylation difference must be inherited from the gametes and stably maintained throughout development. Demonstration of allelic methylation differences is especially critical during preimplantation development as the embryonic genome undergoes generalized demethylation during this period (12). As described later, each of these conditions is met by *H19*.

Initial studies using methylation-sensitive restriction enzymes identified paternal-specific methylation at sites that are located from -2 kb to -4 kb relative to the start of transcription and which could serve as the *H19* parental-specific imprinting mark (Fig. 22.1). These studies (13) used F_1 hybrid embryonic DNA derived from intercrosses between the polymorphic mouse strains C57BL/6J and *Mus musculus castaneus* (*M. castaneus*) and single-strand conformation polymorphism (SSCP) analysis following PCR to determine the parental source of the amplified product. Because the PCR/SSCP assay is limited to CpGs located in methylation-sensitive restriction sites, and only a small number of the 100+ CpGs in this region are found in such sites, this analysis was extended by the bisulfite mutagenesis assay to assess the methylation status of all cytosine residues. In this method, treatment of DNA with bisulfite converts cytosine residues to uracil, but leaves 5' methylcytosine unchanged. Following the mutagenesis of DNA from F_1 hybrid embryos, the DNA is PCR amplified, subcloned, and sequenced. Methylcytosines appear as cytosines on sequencing gels, whereas unmethylated cytosines appear as thymine. The use of strain-specific sequence polymorphisms between C57BL/6J and *M. castaneus* allows the determination of parental identity of the individual subclones.

The bisulfite mutagenesis method provides a more informative and quantitative methylation analysis for several reasons. First, as stated earlier, it directly assays all CpGs within the region defined by the PCR primers. Second, each sequence represents a single strand of DNA that was present in the original sample, and therefore describes the entire methylation profile of an individual chromosome. Third, unlike the PCR-based methylation sensitive-restriction enzyme assay, this technique is quantitative because it determines the number of DNA strands that are methylated at a given residue. Finally, the parental origin of each strand of DNA is unambiguously assigned based on sequence polymorphisms between the two strains of mice used to generate the embryonic DNA samples.

Results of these studies, which are summarized in Figure 22.1 [and described more fully in (14)] examined 59 CpGs in a 2.2 kb distal upstream region located 2 kb from the start of transcription and 9 CpGs in a 350-bp promoter proximal region in DNA from midgestation embryos (Fig. 22.1, striped bars). With the exception of 6 CpG dinucleotides at the 5' end of the 2.2 kb distal region that were equally methylated on both alleles (including *Hpa*II site number 1 that was considered an imprinting mark candidate by the PCR/SSCP assay of blastocysts), the remaining CpG dinucleotides were methylated exclusively on the paternal allele. In contrast, CpGs in the promoter proximal region were preferentially methylated on the paternal allele, but all 9 CpGs were also methylated in a significant portion of the clones corresponding to the maternal allele. A subset of the sites from both regions was also analyzed in blastocyst DNA. Although the distal CpGs were differentially methylated in blastocysts, the promoter proximal region was unmethylated. From these experiments we propose that the region from -2 to

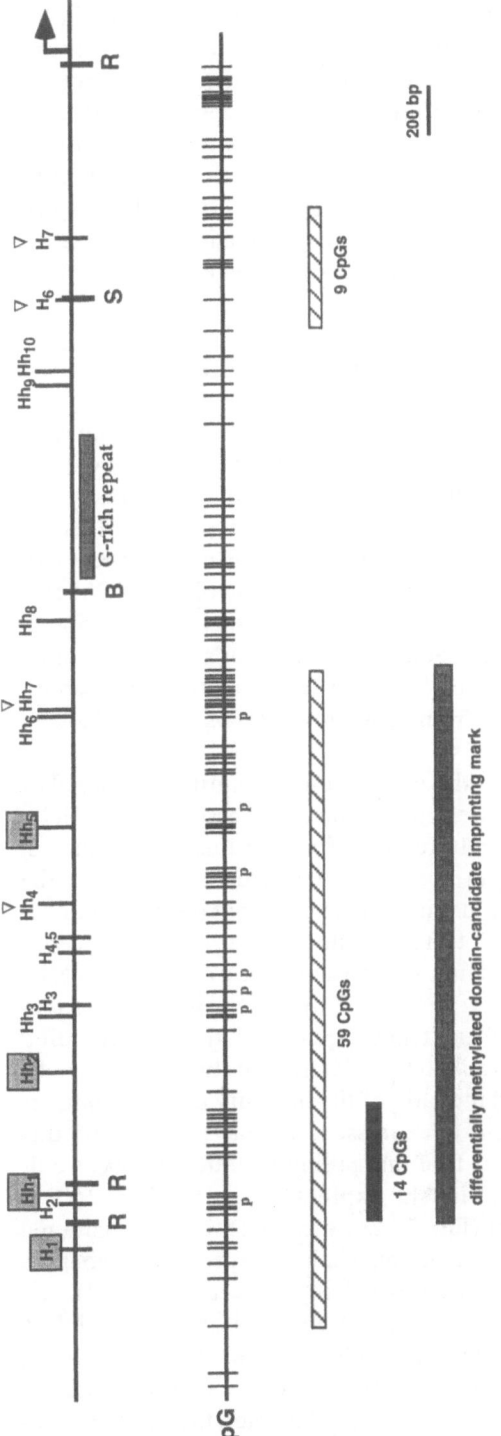

FIGURE 22.1. Location of CpG dinucleotides in the upstream region of the *H19* gene. A 4.6 kb region upstream of the transcription start site (arrow) is depicted on the top line. The methylation sensitive restriction endonuclease sites *HhaI* (Hh, vertical line above gene line) and *HpaII* (H, vertical line through gene line) are indicated on the top line. *HpaII* and *HhaI* sites that were unmethylated in oocytes and methylated on the paternal allele in preimplantation embryos, and are candidates for the imprinting mark, are indicated with a box. The *HpaII* and *HhaI* sites that were assayed but were not candidates for the imprinting mark are shown with an arrowhead. Other restriction endonuclease sites include *Eco*RI (R), *Bam*HI (B), and *Sac*I (S). The second line shows the location of all CpG dinucleotides (vertical lines) found in the upstream region, as indicated by GenBank sequence U19619. Those CpG dinucleotides that are polymorphic between C57BL/6J and *M. castaneus* are indicated with a "p" and were not analyzed either by the PCR/SSCP or bisulfite assay. The two hatched boxes correspond to the regions analyzed by bisulfite mutagenesis of sperm and midgestation embryonic DNA (with number of CpGs shown underneath). The regions designated by the black box (14 CpGs) and the promoter proximal hatched box were analyzed by bisulfite mutagenesis of blastocyst DNA. Although *HpaII* site number 1 (H1) was differentially methylated in gametes and blastocysts, it was equally methylated at later stages of development and is not a candidate for the imprinting mark. The location of the differentially methylated domain (the candidate for the imprinting mark) is designated by a shaded box.

-4 kb relative to the start of transcription acts as a key regulatory domain for imprinted expression and, by all tests thus far, fulfills the criteria of an imprinting mark (i.e., parental-specific differences in methylation that survive the global demethylation that occurs during preimplantation development) (Fig. 22.1). [CpGs outside of the 2 kb region, which are differentially methylated later in development, likely help to silence the paternal allele when transcription of *H19* is increased during later stages of development.] It should be noted that deletion of the 2 kb region on the paternal allele containing the putative imprinting domain results in expression of this normally repressed allele (15).

Effect of Culture Condition on *H19* Expression

Culture conditions clearly influence gene expression in the preimplantation mouse embryo. For example, culture of embryos in commonly used culture media (e.g., Whitten's medium) results in developmental rates that are retarded when compared with embryos that develop in vivo, as well as reduced levels of expression of many genes that have been analyzed (16). Simplex optimization has led to the development of the medium KSOM that supports preimplantation development in vitro at rates that are superior to those obtained by commonly used media (e.g., Whitten's medium) (17). Moreover, for every gene analyzed to date, the levels of transcript abundance are not statistically different from those of embryos that develop in vivo (16).

Culture conditions can influence the expression of imprinted genes. For example, we have observed *H19* expression can be either essentially biallelic or monoallelic, depending on the culture conditions. In these experiments, two-cell embryos were flushed from the oviducts and then cultured to the blastocyst stage in either Whitten's medium or KSOM-containing amino acids (KSOM+aa). Following culture to the blastocyst stage, the RNA was subjected to reverse transcription using oligo (dT) as a primer, the cDNA was then amplified in the presence of [^{32}P]dCTP by PCR using primers that amplify both maternal and paternal transcripts, and the radiolabeled amplicons detected by autoradiography. The electrophoretic mobility indicates which allele is expressed, and the ratio of the intensity of the amplicons indicates to what extent each allele is expressed. We have conducted this experiment several times and always find that preimplantation embryos cultured in Whitten's medium exhibit biallelic expression of *H19* (i.e., *H19* is equally expressed from both alleles) (Fig. 22.2). In contrast, embryos cultured in KSOM+aa essentially maintain maternal monoallelic expression although a small fraction (10%) of the transcripts are paternally derived (Fig. 22.2). Because these assays were conducted on groups of embryos, this paternal *H19* expression in embryos cultured in KSOM+aa could be due to all of the embryos exhibiting some paternal expression or only a fraction of the embryos showing complete biallelic expression. In addition, it should be noted that using a similar approach paternally derived *Srnpn* expression was observed when the em-

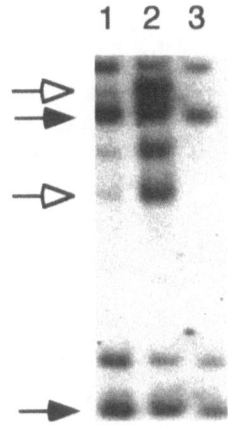

FIGURE 22.2. Effect of culture on *H19* expression. The embryos are products of a cross between females harboring the *Cast* allele and males bearing the B6 allele. (Lane 1) Embryos cultured in KSOM+aa; (lane 2) Embryos cultured in Whitten's medium; (lane 3) Embryos that developed in vivo. Open arrows: position of *H19* amplicon derived from B6 background; closed arrows: position of *H19* amplicon derived from the *Cast* allele.

bryos were cultured in either Whitten's medium or KSOM+aa. Thus, the effect of culture conditions differentially affects the expression of imprinted genes.

We have conducted studies to examine the effect of culture of two-cell embryos to the blastocyst stage in either Whitten's or KSOM+aa medium on the methylation of specific sites within the 2 kb upstream putative imprinting domain. The methylation status of the DNA at the *Hha*I site 5 (indicated by Hh$_5$ of the top line in Fig. 22.1) that resides in this 2 kb domain was assessed as previously described (13) [i.e., DNA from blastocysts was digested with an enzyme (e.g., *Pvu*II or *Hind*III) that cuts outside the region of interest and is then digested with the methylation-sensitive restriction endonuclease *Hha*I]. If the DNA is methylated, the methylation-sensitive enzymes are unable to cut and PCR of this region with flanking primers yields a product. If the cytosine residue is unmethylated, however, the methylation-sensitive restriction enzyme cleaves the DNA, and subsequent PCR of this region does not yield an amplification product.

Results of these experiments indicate that little, if any, of the diagnostic PCR amplicon is detected when the embryos are cultured in Whitten's medium, whereas this amplicon is readily detected when the embryos are cultured in KSOM+aa (Fig. 22.3A). Thus, culture results in a large loss of methylation of this site, presumably on the paternal allele, which is normally methylated. To verify this, SSCP analysis of the DNA was conducted. As anticipated, following restriction with *Hha*I the paternal allele is not detected for embryos cultured in Whitten's medium (Fig. 22.3B, lane 2), but it is detected for embryos cultured in KSOM (Fig. 22.3B, lane 4); as anticipated, little if any of the hypomethylated maternal allele is detected.

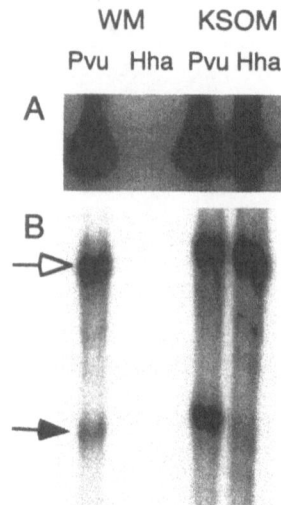

FIGURE 22.3. Effect of culture on methylation status of Hh5 site. (A) The embryos were derived from a cross between females harboring the *Cast* allele and males bearing the B6 allele. The embryos were cultured from the two-cell to the blastocyst stage in either Whitten's medium (WM) or KSOM+aa (KSOM). DNA from the two sets of embryos was then digested with *Pvu*II (Pvu) that cuts outside of the region of interest, or with *Pvu*II and *Hha*I (Hha), a methylation-sensitive restriction enzyme. PCR was then performed with primers that flank the Hha5 site (see Fig. 22.1); a region of the gel is shown. The presence of a PCR product in the Hha lanes indicates that a portion of the original sample was methylated, whereas the absence of a product indicates that the entire sample is unmethylated. (B) SSCP analysis of samples shown in (A). A portion of the PCR sample was used to determine the parental origin of the methylation and a region of the gel is shown. The open arrow is the position of an *H19* amplicon derived from B6 background (i.e., paternal allele); closed arrow, position of an *H19* amplicon derived from the *Cast* allele (i.e., maternal allele).

To determine whether the loss-of-imprinting and changes in methylation resulted from a general effect of the culture conditions on DNA methyltransferase, we assayed DNA methyltransferase activity in the cultured embryos. The amount of DNA methyltransferase activity decreases throughout preimplantation development when expressed as the amount of activity per cell (18); the total amount of DNA methyltransferase activity remains constant until the eight-cell stage after which it decreases. We have previously demonstrated that culture of embryos in Whitten's medium to the blastocyst stage results in the decreased expression of many genes, when compared with culture of embryos in KSOM (e.g., 16). Thus, a disproportionate decrease in DNA methyltransferase activity in embryos cultured in Whitten's medium when compared with embryos cultured in KSOM could result in the Whitten's cultured embryos not being capable of maintaining levels of DNA methylation sufficient to maintain monoallelic *H19* expression.

When compared with embryos that develop in vivo, embryos that develop in either KSOM+aa or Whitten's medium, display similar decreases in the amount of DNA methyltransferase activity per cell; the assay for DNA methyltransferase activity was similar to that described in (18). These results minimize the possibility that the loss-of-imprinting of *H19* that occurs during culture in Whitten's medium can be attributed to either a precocious loss of DNA methyltransferase activity in embryos cultured in Whitten's medium or to the magnitude of this decrease.

The DNA methyltransferase Dnmt1 that is responsible for the bulk of DNA methylation displays a remarkable stage-specific change in intracellular distribution during preimplantation development (19). Between the one-cell and eight-cell stages the enzyme is predominantly located in the cytoplasm. During the eight-cell stage, the enzyme is preferentially located in the nucleus, but the enzyme is again located predominantly in the cytoplasm by the morula stage. Although the molecular basis for these changes and the biological sequelae are not known, we find similar temporal and spatial changes in Dnmt1 localization in embryos cultured in KSOM+aa or Whitten's medium. Thus, the loss-of-imprinting of *H19* in embryos cultured in Whitten's medium cannot readily be attributed to perturbations in these stage-specific changes.

Effect of Culture on Embryo Development

The loss-of-imprinting that occurs during culture under certain conditions could compromise the ability of these embryos to implant and develop to term. In fact, a body of evidence is steadily accumulating that documents that culture of bovine and ovine embryos to the blastocyst stage prior to embryo transfer results in higher incidences of fetal and perinatal loss (e.g., 20). In the bovine, these abnormalities are not observed if the embryos are first transferred to the oviducts of sheep and then transferred at the blastocyst stage to the reproductive tracts of recipient heifers (20). Thus, the abnormalities are likely attributable to embryo culture. Because the culture conditions are most likely suboptimal for these species, loss-of-imprinting may occur during the culture period and could, in principle, contribute to the observed differences in fetal and postnatal loss. The likelihood that human embryos generated in in vitro fertilization programs will in the future be cultured for increasingly longer periods of time prior to transfer to the mother raises the important issue of whether culture of human embryos also perturbs the expression of imprinted genes, and, if so, does this have any consequences on either fetal or postnatal development.

Acknowledgments. The research described in this chapter was supported by grants from the NIH (GM 51279 to MSB and HD 22681 to RMS). MSB is an assistant investigator of the Howard Hughes Medical Institute.

References

1. Bartolomei MS, Tilghman SM. Genomic imprinting in mammals. Ann Rev Genet 1997;31:493–525.
2. McGrath J, Solter D. Completion of mouse embryogenesis requires both the maternal and paternal genomes. Cell 1984;37:179–83.
3. Beechey CV, Cattanach BM. Genetic imprinting map. Mouse Genome 1991;89: 60–61.
4. Neumann B, Kubicka P, Barlow DP. Characteristics of imprinted genes. Nat Genet 1995;9:12–13.
5. Kitsberg D, Selig S, Brandeis M, Simon I, Keshet I, Driscoll DJ, et al. Allele-specific replication timing of imprinted gene regions. Nature 1993;364:459–63.
6. Bestor TH, Ingram, VM. Two DNA methyltransferases from murine erythroleukemia cells: purification, sequence specificity and mode of interaction with DNA. Proc Nat Acad Sci USA 1983;82:2674–78.
7. Nan X, Ng H-H, Johnson CA, Laherty CD, Turner BM, Eisenman RN, et al. Transcriptional repression by the methyl-CpG-binding protein MeCP2 involves a histone deacetylase complex. Nature 1998;393:386–89.
8. Turner BM. Histone acetylation as an epigenetic determinant of long-term transcriptional competence. Cell Mol Life Sci 1998;54:21–31.
9. Li E, Bestor TH, Jaenisch R. Targeted mutation of the DNA methyltransferase gene results in embryonic lethality. Cell 1992;69:915–26.
10. Li E, Beard C, Jaenisch R. Role for DNA methylation in genomic imprinting. Nature 1993;366:362–65.
11. Poirier F, Chan C-TJ, Timmons PM, Robertson EJ, Evans MJ, Rigby PWJ. The murine H19 gene is activated during embryonic stem cell differentiation in vitro and at the time of implantation in the developing embryo. Development 1991;113:1105–14.
12. Monk M, Boubelik M, Lehnert S. Temporal and regional changes in DNA methylation in the embryonic, extraembryonic and germ cell lineages during mouse embryo development. Development 1987;99:371–82.
13. Tremblay KD, Saam JR, Ingram RS, Tilghman SM, Bartolomei MS. A paternal-specific methylation imprint marks the alleles of the mouse H19 gene. Nat Genet 1995;9:407–13.
14. Tremblay KD, Duran, KL, Bartolomei MS. A 5′ 2-kilobase-pair region of the imprinted mouse H19 gene exhibits exclusive paternal methylation throughout development. Mol Cell Biol 1997;17:4322–29.
15. Thorvaldsen JL, Duran KL, Bartolomei MS. Deletion of the H19 differentially methylated domain results in loss of imprinted expression of H19 and Igf2. Genes Dev 1998;12:3693–702.
16. Ho Y, Wigglesworth K, Eppig JJ, Schultz RM. Preimplantation development of mouse embryos in KSOM: Augmentation by amino acids and analysis of gene expression. Mol Reprod Dev 1995;41:232–38.
17. Erbach GT, Lawitts JA, Papaioannou VE, Biggers JD. Differential growth of the mouse preimplantation embryo in chemically defined media. Biol Reprod 1994;50:1027–33.
18. Monk M, Adams RLP, Rinaldi A. Decrease in DNA methylase activity during preimplantation development in the mouse. Development 1991;112:189–92.

19. Carlson LL, Page AW, Bestor TH. Properties and localization of DNA methyltransferase in preimplantation mouse embryos: Implications for genomic imprinting. Genes Dev 1992;6:2536–41.
20. Behboodi E, Anderson GB, BonDurant RH, Cargill SL, Kreuscher BR, Medrano JF, et al. Birth of large calves that developed from in vitro-derived bovine embryos. Theriogenology 1995;44:227–32.

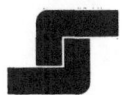

Author Index

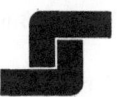

Subject Index

PROCEEDINGS IN THE SERONO SYMPOSIA USA SERIES

Continued from page ii

PROCEEDINGS IN THE SERONO SYMPOSIA USA SERIES

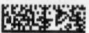